When the Bough Breaks

Parental Perceptions of Ethical Decision-Making in NICU

Winifred J. Ellenchild Pinch

University Press of America,® Inc.
Lanham · New York · Oxford

University Press of America,® Inc.
4720 Boston Way
Lanham, Maryland 20706
UPA Acquisitions Department (301) 459-3366

12 Hid's Copse Rd.
Cumnor Hill, Oxford OX2 9JJ

Printed in the United States of America
British Library Cataloging in Publication Information Available

Library of Congress Cataloging-in-Publication Data

Pinch, Winifred.
When the bough breaks : parental perceptions of ethical decision-making in NICU / Winifred J. Ellenchild Pinch.
p. cm
Includes bibliographical references and index.
1. Neonatal intensive care—Moral and ethical aspects.
2. Infants (Premature)—Family relationships. 3. Birth weight, Low.
4. Decision making. 5. Perinatology. I. Title.

RJ253.5 .P54 2002
174'.24—dc21 2002020407 CIP

ISBN 0-7618-2316-6 (paperback : alk. ppr.)

™ The paper used in this publication meets the minimum requirements of American National Standard for Information Sciences—Permanence of Paper for Printed Library Materials, ANSI Z39.48—1984

To Ellen Jane Lentz, my mother, a most compassionate and caring person, and...

To the parents of high-risk newborns--everywhere.

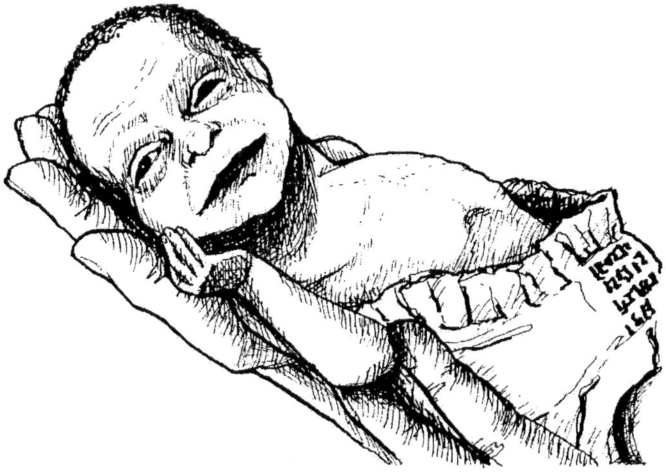

Contents

FIGURES AND TABLES

PREFACE

Rock a bye baby in the tree top,
When the wind blows the cradle will rock,
When the bough breaks the cradle will fall,
And down will come baby, cradle and all.
Attributed to Mother Goose (Lobel 1986)

When you think about this nursery rhyme, it is really a tragic, horrible tale to sing to a newborn in its cradle, especially while rocking the baby to sleep. Yet this rhyme with disaster lurking throughout its innocent singsong rhythm, is truly symbolic of a pregnancy, birth, or early newborn experience gone awry. A baby peacefully nestled in the womb, floating, swaying, rocking in the fluid surrounding it, may suddenly, prematurely, be launched into life on its own. The bough breaks. Prematurity or some other circumstance interrupts the usual pathway to normal babyhood. Literally thousands of errors can occur during fetal life. It is truly a wonder of creation that any of us are born without missing parts and with all parts working correctly. Genetic defects, errors in fetal growth and development, birth trauma, failure to achieve transition to extrauterine life, and even the simple stress of extrauterine life are all hazards from conception onward. The result can be a high-risk newborn.

A high-risk perinatal experience frequently initiates specialized treatment in our health care system. Obstetricians attend to women during pregnancy. When untoward circumstances arise before birth, specific therapy is often instituted. Neonatologists are called in after birth to attend the baby when its status is compromised. Sundry other health professionals including various other physicians, nurses, social workers, laboratory technicians, emergency medical technicians (EMTs), nutritionists, and pharmacists are also involved as the needs of the woman, her family, and the baby are identified at various times during this process as high-risk.

This book addresses a particular aspect of the above drama--the fact that parents are the central feature of the high-risk perinatal experience.

The unvarnished reality of parental experiences is the focus of my work. Parental perceptions are not presented here with an overlay of simultaneous observations and discussions with health professionals or other individuals. Such approaches are reported elsewhere.[a] Only parents were targeted for information about neonatal intensive care in this study in order to avoid diluting the relevance of their experiences. As Anspach (1993) noted, "...there remains a curious imbalance in the literature." Philosophers discuss how decisions ought to be made and we know far more about this dimension than any other. We also know how physicians and nurses think about such decision-making but we know least about the parents.

The parents' stories are neither right nor wrong relative to others' perceptions of the same or similar events. In some cases, we might be tempted to label the parental viewpoint a *misperception* rather than a parental perception. Whether we are in a position to judge or evaluate those perspectives, or ethically, if we *should* evaluate them, is not the focus here. For this book, the parents' perceptions are presented so that readers might consider parental reflections as another set of valid perspectives on the neonatal intensive care unit (NICU) experience.[b] This project report includes a few statistics, but its purpose is to describe in detail the individual parental meanings attached to the more impartial and objective morbidity and mortality rates for high-risk pregnancy and high-risk neonates. This book also includes selected bioethical content, but again the parental narrative in the bioethical material is intended to illuminate the meaning of ethical decision-making for families and their lives during this experience of high-risk care.

As a result of my community health experience and my interest in bioethics, I became attracted to the stories of parents in my practice who had a high-risk infant. Their impressions led me to develop a longitudinal research project, the results of which are described in this book. In some ways, this is also my story as I began the journey through this project as my interest in the topic was caught by parents' experiences in my community health practice. Section I, the Background, is first and includes one chapter. Chapter 1, Getting Started, reviews some of the existing material related to ethical decision-making for high-risk newborns that I consulted as I investigated this area. The review is not exhaustive in that I do not critique of all bioethical debates, discussions, and reports. Such work is available elsewhere and is noted in relevant places throughout the chapter. Rather Chapter 1 includes some history about the development of neonatal intensive care units and then addresses the parents' perspective and its place in the selected bioethical literature, which is more in keeping with the purpose of the project. I actually expand on the background material in the Appendix, The Research Enterprise, to explain the methods employed while attempting to try to better understand what these parents had to say.

In Section II the results of the research project are described and discussed in four chapters. There were various phases to the analysis of the data collected over several years. When this research project began, there were no other studies of ethical decision-making by parents that followed them over a period of time, so in this sense the project was unique.[c] This longitudinal process began prior to the infant's discharge from the NICU (Phase I). The parents were revisited at six months after discharge from the NICU (Phase II) and four years after discharge (Phase III).

The first three chapters of this section (Chapters 2, 3, and 4) include a discussion of the results from the primary analysis of all three phases. A separate chapter represents each phase of the research project. This analysis focused on my goal of understanding and describing the parents' experiences in the NICU and their perception of ethical decision-making across all phases. Each phase of interviewing was analyzed separately and contained its own unique themes (see Table P.1 for a summary).

In the more detailed description of those results presented in these chapters, the organization of the material was modified from the original research reports to avoid repetition. Although all of the content represented in the published research reports is included, the description here is presented in chronological order with the assorted themes embedded in the explanation of the unfolding of events.

Chapter 2 opens with the stories that parents shared with us when they were initially asked to recount their NICU experiences in the predischarge phase: Looking back over these events, what stands out for you? At each of the later two phases of the interviewing, parents were asked to look back over the NICU experience and tell their stories once again. Many recollections were quite similar; sometimes individuals even used exactly the same words to describe an event. Occasionally these later versions differed from the stories given prior to discharge. The remembrances in the later phases need to be simply accepted in the fashion in which they were given, a story now related from a different perspective.

Ethics and decision-making from the parental perspective are discussed in chapters 2, 3, and 4. Although most parents did not perceive themselves to be decision-makers for their infants, various

Table P.1 *Summary of themes and concepts as described in previous research reports*[d]

Phase 1 - **Medicalization of Parenting** (Predischarge): A passive role assumed by parents when the infant was in the NICU

Conflict naming: the parents' description of those events or situations in which they were not sure what was the right thing to do

Content of decision-making: the particular items parents named as targeted areas related to decision-making for the infant

Context of decision-making: the parents' recollection of the circumstances surrounding their decision-making

Information sharing: knowledge acquired for parental participation in decision-making

Infant status: the parents' explanation of the rationale for their infant's admission to the NICU and its subsequent hospitalization

Health care professionals: parental observations about physicians, nurses, social workers, physical therapists, and others who provided care for their infant

Parental recommendations for the future: parents' advice for other individuals who might have an infant in the NICU

Phase 2 **Emerging Ethical Consciousness** (6 months post-discharge): Parents' dawning realization of the scope of decision-making that had occurred and its impact on their present and future lives

Searching for meaning: the parents' process of exploring their experiences in the NICU and attempting to find a suitable rationale for the events they experienced

Communality: parental need for support and meaningful relationships with spouses and children, extended families, neighbors, and the community at large

Contemplation: a growing sense of the importance of control along with the advice they would give to families who now have an infant in the NICU

Table P.1 *Summary of themes and concepts as described in previous research reports* (Continued)

Phase 3 **Life Goes On** (4 years post-discharge): letting go of what might have been and living life to its fullest in the present	
	Processing the story: consigning the NICU events to memory status albeit a powerful and easily accessible one
	Integrating the experience: assimilating the NICU story into the family history and making the infant's life meaningful in the context of the parents' current lives
	Imagining the future: speculating about the long-term effects of this infant on their lives and what they might advise other future parents based on their exposure to the NICU

aspects of the NICU setting and experience relevant to bioethical discussions were explored in order to understand this outcome. Each of chapters 3 and 4 also explores the families' lives during the two intervals after hospitalization: from discharge to six months, and then six months to four years. Finally, parental recommendations for the future as they perceived them at each chronological milestone are reported.

A secondary analysis of the interviews to identify the moral orientation of the parents was also conducted. Identifying moral orientation was an attempt to understand the basis for any decision-making--the *rationale* individuals use to make certain choices out of a whole range of options--rather than a more focused examination of the person's specific *choice*. The results of this task of the project are described in Chapter 5. One of the unique features of this study is this examination of the data using specific strategies to identify the moral orientation of the participants based on the theoretical work of Kohlberg (1958, 1975, 1981, 1984) and Gilligan (1977, 1979, 1982a). The analysis strategy was a modified version of the procedures described by researchers at the Center for the Study of Gender, Education and Human Development at Harvard University, Graduate School of Education (Brown, Argyris et al. 1988; Brown, Debold et al. 1991; Brown, Tappan et al. 1989). All of the chapters in Section II incorporate the various stories of families' lives as well as direct quotes from the interviews conducted with the parents.[e] The stories have been somewhat revised and blended so that no one family can be identified.

However, the stories remain true to the data in that everything described here occurred to some parent at one time or another.

Finally in Section III, Chapters 6 and 7 focus on the meaning of these results. Chapter 6 includes an interpretation and application of the results from all of these phases. The chapter opens with a comparison of the results of this study to an existing theory, namely Reich's Theory of Suffering (1989), and the relationship of this work to his Theory of Compassion (1987c, 1990). Chapter 6 also contains commentary based on a scrutiny of the interview results by gender. Although addressing *parental* perspectives is a critical component of the bioethical parameter of decision-making for high-risk newborns, a certain disservice is rendered by this conflation of information. In the majority of situations, mothers *are* the primary caregivers, and this very important dimension of long-term care for NICU graduates needs to be probed and publicized. Included in the interpretation of the role of mothers as caregivers is some feminist commentary on the NICU situation. At the same time, although some fathers are absent from these families, they should not be neglected. Fathers' roles have not been investigated very frequently so a separate discussion addresses their issues in this chapter. Chapter 7 explores the meaning of the results for the future. The examination includes considerations of technological advancements, the child itself, future family life, and financial ramifications. The discussion includes the implications of these elements both for families and society-at-large. We all face the long-term consequences of decision-making in the NICU as various elements of society impact families and their adjustment, and these families' situations impact us.

An Epilogue is the final segment in the book. Many of us have concerns about families of high-risk infants in stages beyond the four-year postdischarge phase presented here. Although a formal set of rigorously analyzed interviews has not as yet been conducted, several families whose NICU graduates are now older were interviewed. The results provide us with a very small window into their lives and a glimpse of what might be the situation for some of the families in this study as they pass additional milestones in their own futures.

This book, then, is my story as well--the story of my experience with these families as the research project was conceived and evolved over the years.[f] I would ask that the reader keep in mind the fact that this material all passed through my senses as well as those of my research assistant. Although my research assistant conducted most of the interviews there was continuous dialogue between us from first interview to last. We simultaneously implemented the primary analysis of the data across all three phases as the interviews were completed. We regularly met and discussed the meaning of the data as we read and reread the interviews. I alone completed the secondary analysis of the data related to moral orientation as well as the examination of the data by gender and the summaries of the Epilogue interviews. The Appendix, The Research Enterprise provides the details of the process we implemented as well as the documentation and rationale for our decisions. Table P.2 provides a summary of project events.

The modest number of families in the study poses some limitations for the meaning of this data for other parents and families in different situations, although in research parlance our interviews reached saturation, the gold standard for ceasing to collect data in qualitative approaches. A more detailed explanation of limitations is provided in the Appendix, The Research Enterprise. The methodological strategies implemented during the analysis phase, however, provide the strongest possible evidence for the credibility and truthfulness of the data. The conclusions are supported through the various strategies my research assistant and I applied during the research process. Results are further supported by similar findings in other studies. However, the reader is advised to read with these tensions and with the above caveats in mind.

The negativity of many parental comments, as reported previously in research articles based on this project, has been the target of some criticism, which I would like to address. Parents did express a considerable number of negative remarks. This is not to imply that there were no positive aspects to this experience. There are certainly positive observations in previous reports as well as in this monograph. One must keep in mind that experiencing a high-risk perinatal event was an enormous crisis for these individuals and that high-risk events do, relatively speaking, represent a small percentage of the total number of pregnancies and births. Crises and the tragic events surrounding high-risk pregnancies, births, and subsequent care of newborns are circumstances that we would all acknowledge, people generally try to avoid. They simply are negative experiences, something people do not like. Tragedy can beget pessimistic judgments. Parental remarks might also be highly infused with negative perceptions because we allowed them the opportunity to express dissenting viewpoints. We were not caregivers for the child and so there was little risk for parents in being open and honest with us. As indicated by parents themselves during the study, few people wanted to hear their gloomy remarks.

Table P.2 *Chronology of Research Project--Parental Perceptions of Ethical Decision-Making in the Neonatal Intensive Care Unit*

YEAR	EVENT
1985	• Parents in community health case load raise questions about their NICU experiences that appear to have bioethical implications • Literature Review and pilot study conducted
1986	• Society for Health and Human Values (SHHV) regional meeting, presented pilot study
1987	• Association for the Care of Children's Health Annual Meeting, pilot study presented • Health Future Foundation Grant to conduct Phase I (predischarge) and Phase II (six months postdischarge)
1989	• Trigger videotape developed. *Ethical Dilemmas in NICU: The Parents' Perspective* a 7-minute videotape combining photographs of the neonates and parental quotes from Phase I interviews with the parents supplemented by some of the usual sights and sounds of a NICU. Discussion guide available. • SHHV Annual Meeting, Phase I presented including above trigger tape for representation of the data section of the paper. • Background published: "Ethical decision-making for high-risk infants: The parents' perspective." *Nursing Clinics of North America* • Case studies from Phase I utilized: "Parental voices in a sea of neonatal ethical dilemmas." *Issues in Comprehensive Pediatric Nursing*
1990	• Midwest Nursing Research Society Annual Meeting, Phase II presented • University of Maryland/Pi Chapter of Sigma Theta Tau International (STTI), Phase II presented • Grant received from the Nebraska Humanities Council to fund production of full-length video based on Phase I results. • SHHV Annual Meeting, Phase II presented • Premier of video, *I'm Just Your Mother* based on Phase I results • Pilot Study published: "Looking back: Five families share their views of ethical decision-making in the NICU" in *Caring* • Phase I published: "The parents' perspective: Ethical decision-making in neonatal intensive care" *The Journal of Advanced Nursing*[g]

Table P.2 *Chronology of Research Project* (Continued)

YEAR	EVENT
1991	• STTI Regional Assembly, Poster of Phase II displayed • STTI Biennial Convention, Phase II presented • Media Award for video production, *I'm Just the Mother*, STTI Regional Assembly • WOW-TV noon broadcast interview on Phase I, Omaha, NE. • National Center for Nursing Research Grant to conduct Phase III (four years postdischarge follow-up of parental perceptions of ethical decision-making in the NICU)
1993	• Phase II published: "Parental perceptions of ethical decision-making post NICU discharge" in *Western Journal of Nursing Research* • Commentary on methodology published: "Investigator as stranger" in *Qualitative Health Research* • STTI International Meeting, Phase III presented, Madrid, Spain
1995	• Commentary on Phase I combined with results from corollary study of nurses' perceptions of decision-making in the NICU published: "Ethical perceptions of parents and nurses in the NICU: The case of Baby Michael" in *JOGNN* (with Miya, Boardman, Keene, Spielman, & Harr)
1996	• Phase III published: "Ethics in NICU: Parental perceptions at four years postdischarge" in *Advances in Nursing Science* • Ethical issues in NICU, Children's Hospital, Detroit, MI. Presentation combined all three phases of the research project • Ethics and Parental Perspectives of Decision-Making in NICU, University of Pittsburgh, PA. Two presentations, one on the implications of parental perspectives for communication in the NICU and the other on the moral orientation of the parents.
1997	• Midwest Nursing Research Society Annual Meeting, Moral Orientation of Parents of High-risk Newborns presented

Table P1.2 *Chronology of Research Project* (Continued)

YEAR	EVENT
1997	• American Society for Bioethics and Humanities (ASBH) Annual Meeting, Parents and Ethical Decision-Making for High-Risk Neonates: A Feminist Commentary presented. • Sigma Theta Tau International Biennial Convention, Fathers' long-term experiences with high-risk newborns presented.
1998	• Ethical Decision-Making for High-Risk Newborns, Emory University, Atlanta, GA. Presentation based on a summary of all three phases.
1999	• Chronic Illness and the Impact on Families, Panel Member, ASBH Annual Meeting. Presentation based on Phase III.

The reader is asked, then, not to look at this publication as an indictment of an NICU or those health professionals who provide care in such units. One of the dilemmas for health professionals in these units where catastrophe is a daily visitor, is the challenge to work with these infants to the best of their ability while also maintaining their own rationality and sense of accomplishment. If health professionals continually allow themselves to be awash in emotion, feeling the pain, anguish, and suffering of parents and infants every moment, their own integrity could be compromised. What is a crisis for parents however, is the norm for health professionals who work in this area. Gradual loss of sensitivity to the seriousness of events can occur. Several authors have addressed this dilemma for professionals such as nurses and physicians (Bedrick 1992; Berseth et al. 1984; Catlin 1998; Chally 1992; Hefferman & Heilig 1999; Miya 1989; Miya, Boardman et al. 1991; Sanders et al. 1995). The perspectives of professionals providing care in the NICU were *not* the focus of this project. However, some commentary about a balancing of needs among patients, parents, and caregivers is presented in Section III.

Finally, a word about the topic of high-risk infants in general. The unusual situation frequently seizes our attention. This book is no exception. The results that represent the majority of families, the themes, concepts, and categories of data emerging from the data and dominating the discussions are clearly designated. A whole range of perceptions is included here. However, the challenging situations, whether they are tragic or dramatic, are the ones that will stand out in the discussion. The reader must remember, some of these situations are not necessarily the rule but can be an exception. In my opinion, it is to the dilemma or the less than optimal outcome that we must direct our concern as ethical health care professionals and as responsible members of society. When a high-risk pregnancy, birth, or subsequent newborn experience results in a good outcome with no residual sequelae or problems, then we need not worry so much about the family and its adjustments or the integration of the new member.[h] Therefore the more devastating experiences and outcomes are an important element in certain sections of this book. It is to the adverse situation that we must direct our energies in order to critically examine what we are doing in our delivery of health care and ask ourselves if practice should continue in this manner. Or, if unfavorable circumstances from the parental perspective continue, then we must determine a better way to provide optimum health care for those for whom the experience is less than optimal.

I have come to view the unfortunate situations for high-risk newborns as the shadow side of neonatal care. There is a strong reluctance to acknowledge this dimension of health care and to discuss it. The media prefers featuring the "miracle" baby who survives against all odds, the one who is restored to a normal status after a harrowing birth or multiple newborn problems. Newman describes a baby who does not improve despite innovative NICU care as "a hidden dimension of our society's experience because it simply does not fit into our cultural universe" (in Layne 1996, p. 642). Layne, a medical anthropologist, labels such aversion as culturally sanctioned silence. This silence prevents public discourse and hampers the enrichment of society in ways which could ultimately benefit all of us but especially parents of NICU babies.

This book was written to concentrate particularly on the parents of high-risk newborns. I have not attempted in this report, as noted above, to provide a balanced perspective in terms of all possible persons involved in decision-making in the neonatal intensive care nursery where the infants were first hospitalized. I hope that the book stands as an advocacy gesture for these parents. The parents' role in decision-making is seriously debated in the literature, and some of this aspect will be discussed in Chapter 1, Getting Started. I observed that the parents' perspective was not given sufficient emphasis when I first began to develop an interest in this area. I believe this study serves to partially fill the void.

I must also be clear in stating from the start that I am not suggesting a particular philosophy of intervention for high-risk infants: not treating them or leaving them to die, actively ending an infant's life, or implementing treatments aggressively in all cases across the board. Advocating a specific level of intervention is a possible conclusion to which some readers may leap.[i] Rather I am sharing these stories and my experiences with these families so that both health professionals and the general public understand the meaning of the decision-making that occurs in the NICU--especially the meaning for families who have to live with the outcomes of such decision-making. Eventually we are all connected to these outcomes since we live in community with one another and collectively work to provide the necessary societal supports for these families and their children. Presently it is not clear that we are ready to take a shared responsibility for these community members seriously, yet technological developments are enabling more and more marginal newborns to be treated. Reproductive therapies are capable of increasing the number of high-risk pregnancies. Justice does not seem to be served when monumental efforts are made to save and treat infants while at the same time the general public votes to decrease or eliminate various benefits that are essential for such families and their children to survive postdischarge. Families can be left wanting as they struggle to provide for and live with their infants who have special needs. We should take suitable action to support the baby's family both before and after discharge. Support seems to be a missing or at least a weak link in these parents' high-risk experience and subsequent adjustment at home.

This book does not have to be read in the order in which it is presented, and some sections could be skipped initially, depending upon the reader's goals. For those readers simply interested in the results, Section II--Understanding the Parents' Experience with High-Risk Infants, can be read independently of the Background section, and the closing Section III, Contemplating the Parental Perspective. Reading Chapter 1, Getting Started, and the Appendix, The Research Enterprise, assists in putting the project in context but this material is not absolutely necessary in order to understand the parents' commentary. The description of the research enterprise obviously targets readers who are interested in the framework for the research process--various procedures, tasks, and strategies employed to conduct the study. The most thorough understanding, of course, will result from a perusal of all sections. Whatever you decide, come and share my exploration of the world of the NICU as the parents lived it.

Notes

[a] For example, see ethnographic studies or journalistic accounts such as Anspach (1993), Frohock, (1986), Guillemin and Holstrom (1986), Gustaitis and Young (1986), Levin (1986), and Lyon (1985).

[b] Although the unit can be identified in a shorthand manner by pronouncing the initials (*NICU=en-eye-see-you*), pronouncing the first three letters (*NIC*) together followed by the *U* (*nik'you*) is used more frequently by health professionals working in the area by my observation.

[c] A number of studies were published that followed the developmental status of NICU graduates on a long-term basis including physical abilities and such characteristics as likelihood to graduate from high school. Only one project out of the University of Kansas, examined parental perspectives in cases of children with spina bifida postdischarge. At the time of data collection some children were older (age range: less than 1 year, *n*=3, to 19 and older, *n*=4). However, parental perspectives were only sought at this one time and parents were identified through a follow-up clinic rather than at the birth of the child (Barber, Marquis, & Turnbull 1992; Evans 1989)

[d] Bold words and phrases are the names of the concepts and themes.

[e] The assurance of confidentiality and the use of direct quotes and detailed description are certainly of grave concern and create a obvious tension for qualitative investigators (see Davis 1991). A number of expressions, descriptions, and explanations by parents were not unique to a single individual. So identifying the specific person to whom the quote should be attributed is not always evident. See the Appendix, The Research Enterprise, for a specific example. As I read all of the interviews for the secondary analysis, the similarities among selected interviews was even more apparent.

[f] On the basis of the advice I received from the initial copy-editor who read a portion of this monograph, I decided to use personal pronouns when describing my experiences rather than the cumbersome *the author*, *the investigator*, or a similar phrase. However, when the experience involves both my research assistant and myself, *we* is used.

[g] There is an error in this publication. The number of fathers participating in the project is incorrectly noted in this article, page 713. Table 2 figures are also incorrect, page 715. The correct number of fathers is 19.

[h] There is both debate about this approach and some dissenting research results. At least one family in this study with good outcomes for their twins was distressed because of the lack of familial support. Penticuff (a consultant in the research project) observed in her research and clinical experience that the critical difference for mothers coping with the outcomes for their high-risk infants was not the degree of residual limitations in the child but rather the presence or lack of support in their caregiving for the child.

[i] Our work was misinterpreted in some cases. In a dissertation written subsequent to at least one of our reports in *Issues in Comprehensive Pediatric Nursing*, the student wrote, "Several authors have argued for treating all newborns regardless of

premature or handicap (Pinch & Spielman 1989[b]; Caplan & Cohen 1987)." From my perspective, this is a totally erroneous interpretation. Without an exact quotation from our work, it is difficult to uncover the rationale for such a conclusion. Given what I believe to be a clear position relative to advocacy for parental involvement in decision-making, which would lead to a possible wide spectrum of decisions for a neonate, plus subsequent interpretation of our work by others in this same light, it would seem that Davis (1994) was incorrect in making this statement The report in *Issues...* was a discussion of "the family's perception of the consequences of intervention" in the NICU (p. 424). There was no place in the article where any position was taken by us, relative to the treatment of infants in NICU, for or against.

ACKNOWLEDGMENTS

Many people need to be credited for the assistance they provided during the writing of this book. I hardly know where to begin and I am fearful that I will miss someone. The order of my thanks does not necessarily reflect the importance of various people. Funding to conduct the research and administrative support for a sabbatical were certainly critical to the process. Initially Health Future Foundation of Creighton University provided a grant enabling me to conduct Phase I and Phase II of the project. Next the National Institute for Nursing Research funded Phase III of the project (#1-R03-NR02819-01). The Nebraska Endowment for the Humanities and the Graduate School, Creighton University (Dr. Michael Lawler, former Dean) funded the video production. Production of the video was also partially underwritten by the Biomedical Communications Department, Creighton University.

Several administrators were instrumental in supporting my request for a sabbatical (calendar year 1996) as I hold joint appointments in the School of Nursing and the Center for Health Policy and Ethics. The following individuals are included in that category: Dr. Shirley Dooling, former Dean, School of Nursing, now deceased; Dr. Joan Norris, Associate Dean and Dr. Edeth Kitchens, present Dean, both in the School of Nursing; Dr. Charles J. Dougherty, former Director, presently President of Duquesne University and Dr. Ruth Purtilo, present Director at the Center. Other administration and staff support includes reference librarians, work-study students, and other university personnel who were most helpful in their assistance during the process but especially Rita Nutty, Oscar Punla, Joy Steward, and Jamie Waters. After the production of the "trigger" tape based on parents' quotes, Charles A. Lenosky currently Director of Media Services, encouraged me to produce a full-length video based on my research. This dream also materialized with support from Chuck and the production crew.

I am particularly grateful for libraries in general, and each of their staff. Although I most often depended upon the university libraries for my references, the public library system as well as those libraries that responded to interlibrary loan requests were all important. For those of us whose laboratory is the library and whose tools are the written word, I cannot express enough thanks for the funding that provides for the existence of libraries and for the dedication of the staff of those institutions who are always willing to provide their assistance. They deserve a special tribute.

I also thank my family for bearing with me. My husband, Lew, has been most supportive of all of my professional endeavors during our 40+ years of marriage but writing a book extracts a particularly heavy toll. Our children and their spouses also understood the importance of this goal and encouraged me while I was deeply engaged in the process: Karen and Rob Hentz, Heather and Jim Conway, and Nathan Pinch. The results of this work make me particularly thankful for healthy grandchildren who did not need a NICU--Jake and Sara Conway.

An extra special thanks goes to Margaret L. Spielman who has been a valuable colleague, faithful Research Assistant, friend, and source of support. Although Ms. Spielman retired from her faculty position prior to the completion of the research project, she continued to be actively involved in the tasks for its entire duration. Her involvement included periods in which she was paid as well as those many hours she voluntarily carried out important tasks. She also read major portions of numerous drafts of the book. I really could not have completed the project without her.

I reached several points in the project when I felt "stuck" and the copy editing assistance of Ms. Laurie Lieb was especially important at one of those points. She really pushed for clarification in her review of Chapters 2, 3, and 4 as I prepared a prospectus for the book. Ms. Sandy Benson helped put Chapters 1, 5, 6, 7, Epilogue, and the Appendix in shape and tighten up the presentation. Dr. Joan M. Lappe, Dr. Eleanor Howell, Dr. Judith Kissell, and Ms. Su Reinarz each read early drafts of individual chapters. Dr. Jos Welie suggested the inclusion of additional family stories for an Epilogue.

Then there are possible mistakes. Any errors in the text are solely my responsibility and not anyone else who so generously and willingly volunteered their expertise. I apologize for any inaccuracies that occurred. I tried very hard to check and recheck sources, read and reread the material many times; information is documented extensively.

I would welcome information from readers about any oversight and I would appreciate the source for any contradictory information.

Last, but certainly not least, are the parents of the high-risk neonates who were willing to open their hearts and homes to us. This includes but is not limited to the parents who were participants in the research project. Many other parents contributed their support and insight. Through word-of-mouth, parents became aware of the project and several called, wanting to become part of the study. Although formal participation was not possible for the research study itself, we had meaningful conversations that provided additional support for the importance of the study and the validity of the results. Parents who volunteered for the Epilogue graciously shared their on-going experiences with the high-risk graduate beyond those years represented in the research project. The labor intensive research process and the toil necessary to write this book all seemed worth while every time a parent remarked, "How did you know that?" "You are right on target!" "That is exactly what happened to me!" or "You must be sure and tell other parents" when they became aware of our results. The completed book is my tribute to the parents in my study and is dedicated to all parents of high-risk neonates.

CHAPTER 1

Getting Started

I sat at the kitchen table with Carol.[a] Her infant was encircled by her arms and supported on her lap. The apnea monitor was on the chair next to Carol and the tube for the baby's feeding protruded from his nose and ran up to a bag hanging from a stainless steel pole next to her chair. The woman--Carol is not her real name--was exhausted and depressed. The small infant in her arms was not the child she had expected. In Carol's dreams during pregnancy, throngs of Pampers and Gerber babies tumbled about her as she sat in the middle of a meadow filled with a dazzling array of spring blooms. Even in her waking moments during the pregnancy, Carol envisioned herself rocking a plump, gurgling newborn whose smile sent her into ecstasy.

Carol tried not to be seduced by these fantasies because she did not want to jinx the pregnancy. She acknowledged the possibility that something could go wrong. She legalistically calculated in her mind just how much anticipation and preparation she could allow herself without tempting vengeful, jealous gods. Her strategy had not worked. Her situation was the nightmare of all nightmares. Labor pains had started early and could not be stopped. She felt as if she had spent endless days on bedrest. Medications were ordered to halt the cramps and Carol thought she would go crazy. Once she even considered suicide. After the delivery the baby was whisked off to a special nursery which she later learned was the neonatal intensive care unit (NICU, pronounced nik'you).

When Carol first saw the baby, it was a jarring experience. How could this tiny, skinny, almost inert object, connected to all sorts of tubes and lines, be her child? She and her husband just looked at one another. He quickly and quietly wheeled her out of the nursery on that first visit because they both had to cry. Carol and hope were constant companions over the next few months. There was hope that the baby would live, but there was also hope that he would die. Most of the time Carol hoped for a miracle to cure her baby and erase the pain and suffering she saw. The sense of the baby's pain and suffering allowed a different hope to surface occasionally and urged her to envision the baby simply giving up and dying. She felt joy and happiness at his progress along with guilt and self-recrimination when she longed for her own child's demise.

The NICU experience passed. Whatever emotional upheaval Carol faced during those weeks moved to the background now, to be replaced by her reactions to the responsibility of caring for this child herself. With a mask of confidence that would later haunt her, Carol left the hospital with her husband and the baby. Total responsibility for this fragile, sick baby overwhelmed her at first. Yes, her husband was kind, considerate, understanding, and supportive--but he had his own tasks, his own role--and he left home every day to go to work. Carol had to feed, bathe, dress, medicate, and comfort this baby--all day and many times at night as well. The baby had a favorable prognosis but in the meantime apnea monitors and tube feedings were not part of the dream homecoming.

Friends and family were not prepared or equipped for Carol's situation. At first they did not know what to say to her when her pregnancy was obviously over and there was still no baby at home. Family members did stop by, but later, when the baby was home, they were hesitant to touch him or ask to hold him. Some tried to ignore the situation altogether and found any topic under the sun to talk about rather than this newborn or his mother's concerns. Some neighbors and friends simply ignored Carol and her husband. About three weeks after they brought the baby home, cabin fever struck a desperate blow and Carol went to the grocery store with the baby. The trip was a complete fiasco. The equipment was not too difficult to manage but people's responses cut through Carol's heart like a knife. Many people stared, but actually it was worse when others did not even see them. Invisibility was terrifying to Carol.

So Carol continued her life as a mother meeting the demands of her newborn. As a community health nurse, I made home visits as part of the follow-up procedures for these high-risk infants. Carol liked to talk. She had survived the extended hospital stay of her infant and all of the ups and downs it entailed. Now she wanted to know why? Why her? Why this baby? Why now? Why had it all turned out this way? No easy answers were forthcoming for her as she endlessly reviewed the events around conception, pregnancy, and birth. She kept asking herself, "What did *I* do that was wrong?"

As weeks turned into months, Carol vacillated between a combination of pleasure in having her baby home and marvel at his slow but sure progress, and anger tinged with impatience when the path to normalcy became tortuous or blocked. Carol insisted that she was not fully prepared for these events nor for those that possibly lay ahead. It was not a matter of being informed. She heard what health professionals told her and could discuss the status of her son, the treatments, and his prognosis. What she had not realized or internalized was the meaning of this information for her own life, her marriage, and day-to-day living with her baby, as well as all future goals.

Providing holistic care for Carol therefore meant more than implementing technical skills and providing psychosocial support. I really wanted to understand her situation and the experiences she had with her child, what she anticipated, and what in fact ensued. High-risk newborns and decision-making in the neonatal intensive care unit were of major interest to scholars in bioethics, as I had learned in graduate school. Carol and other parents like her prompted me to pull out my bioethical materials related to high-risk newborns.

Some would call the survival of Carol's baby a modern *miracle*. Several decades or even a few years ago, Carol's baby might not have survived. Before exploring the bioethical issues of Carol's situation and similar ones in the NICU, it would be helpful to understand the context in which this baby began his life.

Societal Factors Predating Neonatal Care

Neonatal intensive care has a relatively short history. The formalization of high-risk care did not begin until the 1960s. However, at least three earlier developments during the 20th century set the stage for the evolution of the neonatal unit. First professionals and society as a whole had to acknowledge the intrinsic worth of the object of our treatment--not just a newborn, but a medically needy child (Zelizer 1985). Second, before specialized care of the newborn could be shaped, physicians needed to have access to these infants (Wertz & Wertz 1977). The third change related to the role of effective procedures and technology as they were applied to fragile infants.

The Intrinsic Worth of a Child

There has long been a public fascination with tiny babies and multiple births, as well as a certain degree of repulsion for abnormality. A most gripping photograph of a newborn in my study shows an infant so small his entire body is held completely in the nurse's hand. The observers' attention is riveted on the juxtaposition of an adult palm and a whole infant's body. To make this fascination concrete, one need only remember the media coverage of unusual births and infants: the Dionne quintuplets and decades-long interest in them, several cases of conjoined or Siamese twins, tiny babies on display at Expositions and Fairs in the early part of this century continuing through the more recent birth of several sets of septuplets. On the other hand, many handicapped children continue to be institutionalized or hidden from public view not only because of the parents' inability to provide home care but also because of the shame or guilt families feel about the appearance and/or behavior of the child (Fiedler 1984).

Deciding whether resources should be invested in these specific children, however, is different from being fascinated with them. There had to be a collective, although possibly unspoken, societal agreement that such children deserved special treatment. Children did not always have intrinsic worth; they were valued for many different reasons. Philippe Ariès in *Centuries of Childhood* (1962) noted a *discovery* of childhood as a separate stage of life prior to the 20th century in Europe. Instead of the perception of children as miniature adults, features particular to different age groups were recognized. Rather than children engaging in real labor, they garnered special privileges in various stages of childhood.

In the past, parents were often reluctant to invest interest in or attachment for a child who might early succumb to disease. At many times in history, children were valued more for their contribution to family life than for any actual pleasure they gave their parents. Small children were expected to complete chores around the house that were necessary for the full functioning of adults who often worked from dawn to dusk. Older children in rural areas were obligated to assume responsibilities for animals or fields of crops. In more urban areas, arrangements were often made for children to be apprenticed to skilled workers, or they were simply sent to factories to work.

Family life grew in importance and of course, raising children can be part of family life. Families could be seen as a place where children can feel secure and protected from the ills of society or the vagaries of adverse adult actions and behaviors. The perspective of children's inherent worth also gradually evolved as hazards of childhood were slowly conquered. Adults began to view children as individuals in their own right, not as possessions to be exploited.

Between the 1880s and the 1930s in the United States, a most profound change in the concept of the child occurred. For those between the ages of newborn to 14 years, economic value was gradually replaced by more sentimental value (Zelizer 1985). Several factors contributed to the complex process of change. Zelizer noted six factors: the mortality rate for children improved, child labor legislation was enacted, the morality of insurance policies for children was debated, wrongful death cases of children were won in the court system, adoption practices changed, and the sale of newborns through black market strategies flourished. As Zelizer very bluntly pointed out, children today are economically worthless but emotionally *priceless*. Children are also expensive, requiring real dollars and cents from the family's income. In the case of the critically ill newborn, expense can amount to hundreds, thousands, and even millions of dollars. Society not only altered its customary view of children, but also came to believe in making substantial financial investments for compromised infants.

Physician Access to the Imperiled Newborn

At the turn of the 20th century and for some years to follow, home births and midwife delivery dominated the obstetrical scene. In this period, any sort of formal medical intervention for a newborn was not likely to occur. Even in physician directed deliveries of premature infants, the care of the newborn was the mother's responsibility (Baker 1996). Physicians had yet to develop a scientific interest in newborn care. A significant number of hospital births under the physicians' authority was necessary for medical interventions to be directed at the infant and professional care instituted.

Initially urban women sought physician monitoring during pregnancy and sometimes selected a hospital birth (Wertz & Wertz 1977). Gradually more and more women gave birth in the hospital, and hospital deliveries steadily extended to rural women as well. Physician-controlled pregnancy gradually resulted and specialization evolved, sometimes referred to as the medicalization of pregnancy (Barker 1998). Not only did physicians target the childbirth process but other medical practitioners also confined their practice area to children and the specialty of pediatrics evolved. Later, of course, when NICUs were established and neonatal care emerged, further specialization developed and training for neonatologists began in the 1960s.

Technological Intervention for the Endangered Newborn

As a third consideration, physicians required some effective means to improve the course of the baby's development as they cared for infants. One could not simply watch and wait, although that too continues to be a dimension of high-risk care. A total watch and wait approach could take place in the home, and it did. Babies sometimes were warmed, resting on oven doors or swaddled and tucked into a shoe box or bureau drawer. To legitimatize hospital care, some sort of practitioner action had to be part of the care that could not be provided in the home. Even more specifically, devices were needed that generally were not available in the home setting, or that required special training to operate. Eventually these interventions had to meet some sort of standard leading to a label of *successful.* Technology or procedures must be available, admired, and desired. Finally, certain babies had to benefit from these interventions.

The use of innovative devices and protocols for the treatment of compromised infants became centralized. When women began to deliver children in the hospital, special nurseries for sick newborns were formed and premature nurseries were organized (Baker 1996; O'Donnell 1990). Separation of newborns with special needs was a practical decision, not only in terms of the infants' increased requirements, but also to safeguard healthy newborns. As sophisticated technology was utilized and close monitoring was required, specialized nursing care was also ordained. The adult intensive care unit provided many valuable lessons for those who were seeking advanced, effective interventions for the child and newborn.

Once these three phenomena were in place--valuing the newborn, hospital birth, and technological success--then the intensive care nursery could become a reality. Some highlights of the NICU's history serve to advance our understanding of the context of the neonate's initial life experiences. Following the discussion of the NICU history, the state of the art of bioethics related to high-risk newborns will be reviewed. For example, bioethical concerns surface when there is disagreement about whether the possible treatment is desirable or *good*, whether we *should* or *ought* to use all or part of the interventions available to us. Related to using technologies and procedures are decisions about when it is morally permissible to stop them. In addition, moral problems arise about the social implications of intensive care--who bears the burden, what regulations (if any) might be imposed. Following closely on the heels of such considerations is the ultimate question of *who* shall make all these decisions. Given the emphasis here on parents, this last consideration is crucial.

History of Neonatal Care

The premature baby has long challenged the ingenuity of midwives and physicians. About 7% of the infants born each year fall into the premature category[b] (approximately 280,000 out of a total of almost 4 million births) (Births 1998; Fertility 1999). Additionally, some 3% of births (150,000) have major birth defects (genetic, chromosomal, or environmentally related anomalies) requiring specialized care (Fertility). Monumental accomplishments mark current practice including the long-term survival of several infants weighing less than 500 grams (about 17.6 ounces) (Amato & Schneider 1991; Muraskas, Carlson et al. 1991; Muraskas, Marshall et al. 1999; Sherer et al. 1992).[c] However, until around 1960, little in the way of standardized, efficacious treatment was available or applicable to the imperiled newborn (Lyon 1985). Imperiled newborns, in addition to premature infants, include newborns born at term who developed problems in utero or in the transition to extrauterine life.[d] In the years when few births occurred in hospitals, sick or premature infants may have lived only a few hours and little regret may have accompanied some of these outcomes (Anspach 1993). Premature babies as well as those with disease or disability were consigned to a natural death since effective interventions were simply not widely available (See Table 1.1 for a summary of selected events in the history of NICUs)

As the years passed, physicians monitored an increasing number of pregnant women, and by 1939, half of all women delivered their children in hospitals (Kett 1984). The medicalization of childbirth expanded as more birth experiences moved from home to hospital and medical interventions escalated. As medical care provided more solutions to problems of pregnancy and childbirth, the search for scientific, medical answers to newborn problems was predictable.

Table 1.1 *Selected Highlights of Neonatal Intensive Care Development*

DATE	EVENT
1878	• Tarnier develops the first incubator or warming chamber (Anspach 1993)
1898	• Dr. Martin Couney, the Incubator Doctor, made his first visit to the U.S. to exhibit his premature babies--last exhibit in 1950 (Silverman 1979)
1900	• Budin wrote the first textbook on care of the premature infant, which consisted of a collection of 10 of his lectures (Silverman 1979)
1920	• Dr. Julian Hess patented the Hess incubator
1922	• First special care unit for premature babies at the Sarah Morris Hospital in Chicago (Murray & Caplan 1985; Plass 1994)
1929	• Role of surfactant in respiratory functioning identified
1930	• Drinker infant respirator installed in Philadelphia Lying-In Hospital to provide continuous respiratory support for premature (O'Donnell 1990)
1950	• Allen and Diamond develop the ability to provide exchange transfusions (Queenan 1985)
1951	• High concentrations of oxygen found to cause retrolental fibroplasia (Lyon 1985)
1952	• Danish clinician called on anesthesiologist during polio epidemic, who introduced positive pressure breathing to save children's lives at Blegdam Hospital in Copenhagen. Forerunner of ventilator (Wildes 1995)
1953	• First modern use of mechanical ventilation of the newborn (Cassani 1994)
1958	• Phototherapy discovered as a treatment for hyperbilirubinemia (Lyon 1985)
	• Development of the ventricular shunt (Anspach 1993)
1962	• Establishment of National Institute of Child Health and Human Development (Historical resources, n.d.; Weir 1984)
	• First NICU established at Vanderbilt Medical Center in Nashville, TN (Harms & Giordano 1990)

Table 1.1 *Selected Highlights* (Continued)

1963	• Birth of the Kennedy son who was diagnosed with "ideopathic respiratory distress syndrome" which alerted the public to the status of neonatal care (Harris 1995)
1965	• Premature nursery becomes the neonatal intensive care nursery (Krollman et al. 1994)
	• Necrotizing enterocolitis reported by Mizrahi, Blanc, and Silverman (Queean 1985)
1966	• Speciality of neonatology established (Lyon 1985)
1968	• Total parenteral nutrition available (Krollman et al. 1994)
1970	• Regionalization and transportation of risky infants to experienced staff and sophisticated equipment (Harris 1995)
1971	• Contiuous positive air pressure (CPAP) introduced by Dr. George Gregory (O'Donnell 1990)
	• First use of extracorporeal membrane oxygenation (ECMO) [e] on a premature (Herschl & Bartlett 1998)
	• Prenatal lung maturity test devised (Lyon 1985)
1972	• Neonatal nursing care recognized (Krollman et al. 1994)
	• Neonatal temperature control with radiant heat (Queenan 1985)
1974	• First perinatal outreach program established by Children's Hospital, Denver CO through a grant from the National Foundation March of Dimes (Gardner 1994)
1975	• Speciality of perinatology established (Lyon 1985)
	• Neonatologists first certified (Bucciarelli 1994; Horbar & Lucey 1995)
1976	• 125 NICUs in North America (Horbar & Lucey 1995)
1981	• Initial trials of the Nellcor pulse oximeter to better monitor respiratory function (Cassani 1994)
	• Open fetal surgery first performed at the University of California at San Francisco for urinary tract obstruction (Fetal firsts 1997; Harrison et al. 1982)

Table 1.1 *Selected Highlights* (Continued)

1981	• Neonatal surfactant therapy proposed by Fujiwara, Morley and Jobe (Queenan 1985)
1982	• *Neonatal Nursing* first published for specialists in the nursing care of prematures (O'Donnell 1990)
1983	• 1509 physicians practicing neonatology (Horbar & Lucey 1995) • First year for certification of neonatal nurse practitioners (Waltman & Schenk 1999)
1984	• Founding of the National Association of Neonatal Nurses (Merenstein 1994) • Two hundred programs and more than 800 certified perinatal and neonatal specialists reported (Weir 1984) • Mechanisms of gas transport during ventilation by high frequency oscillation reported (Chang 1984)
1985	• 600 hospitals provide 7500 neonatal intensive care beds with about 1200 pediatricians trained in neonatology (Murray & Caplan 1985)
1989	• Cryosurgery for retinopathy (Krollman 1994) • Perflurochemical liquid first used for ventilation with human neonate (Weis & Fox 1999)
1993	• Laser surgery for retinopathy (Krollman et al. 1994) • EXIT (ex-utero intrapartum treatment) developed for various types of airway obstruction in the fetus (Fetal firsts 1999) • 528 physicians in neonatal training programs and 2498 board-certified neonatologists (Horbar & Lucy 1995)
1995	• 3000 neonatologists are active in the U.S. 500 hospitals report housing a NICU accounting for 12,000 beds in one report (McCormick & Richardson 1995) • 700 units including both level II and level III nurseries are cited in another report with 3740 individuals interested in neonatology (Horbar & Lucey 1995)

Fundamental Needs of the Compromised Newborn

The first factors critical to the survival of fragile newborns involved the basic means to keep them warm, prevent infection, support respirations, and provide nourishment. These four factors combined to form the driving force in developing successful strategies to save the lives of these infants. The temperature regulation challenge first benefited from Dr. Etienne Stephene Tarnier's *warming chamber*, which was devised for him by M. Odile Martin of the Paris Zoo in 1878 (Anspach 1993; Guillemin & Holmstrom 1986; O'Donnell 1990; Plaas 1994; Silverman 1992). This first device was a modified poultry incubator called a *Lion Incubator* installed for use in the Paris Maternité Hospital.

A somewhat carnival-like atmosphere surrounded the early publicity about the infant incubator. Dr. Pierre-Constant Budin, a French obstetrician and associate of Tarnier, displayed six incubators containing premature patients at various expositions and exhibits throughout Europe (Anspach 1993; Silverman 1992). Dr. Martin A. Couney, a student of Budin, transported this strategy to the United States and between 1889 and 1940 demonstrated the care and feeding of infants at various fairs and expositions. Mexico and South America were sites of similar exhibits.

In the meantime, Dr. Julian Hess patented an incubator in 1920 and subsequently established the first special care unit for premature babies at the Sarah Morris Hospital in Chicago (Murray & Caplan 1985; O'Donnell 1990; Plaas 1994). By the 1940s, premature nurseries were being set up in various hospitals and medical centers across the country (Jonsen 1991; Guillemin & Holmstrom 1986).

Infection was recognized as a threat decades before NICUs were established. An initial strategy to combat infection was the isolation of newborns; syphilitic newborns were among early examples of separate care (Baker 1996). The later advent of antibiotics contributed to the solution of the infection problem. Although certain decayed materials and molds had been used for centuries as primitive medicinals, the connection of microbes, infection and the effectiveness of molds in treating disease was not made until the 19th century. Only after the isolation of substances like penicillin (1939), actinomycin (1940), and streptomycin (1944) was there systematic employment of and research related to these products. Appropriate use of antibiotics and dosage titration for premature infants and newborns followed. The conquering of infection was not without hazard. Serology, symptomatology, therapeutic dosages, and serious side effects all posed significant challenges along the way in neonatal care (Korones 1976).

Subsequent Treatment Developments

Premature babies continue to be treated in special nurseries as do those with congenital problems, life threatening genetic defects, and other medical problems. Initially, treatment was rather basic, as attested to in the previous discussion of warming and infection, and achievements varied. More successful medical interventions occurred after World War I (Cohen et al. 1987). War needs were the motivation for scientists to develop technology that could be applied later to peacetime medical care. One significant development was the fabrication of materials such as Plexiglas and plastics. Additionally, the accomplishments of adult intensive care units stimulated physicians to apply the same concepts of care to newborns: skilled, high ratio nursing care and the application of the latest medical innovations.

Lung and other elemental problems haunted pediatricians for some time. Ventilatory assistance, an increased understanding of the iatrogenic effects of oxygen,[f] and a breakthrough in the treatment of jaundice all catapulted successful high-risk newborn care forward. Scientific knowledge and various inventions were decisive for the improvement of respiratory function as well as other problem areas such as nutrition, congenital anomalies, and other iatrogenic conditions in the premature newborn.[g]

One necessary ingredient for the correction of respiratory difficulty grew out of the discovery of positive pressure breathing during the polio epidemic of 1952 (Reiser 1993). Donald and Lord described mechanical ventilation of the newborn in 1953 (Cassani 1994). A team at the University of California at San Francisco headed by George Gregory, an anesthesiologist (Lemburg 1997), reported success with CPAP (continuous positive airway pressure, not mechanical ventilation) for prematures with respiratory distress syndrome (RDS) in 1971 (Lyon 1985). This discovery, along with positive end expiratory pressure (PEEP), combined to lower the mortality rate for RDS to 20% during the 1970s.[h]

Surfactant and its role in respiratory functioning was another such scientific breakthrough first described by Kurt von Neergaard in 1929 but left idle for more than two decades (Lyon 1985). Interest in surfactant was renewed in the late 1950s, and progress raised the hopes of those in neonatal care. Experimental surfactants became available in the late 1980s and were approved by the Federal Drug Administration in 1990 (Muraskas, Marshall et al. 1999). Later, scientists developed artificial surfactant and research in liquid ventilation ensued.[i]

The French, besides devising a method of warming premature infants with incubators, also designed a method of feeding babies too weak to bottle-feed (Baker 1996). Gavage, the insertion of a tube through the nose into the stomach in order to introduce a diluted milk feeding or breast milk, substituted for normal sucking and swallowing (Lyon 1985). Gavage feeding continues to be used, but formulas have become quite sophisticated in their replacement of natural nutrients for the underdeveloped gastrointestinal tract of the premature or the special needs of an impaired newborn. Intravenous or central lines accessing the circulatory system are another modern alternative for meeting nutrition requirements.[j] Such access can provide not only the water with glucose (sugar) that numerous patients frequently receive but total parenteral nutrition can be delivered via the central line. This means that infants unable to take nourishment by mouth or whose gastrointestinal tract will not tolerate breast or bottle feedings can acquire proper nutrition. Although long-term use is possible, it too is not without iatrogenic problems--liver damage and possible need for liver transplant (Barr 1998).

Prevailing Philosophy of Care

Rescue can be used to characterize the early years of most premature care (mid-1940s to 1970s) or a physician's own philosophy of care (Jonsen 1991; Lyon 1985; Silverman 1981, 1992). At least one bioethicist views much of medical practice as rescue, making the neonatal unit no different than any other arena of care (Minogue 1996). But compromised babies were a special challenge to early staff personnel who were in charge of the infant's hospitalization. Few protocols and standards of care existed in the early days of the NICU. Physicians simply moved quickly and used whatever means were available on prematures and other newborns with medical problems. Personnel were especially motivated when such compromised infants breathed spontaneously or initially survived without aggressive therapy. The infant's *fight for life* was taken as a sign to facilitate in any way possible, the functioning of the newborn's various systems.

Originally most if not all of the care provided for extremely small newborns or those with congenital anomalies was at least somewhat experimental. Each new lower birth weight or gestational age presented a type of challenge which the staff attempted to meet by getting the infant to survive longer or grow bigger than the previous attempt. Usually, all theories of care were exhausted before the medical staff decided a specific case was hopeless. In this manner, a regimen for treatment was created. Although treatment was *experimental*, physicians were reluctant to experiment. In other words, there was not a strong desire to randomize and treat these newborns according to an evolving protocol. Instead physicians felt pressed to move promptly, apply as many treatments as appropriate, and save as many lives as possible. Some judged this to not always be a prudent manner in which to act. A friend of author Lyon (1985) noted that medical interventions in the neonatal intensive care unit were merely turning previous "miscarriages...into lifelong heartaches." Some believe that the *rescue* imperative continues to haunt the practice of neonatology and the care of newborns in the NICU today (Simpson 1999; Stevenson & Goldworth 1999). Health care professionals often feel reluctant to deny the use of any potentially useful treatment (R.H. Clark 1996).

Morbidity and Mortality

The success of neonatal units can be demonstrated in one way by the decreasing mortality and morbidity rates for newborn infants. Statistics are usually discussed in terms of infant weight or gestational age. Generally speaking, the smaller and more sick the infant, the greater the residual sequelae and the higher the death rate. In 1950 it was rare for infants weighing 1000 grams or less to survive (Avery 1994). In the mid-1960s, 28-week infants were not even admitted to the premature nursery because they were believed to be nonviable (Krollmann et al. 1994). In 1969, 50% of infants between 1000 and 1500 grams lived to be discharged while only 20% of those between 750 and 1000 grams survived, and a mere 4% of those under 750 grams managed to overcome initial travesty (Lyon 1985).

Over the next two decades or so, the overall death rate for premature infants dropped 55% (Lyon 1985). In 1976 the World Health Organization defined fetuses weighing less than 500 grams as nonviable (Hack & Fanaroff 1986). By the mid-1980s, 85% to 90% of the 1000 to 1500 gram infants survived, as did 50-75% of those between 750 and 1000 grams, and 25% of those below 750 grams (Lyon). Eighty-nine percent of infants over 29 weeks gestation survived without major disability, while 50% of infants 25 weeks or less were without major disability (Mellien 1992). The rarity of the smaller weights must be acknowledged as well. Only 0.6% of live births weigh less than 1000 grams (Paneth 1992). A single case of survival of a 440-gram, 25-week neonate was described in 1984, and, as already noted, several small newborns made history in the 1990s (Mellien; Sherer et al. 1992).

However, lower weight infants are surviving longer now.[k] Infants weighing less than 1000 grams were 29 times more likely to survive in 1983 than in 1960. The most significant differences in mortality, however, are in infants weighing more than 1500 grams, and those born between 28 and 34 weeks gestation. By 1990, the overall neonate mortality rate had declined 78.5% from rates reported for 1940 (Avery 1994). In 1993, the United States ranked 22nd worldwide in infant mortality, but the weight-specific survival rate in the U.S. was the highest of any country (Inglis 1994).

*Re*hospitalization is a greater problem for the low birth weight baby than for a normal newborn (Hurt 1984). Normal babies had a repeat hospitalization rate of 8.4% while the former NICU patient rate was 19% in 1980. Postdischarge mortality was 10 times as great for NICU babies as for normal newborns. Additionally, in 1984, between 2300 and 17,000 children were estimated to be dependent on life-saving technologies, including ventilators (Task force 1988). Many of these children were graduates of a NICU experience.

Babies of lower birth weight (1000 grams or less) often continue to have problems in childhood (McCormick et al. 1992). In a 1992 study (Schlomann), these children showed developmental difficulties, attention deficits, and more frequent illnesses resulting in school absences. A 72% handicap rate was reported for infants who had required mechanical ventilation during their neonatal period. A study in 1994 reported school-age outcomes for children with birth weights under 750 grams (Hack et al. 1994). These children were found to be at high-risk for diminished cognitive ability, decreased psychomotor skills, and poor school performance. Low birthweight infants (less than 2,500 grams) were found to be more likely to use special education services when they attended school and were more likely to repeat a grade, adding to the cost of their education (Lewit et al. 1995). More recently, newborns weighing less than 5.5 pounds were found to be less likely to graduate from high school by age 19 (53.5% of graduates who were normal newborns versus 15.2% of siblings who had been low birth weight) (Conley & Bennett 2000). There appears to be a finite limit to the survival of an intact, reasonably functioning infant. However, what exactly defines this limit is difficult to determine.

Arbitrary cutoffs based on gestational age or weight will not work in the view of some experts (McCormick 1994). Rather neonatologists continue to assess individual infants and make decisions based on vitality and viability rather than on a simple calculation of gestational age and weight.

Levels of functioning and self-perceived quality of life of extremely low-birth-weight (ELBW) infants at adolescence can be in marked contrast to an outsider's perception (Saigal, Feeny et al. 1996; Saigal, Stoskopf et al. 1999). In a study of ELBW infants, now adolescents, morbidity and quality of life measurements were lower than a matched group of children. However the adolescents own view of their quality of life, those with a history of ELBW, was quite satisfactory and much the same as other adolescents. Even more interesting was the finding that health professionals were less accepting of disability in a series of hypothetical cases than either parents or adolescents who were ELBW.

Monetary Considerations

Specialized infant care requires significant financial investment. Among all types of hospitalization, neonatal care can be the most costly (Murray 1985b). The United States (U.S.) Office of Technology Assessment (1987) stated that while 8% of admissions were accounted for by neonatal admissions, they required 25% of the hospitals' costs. All sorts of statistics are available for the cost of NICU care, and their common theme is that the bills for such care are high. The cost of NICU care may be acknowledged, but it is rarely questioned. The NICU continues to be an area of health care where pressure to curtail spending is *not* exerted. Overall, an assumption of unlimited resources has been observed (Schlomann 1992).

In the late 1960s, a modest figure of $100 per day for a 3-4 week stay was given ($100 for 1968 = $508 for 2001) [1] (Hack & Fanaroff 1989). The U.S. Office of Technology Assessment (1987) cited average hospital costs in 1987 for low birthweight (1500-2500 grams) infants ranged from $12,000 to $39,000 while costs for a very low birthweight (1000-1500 grams) survivor ranged between $31,000 and $71,000. Based on a 1998 project on shifting NICU cost to aftercare, daily charges for NICU were calculated at about $2,500 (Chan 2000). Costs for individual cases with borderline health status can reach hundreds of thousands or even millions of dollars (Guillemin & Holmstrom 1986; Weir 1992). Although most reports use *costs* and *charges* interchangeably, in the majority of cases figures reflect what is charged by the facility. Rarely is the actual cost calculated.

In 1985, $1.9 billion was spent on high-risk infants ($3.12 billion in 2001 dollars) (Harms & Giordano 1990). Costs of intensive care have been estimated to run about three times those for other patients (Wildes 1995). In 1986, for an average hospitalization of 137 days, the average cost of intensive care amounted to $158,000 (Hack & Fanaroff 1986; Harris 1995). In 1987 the United States spent $3 billion on NICU care ($4.6 billion in 2001 dollars), while an estimate for 1978 was only $1.5 billion ($4.1 billion in 2001 dollars) (Frohock 1986). By 1995 the figure was $4 billion for low-birth weight infants (billion in 2001 dollars) with roughly half going to the very smallest (Lewit et al. 1995).

A report in 1986 emphasized the differences in cost relative to the age of the neonate; smaller, younger infants escalated the costs of treatment. As one article noted, we moved from Baby Doe to Baby Dough (Peabody & Martin 1996). Infants over 29 weeks gestational age had initial hospitalization bills half the amount of infants born at 25 weeks or less (Mellien 1992). Another report, found a similar difference by weight: 500-999 gram survivors averaged $200,000 in initial hospitalization charges while the 1000-1499 gram infants averaged $100,000 ($354,618 and $177,309 respectively for 2001 dollars) (Boyle et al. as quoted in Menzel 1990, Note#5, p. 113). One state report also released during the mid-1980s noted an average charge for initial hospitalization of $7850 ($12,924=2001 dollars) per neonate, compared to $32,900 ($53,998=2001 dollars) per severely ill neonate under 1000 grams (Imershein et al. 1992). For a 500-999 gram infant in 1990 an average of $200,000 ($270,237=2001 dollars) was cited and for a 1000 to1499 gram newborn, $100,000 was the average charge (Menzel 1990; Paneth 1992). In a 1993 report, the average charge for the surviving neonate's hospitalization when weighing between 500-600 grams was $1 million (Paneth 1995).

A Canadian economist, Robert Evans, discussed an interesting phenomenon related to the cost of high-risk newborn treatment (1987). Dr. Evans based his observations on statistics covering a 20-year span from the late 1960s to the late 1980s in British Columbia. Efforts had been instituted to reduce pediatric costs, and indeed these efforts were successful overall. When the figures were examined in detail, pediatric surgical care actually accounted for the decrease while medical admission costs remained stable. Even more to the point, when medical care was further analyzed by differentiating the costs by including patients 1 to 14 years of age, rather than 0 to 14, it was found that even the cost of medical admissions had decreased. When medical care included sick newborns 0 to 1 year, this expense alone prevented the medical side of pediatric care to reflect any cost saving.

A counter argument was developed supporting the financial investment in NICU care on the basis of distributive justice (Meadow et al. 1996). Mortality rates and length of stay for NICU babies and adult ICU patients requiring mechanical ventilation for respiratory failure were compared. They concluded that ICU adult patients who died used more resources than the NICU babies. Additionally, the longer NICU patients remained in the unit the more likely they would be discharged while the reverse functioned for the adults.

A focus on initial costs, however, disguises the overall financial requirements for these sick newborns and even the above study did not consider this element. Certainly, the need for professional interventions in the care of some of these children does not end at discharge from the NICU. About 5% of children or 3.3 million live with either a long-term disability or limitation related to a chronic condition (Newacheck 1990). The U.S. Office of Technology Assessment reported that out of 100 very low birthweight infants, 27 will die, 16 will be seriously disabled, and most of the remaining 57 will be normal (1987). Some may develop mild learning disabilities. Lyon (1985), when discussing post-acute care expenses, noted that $2.3 billion (2001 = $3.8 billion) was spent on the rehospitalization of birth-impaired children and adults in 1985, while $350 million (2001 = $575 million) was utilized for their office visits. Nearly half of office visits to physicians are accounted for by only 10% of the high-use children's cohort (Newacheck). Children ages 1 to 15, born with low birthweight (7% of children in that age group or 3.5 to 4 million total), were estimated to cost $5.5 to $6 billion more than if they had been of normal birth weight (Lewit et al. 1995).

On an individual basis, a child with Trisomy-21 (Down syndrome), if institutionalized in 1984, would generate costs of $1.5 million (2001 = $2.5 million) over a lifetime of about 50 years (Lyon 1985). In general, families pay only about one fifth of these expenses out-of-pocket (Newacheck 1990). Some expenditures are met by parents' private insurance policies, but the remaining support comes from public insurance, special federal and state programs, and service organizations. Although financially supporting the care for these infants is important, such needs do not entitle the infant to infinite resources (Fost 1999). Another seldom discussed financial repercussion of long-term disabilities is the lost contribution to society by individuals who may never work or contribute to the life of the community yet proportionally use more resources.

At the other end of the spectrum is the prevention analysis of financial implications. Effective means to prevent premature birth and the need for NICU care could make a significant difference economically. According to the 1985 report of the Committee to Study the Prevention of Low Birth Weight at the Institute of Medicine, an investment of $12 million (2001 = $19.7 million) in prenatal care could save upwards of $40 million (2001 = $65.7 million) in health costs during the first year of life (Schlomann 1992). Put a different way, the estimated *total* cost of prenatal care for one woman is less than half of the *daily* cost of one day in the NICU (Anspach 1993).

Another more controversial strategy to decrease admissions to the NICU is genetic screening. An account from the United States Centers for Disease Control and Prevention estimated that mass screening for spina bifida and the prevention of such births would save more than $4 million (2001 = $6.5 million) based on testing a hypothetical cohort of 100,000 women. However, this is grounded on an unrealistic assumption and morally questionable situation that all fetuses would be aborted if the neural tube defect was found and could not be corrected (Lyon 1985).

Fetal therapy is an option that has the potential to reduce the length of stay and possibly even admission rates to the NICU, which ultimately affect costs for compromised infants. Since 1963, intrauterine transfusion for Rh hemolytic disease has developed and become standard treatment.[m] Surgical interventions for congenital hydronephrosis and obstructive hydrocephalus were implemented in the early 1980s (Fletcher & Jonsen 1984).[n] Other surgical possibilities include transplants, correction of spina bifida and diaphragmatic hernia.[o] A remarkable photograph of a fetus reaching out of the uterus and grasping the surgeon's hand during the procedure to correct spina bifida, reverberated around the world on the internet and captured the interest of millions (Holding hands 1999).[p]

The People and the Place

The first neonatal intensive care unit, as distinguished from a premature nursery, was started at Vanderbilt Medical Center, Nashville, Tennessee, in 1962 (Harms & Giordano 1990;). By 1965, 16 such units existed, and the number increased rapidly over the next few years (American Hospital Association [AHA] 1988, 1992; Robert

Wood Johnson 1985; Tooley & Phibbs 1976). Regionalization and transport services were used as a combined approach to consolidate services, provide experienced staff, and apply sophisticated technology for the treatment of at-risk infants (Harris 1995).[q] More and more medical centers created their own units, and by 1973 most larger hospitals contained a NICU (Lyon 1985). In 1980 there were 600 NICUs in the United States. A 1984 report showed that 0.9% of hospital beds were devoted to pediatric and neonatal intensive care units (Wildes 1995) and for 1988, 703 hospitals with 11,020 bed offered Level III services (Bucciarelli 1994). In 1993, 794 units with 13,873 beds were reported (AHA 1994-1995). In 1962 the National Institute of Child Health and Human Development was established, indicating interest in child welfare at the federal level (Historical resource, n.d.). This effort moved neonatology nationally beyond its early emphasis on prematures to an expanding range of medical problems in newborns.

With the advent of research endeavors such as those related to respiratory problems, care of premature infants by physicians became a subspecialty called neonatology. The movement enlarged as these physicians focused on an ever-increasing range of medical problems in newborns, including congenital anomalies and other disabilities. They no longer limited themselves to the premature but instead included all high-risk newborns. By 1975, neonatology became a subspecialty with board certification; 355 physicians passed the first qualifying examination. In 1991, 103 training programs for neonatology had been approved (Bucciarelli 1994; Lyon 1985). More than 1200 certified perinatal and neonatal specialists served the NICUs (Murray & Caplan 1985), and by 1993, the number of specialists had increased to 2,610 (American Medical Association [AMA] 1994). In addition to neonatologists, a variety of other physicians--including cardiologists, radiologists, surgeons, ophthalmologists, neurologists, and pathologists--participated in the care of high-risk newborns as needed.

Korones recognized the importance of neonatal nursing care for the successful outcomes of infants in his classic textbook, *High-Risk Newborn Infants*, first published in 1972 (Krollman et al. 1994). The journal *Neonatal Nursing* began publication in 1982 for nurse specialists in the care of prematures. Then in 1984, the National Association of Neonatal Nurses was founded (Merenstein 1994). Other allied health personnel were also part of the team responsible for carrying out procedures and monitoring the status of the neonate. Social workers, child life specialists, respiratory therapists, physical therapists, pharmacologists, laboratory technicians, and pastoral care personnel can all be involved in infant care and extended interventions for the family.

In addressing various factors in the NICU setting, we have yet to consider the parents of this infant. In the early days of the incubator sideshows, infants were completely handed over to physicians and nurses by hospitals or foundling homes operating on behalf of the parents (Lyon 1985). Once the infants were sufficiently strong and healthy, they were returned to the parents, but sometimes with great difficulty. Parents were not as appreciative of the baby's survival as expected. Zahorsky, a St. Louis pediatrician, called this phenomenon of withdrawal or rejection by parents *hospitalism* (Silverman 1979). Even within hospitals, parents were routinely excluded from visiting nurseries when special units were first established. This exclusion was based on the staff's understanding that a visiting parent would only increase the dangers of infection for the compromised newborn. However, a study in 1970 showed that the "presence of mothers did not increase the risk or occurrence of infection" and visitation rules were revised accordingly (Harris 1995). One report noted the distinction in these rules between mothers and fathers, pointing out that fathers did not obtain a *non-visitor* status in the NICU until 1974 (Krollman et al. 1994). The idea that an emotional investment by parents in the neonate was necessary for the ultimate health of the child was an even later development. The research on maternal-infant bonding in the 1980s provided the basis for the impetus to facilitate parental contact with the newborn rather than thwarting it (Klaus & Kennel 1982).

The first support group for parents was established in 1975 at the University of Utah Medical Center. In 1982, Parent Care, Inc., an international organization dedicated to improving the NICU experience for babies, families, and caregivers, was established (Plaas 1994). Specialty support groups were also founded for mothers of twins, mothers of triplets, or as some groups have evolved, for mothers or parents of multiples.

An increasing emphasis on fathers and their role with high-risk neonates is more recent. A National Fathers' Network was formed in the 1990s, funded by a SPRANS grant from the Maternal and Child Health Bureau (National Fathers 1992-1993). The network was devised to act as an advocate for fathers of children with special needs. Also, a monthly column, "Fathers' Voices," was published in *Exceptional Parent* magazine (May 1996). Finally, in this age of the information superhighway, the internet has many sources for networking, support, information, and advice related to the high-risk newborn, the NICU, and caring for a child with special needs.[r] Evaluating those sources can be most challenging, as not all of them are not equally valid or reliable.[s]

By examining the confluence of these developments, we can see how multiple elements contributed to the formation of one of the most sophisticated, complex, labor-intensive units in the hospital. A large dimension of high-risk newborn care is highly dependent on the most advanced, complicated technology which is able to substitute for the neonate's underdeveloped bodily systems. The expertise of many professionals combine to address the needs and solve the problems of compromised newborns. However, even knowing details of these elements does little to prepare anyone for a first visit to the NICU. The tiny size of these infants contrasted with the multiple devices that keep them alive can be shocking for the uninitiated. Within this milieu, many decisions must be made. What is done, how treatment is accomplished, and who makes the decisions lead to another dimension of concerns--not simply what we can do, but what we *should* do, when we *should* stop, and *who should* be responsible for decision making.

Bioethical Issues in the Neonatal Intensive Care Unit

Modern bioethical debate and discussion about high-risk neonates spans only a few decades.[t] The bioethical exploration of treatment decision-making begins with what is available and what is possible, who is involved, and then moves on to examine what *should* be done, why it should be done, and which decision ultimately prevails. Examination of the bioethical dimension of intensive neonatal care is the search for and judgment about the good and the bad, the right and the wrong (Hospers 1972). Contributing to this search is the set of various values, beliefs, and traditions, and the sense of moral responsibility of the individuals involved in the situation (Frazer et al. 1992). Interest in the issues certainly affects those directly involved in the infant's care such as the health professionals and the parents, and may also extend to others, both in the acute care hospital and in the community at large. It can be as broad as the boundaries of society (See Table 1.2 for a summary of selected factors related to bioethical debate in the NICU).

The inability to predict outcomes with certainty during most of the time premature and intensive care nurseries have existed, means that many, if not all treatment decisions have ethical implications (Caplan

Table 1.2 *Major Issues Related to Neonatal Bioethical Decision-Making*

DATE	EVENT
1956	• Tjio and Levan demonstrate presence of 46 chromosomes (Queenan 1985) • Aminocentesis for bilirubin in Rh immunization used by Bevis (Queenan)
1958	• Obstetric use of ultrasound by Donald (Queenan)
1963	• Infant boy born at Johns Hopkins Medical Center, Baltimore with Trisomy 21 and duodenal atresia. Surgery for the atresia was withheld and he was not fed. He died 15 days later (Sparks 1988) • Intrauterine transfusion for Rh immunization by Liley (Queenan)
1968	• Treatment of a viable, aborted fetus (Maxwell 1968)
1969	• Initial discussion of treatment decision-making for congenital anomalies (Rickham 1969) • Hastings Center established for the discussion, debate, and pronouncement on ethical issues, including those related to infants and children (Callahan 1984)
1970	• Experimentation targeting neonates first described, focusing on nutrition problems (Mann 1970)
1972	• Film produced by Joseph P. Kennedy Foundation based on 1963 case from John Hopkins Medical Center, *Who shall survive?* (Sparks 1988)
1974	• *Maine Medical Center v. Houle* one of the first cases of forgoing treatment to be determined by the court (Paris, Ferranti & Reardon 2001) • Duff and Campbell published their report in *The New England Journal of Medicine* on 299 deaths in the Yale-New Haven Hospital intensive care nursery, of which 43 resulted from withdrawal of treatment
1974	• National conference in San Francisco organized to explore the ethical issues and policy implications of neonatal intensive care (Jonsen & Garland 1976)
1976	• Symposium on selective nontreatment of infants, Center for Bioethics at the Clinical Research Institute, Montreal (Weir 1984)

Table 1.2 *Major Issues* (Continued)

1978	• *Encyclopedia of Bioethics*, first edition published, which included an entry on Infants. This discussion addressed aspects of care, ethical issues, infanticide, and public policy • Steptoe and Edwards successful development of *in vitro* fertilization
1982	• Bloomington, Indiana: Couple allowed newborn with Trisomy-21 to die of treatable condition (Tracheo-esophageal fistula). Became known as the Baby Doe case
1983	• *Baby Doe* federal regulations devised, an attempt to prevent discriminatory treatment of infants with handicaps (Steinbock 1984) • Long Island: Baby Jane Doe case of newborn with meningomyelocele, anencephaly, and hydrocephaly whose parents refused surgery but allowed other therapies. A self-appointed lawyer intervened to compel implementation of more aggressive treatment
1984	• Cardozo School of Law Conference "Which Babies Shall Live: Humanistic Dimensions of Care of Imperiled Newborns" • Buster Bustilllo succeeded in embryo transfer (Queenan)
1985	• Child abuse regulations connected compliance with infant care regulations to federal funding for child abuse programs (Murray 1985a)
1986	• Supreme Court struck down the Baby Doe regulations (Lantos 1987)
1987	• Report published by Hastings Center from a project begun in 1984 to examine the moral dilemmas of neonatal intensive care (Caplan & Cohen 1987)
1992	• Harrison's (1993) Parent-Physician conference to develop *Principles for Family-centered Neonatal Care*
1993	• Separation of the Lakeburg conjoined twins
1995	• Gregory Messenger, MD was acquitted on charges of manslaughter for the removal of his premature son from a ventilator (*People v. Messenger* 1995)

Table 1.2 *Major Issues* (Continued)

1996	• American Academy of Pediatrics' Committee on Bioethics published *Ethics and the Care of Critically Ill Infants and Children* in which they recommended that parents and physicians "make reasoned decisions together about critically ill infants" (G. Clark 1996) • Initiation of the European Union Collaborative Project on Ethical Decision Making in Neonatal Intensive Care (EURONIC) (Cuttini et al. 2001)
1997	• Birth of the McCaughey septuplets
1998	• Birth of the Chukwu octuplets
2000	• *HCA v. Miller* tested the physician's decision to save the life of a viable newborn (Paris et al. 2001)
2001	• Neonatal End-of-Life Palliative-Care Protocol proposed outline the needs of the various players in order to provide a pain free, dignified death (Catlin & Carter, 2001)

& Cohen 1987). A bioethical dilemma is created when various solutions appear equally good or bad, and priorities seem difficult, if not impossible to set. Conflicts also arise when the people involved place significantly different values on the possible actions (Brody 1981).

Exemplar Debates

Little ethical debate accompanied the commercial use of infants in the carnival-type displays of incubators, in the early 1900s. No great public outcry or debate arose around the removal of these newborns from hospitals or parental care. Apparently their possible survival was so marginal that no one thought to question the infants' use in the demonstration of neonatal equipment.

Attention to the ethical dimension of neonatal care waxes and wanes, especially in relation to individual cases that attract the media spotlight. For example, in 1971, the case of a newborn with Trisomy-21 at Johns Hopkins Hospital created interest among several ethics scholars.[u] The infant had duodenal atresia, a repairable defect,[v] but surgery was declined and the infant died (Cooke 1973; Dyck 1973;

Fruend 1971; Gustafson 1973). The story of the decision-making related to this neonate was the focus of a film produced by the Joseph P. Kennedy Jr. Foundation.

Another intense public debate arose in 1982 over what would become known as a Baby Doe case (Annas 1983; Lyon 1985). Baby Doe was the pseudonym used to preserve the infants' anonymity in these cases. The situation, in Bloomington, Indiana, involved a parental decision to not treat a child with Trisomy-21 and other pathologies including esophageal atresia.[w] The decision to not treat this Baby Doe led to a passionate public response, which in turn influenced federal officials. The federal answer was posed in the form of rapidly developed government regulations to prevent discriminatory treatment of handicapped infants. The proliferation of Baby Doe type cases targeted by the media, fueled public questioning of forgoing treatments for fragile newborns (Donley & Buckley 1996; Moskop & Saldanha 1986).[x]

Using a section of the Rehabilitation Act of 1973, the Department of Health and Human Services (HHS) issued warnings to medical institutions that received federal funds. The memo reminded these hospitals that they were in violation of federal law if they withheld treatment or nourishment from handicapped babies. Not only were treatment decisions for Trisomy-21 children affected, but the regulation was extended to virtually all newborns, even those with enormous problems requiring multiple interventions with little hope of a good outcome. But decision-making was not always clear. Although the regulations undeniably impacted prejudicial treatment for Trisomy-21 children, the most difficult cases were low birth weight babies and those with complex life-threatening problems (Jonsen 1991). The outcome for many infants was clouded by uncertainty. Given the mandate of the Baby Doe regulations to treat the handicapped, an aggressive approach to newborn care lawfully infiltrated every infant's treatment. Posted regulations were a powerful message to parents, families, and staff to treat, treat, treat. Given the litigious nature of our society, aggressive care was further reinforced (Kinlaw 1996). Additionally the ability to *do something* was increasing exponentially--technological advancements and increasingly available medical interventions expanded the armamentarium of the physicians. Undertreatment was replaced by overtreatment (Fost 1999). Many health professionals struggled with deciding how to treat, as they encountered lower and lower birth weights and resuscitation at birth became routine. They also questioned how long to aggressively intervene before procedures could legitimately be labeled futile. Agonizing decisions were made for these neonates. Although the Baby Doe regulations were eventually struck down, the mandate to treat continues to permeate decision-making.

The more recent separation of the Lakeberg conjoined twins also garnered widespread media attention (Dougherty 1995).[y] The twins shared a heart so the surgical procedure required the death of one twin (Amy) and the survival of the other (Angela). Several ethical questions were raised by this event. Among them was the issue of sacrificing one life for the benefit of another. There was little hope of success even for the baby who received the heart and Angela did die 9 months later. Another issue was the allocation of scarce resources; the cost of care was estimated at $1.2 million in 1995.

The Johns Hopkins infant, Baby Doe, and the Lakeberg twins are all relatively contemporary cases. However, ethical concerns about newborns, especially impaired or handicapped infants, existed prior to the development of specialized care despite the lack of ethical debate for the exposition preemies. For centuries, discussion and debate centered on infanticide (Kohl 1978; Piers 1978; Weir 1984).

Infanticide

There has long been interest in determining the acceptability or unacceptability of children. Societies have invariably set standards for what is normal and acceptable for a human, what is abnormal but still acceptable or even lauded, and what is abnormal and unacceptable. Those standards were applied either formally or informally, beginning at birth to determine group membership and identity (Koch 1999). Although not practiced widely in modern times, infanticide was sanctioned at times in the past for various reasons (Turnbull 1986; Weir 1984).

Infanticide served over the ages as a religious sacrifice, a system for sex selection, a means of population control, a method of birth control, a way of relieving economic crisis, and a solution for the removal of weak or abnormal infants. Gradually, as the result of many factors, but especially the practice of Christianity in the first century, infants were included in the valuing of all humans and infanticide was perceived as sinful. Sanctity of life, however, never achieved inviolate status (Koch 1999; Tooley 1983). In the Middle Ages, an important distinction was made between actively killing an infant and simply allowing it to die.[z] Children in the 18th century were abandoned to foundling hospitals in greater numbers than the dedicated personnel could handle. Many of these children died.

Through the ensuing years, the Christian perspective, even when supported by secular law, did not completely eliminate the practice of infanticide nor bring about its complete disapproval. In England, for example, statutes distinguished between homicide and infanticide, with the applicable punishment less severe for the latter. In the United States no such distinction existed. Aside from a religious failure to condone infanticide, what other factors influenced the infant's destiny? If the infant was male, normal in physical appearance, a member of the ethnic majority, and legitimate,[aa] infanticide was not a likely alternative.

Conceptually, some infanticide continues in our current society. For example, stories of young women giving birth in a bedroom or a bathroom and then attempting to dispose of the newborn are not unknown. Newborns have been abandoned in various places, sometimes with the apparent hope that they will be found and cared for, but other times with the obvious intention of causing their demise (Abandonment case 2000). A poignant feature in an issue of *People* magazine traced the stories of several adults who had been abandoned at birth (Jerome et al. 1997). In 1969 Resnick conducted a psychiatric review of 131 cases of filicide, and although not all involved newborns, the largest group included those between 24 hours and 6 months of age. Resnick developed a classification system based on the motive for filicide and, interestingly enough, altruistic motives exceeded all other categories.

Selective treatment of newborns in hospitals was briefly identified with infanticide. The first edition of the *Bibliography of Bioethics* only categorized articles about newborn care under the heading of *infanticide* (Walters 1975). That heading was dropped in the next year's edition and has not appeared since that issue.

Decisions in the neonatal unit, however, mirror the major issues in the history of infanticide (Weir 1984). For a variety of reasons, questions are raised about whether or not some neonates ought to be treated, how aggressive treatment ought to be, when treatment can stop, and who makes these decisions. The private nature of hospital care and the authority of a respected professional--the physician--have made decisions for neonates usually less accessible to public scrutiny and legal sanction. What is done, or in the case of nontreatment what is not done, and who makes the decision have significant implications for continuing concern in bioethics about neonatal care.

The Initial Controversies

The earliest years of neonatal intensive care (pre 1970), produced few ethical analyses. The newborn with Trisomy-21 concurrent with other anomalies, seems to have garnered attention initially for several reasons. First, the medical treatment for a problem such as duodenal atresia carried a low risk--it was a routine measure, yet parents requested or physicians suggested that treatment not be instituted. Withholding treatment was associated with the belief that a child with Trisomy-21 would not only impose burdens upon the family, but the child itself would suffer more in living than in having its life ended very early. This value judgment was applied to children with varying degrees of mental retardation, not just the severely retarded.

Two ethicists, Bard and Fletcher (1968), posed a strong utilitarian argument for nonvoluntary euthanasia of children with mental retardation, particularly those with Trisomy-21.[bb] Applying a quality of life principle, they determined, with some opposition, that the individual with Trisomy-21 lacked sufficient qualities to be considered a human person. Debate evolved around the personhood focus, and that argument was employed in other neonate cases especially as smaller and smaller infants were resuscitated.

Cases of spina bifida formed another category of medical problems analyzed by ethicists (Fernadez-Serrats et al. 1968; Success and failure 1969; Zachary 1968), as did prematurity and surgery (Maxwell 1968; Rickham 1969; Success and failure). In addition to Bard and Fletcher, scholars like Ramsey (1970), Kelly (1958), Curran (1970), and Häring (1968) contributed to ethical analyses. One kind of argument was framed in the context of whether or not treatment was morally required. Generally extraordinary treatments were said to be not morally required, while ordinary treatment would be morally required. The categorization of extraordinary versus ordinary was based not on an intrinsic element of the treatment, but rather on the degree of burden it inflicted upon the person for whom it was prescribed, or the person's family.[cc] Other arguments were drafted using the principles of direct versus indirect means, allowing or causing, or withholding versus withdrawing treatment (Caplan, Capron et al. 1987). Only a few analyses addressed the question of who should decide (Asch et al. 1987). In reality, aggressive treatment for many infants continued, regardless of the ethical arguments. The health professional ideal of saving as many infant lives as possible appeared to be the norm unaffected or only nominally influenced by the bioethical debate.

A number of events besides the Baby Doe cases put the ethics of neonatal care in the public limelight. A significant contribution to the public dimension of bioethics and high-risk newborn care was an article by Duff and Campbell (1973) in the *New England Journal of Medicine*, which was one of the earliest professional discussions about treatment decision-making in the special care nursery. The physicians described decision-making in the Yale-New Haven Hospital from 1970 to 1972. During those years, treatment was withdrawn from 43 newborns, who were allowed to die (11% of a total of 299 deaths). In the same issue of the journal, Shaw, a pediatric surgeon, also cited cases in which infants were allowed to die (1973). These reports caused a stir, not necessarily because infants with severe problems died, but rather because the issue was publicly addressed and the circle of interested parties was significantly expanded. The insular nature of medical practice was breached and this development surprised many people. Decision-making within the bureaucratic institution in which medical care was delivered to high-risk infants shifted from a private process to one that could encompass whole health care teams. The decision-making process could vary depending upon the setting and the participants.

In summary, theologians, philosophers, health professionals, and others all contributed to the debate about handicapped newborns. In terms of treatment, concerns often centered on possible discriminatory treatment of handicapped newborns and the resulting neglect (Jonsen 1991; Hauerwas 1975; Klitsch,1983; Ragatz & Ellison 1983; Ramsey 1978). This debate both preceded and paralleled the Baby Doe cases of the 1980s and the subsequent federal legislation to prevent discrimination. As more sophisticated treatments were developed, additional questions were raised about the use of those procedures and any rationale for the decision either to treat or not to treat. The strategy of treating all infants with nearly every available intervention was systematically questioned as ethical debate grew throughout the 1970s and mushroomed during the 1980s. Some of the questions arose from unsuccessful outcomes, especially in marginally viable newborns. Pain and suffering were considerations as various individuals struggled with determining reasonable expectations for the kind of treatment and degree of aggressiveness that was ethically required (Butler 1989). These debates generally fell under the rubric of discussions, which were labeled the extraordinary/ordinary treatment controversies. Given the unpredictability of outcomes for many early interventions, the question of whether experimentation was ethically acceptable was debated as well.

Typically, the early decades reflected that medical decisions may not have been made for the *right* reasons; that is, they may not have been based on the strongest possible ethical grounds. Hence much of the ethical debate involved framing discussions within a process of inquiry that demanded examination of possible discriminatory action. Were infants not treated when their mental status was predicted to be below normal, even slightly below normal? Was it ethical to deliberate quality of life in relation to the infants' treatment? If infants were not treated, would it be more merciful to end their lives--the question of euthanasia? Were family concerns allowed to have too much impact on the medical care of and decisions for the infant? On the other hand, what about parents who were not involved in decision-making? How influential was the public voice? What was community responsibility relative to attitudes and resources for a handicapped child? Who should ultimately make decisions? Although the infant is dependent upon physicians and other health professionals initially during hospitalization, many years of dependency on and support from the family will be required after discharge.

More Recent Deliberation

Some contributions to neonatal bioethics since the late 1980s can be categorized by utility. Jonsen (1991) chose this term because he saw the ethical focus shifting from concerns of discrimination to one of maximizing the good. Concern about the economics of the neonatal unit surfaced in the late 1980s and continues to the present. Outcomes for neonates treated in the NICU became integral to the bioethical debate as studies were completed on long-term development of these infants (Brooten et al. 1986; Ferrara et al. 1989; Fischer & Steverson 1987; Hack & Fanaroff 1989; Lantos et al. 1988; McCormick et al. 1992; Saigel, Szatmari et al. 1990).

Jonsen (1991) used the anencephalic infant as a model to represent this era, a parable of utility for discussions about the prudent use of resources and avoidance of waste. Transplanting viable organs from an anencephalic infant whose own life is doomed transforms a sense of waste into a more optimal outcome for another child. Many parents of anencephalic infants seized such an opportunity and even requested, unsolicited, that these infants' organs be given to another sick infant.

Although anencephalic newborns' organs were used for transplantation for a short time, the practice was quickly curtailed. A major portion of the brain and skull are missing in these infants, but since brain-stem activity is present, determination of death for timing of the removal of organs posed a problem. Infants were often able to breathe and possessed a sucking reflex. They did not always need extensive technological support. Most important, they did not immediately meet the standards for determining death--cessation of breathing, heartbeat, and/or brain activity. In some anencephalic infants, other congenital problems existed, preventing the donation of certain vital organs (Capron 1987).

In general over the course of debate about the ethics of neonatal care, myriad topics were targeted and various orientations were represented (Bailey 1986; Berseth 1987; Clancy et al. 1992; Ellison & Walwork 1986; Klitsch 1983; Kuhse & Singer 1987; Marchwinski 1988; Martin 1985; Reedy et al. 1987; Sims-Jones 1986). Discussions centered on such issues as:

- quality of life including infant outcomes
- lung viability and whether or not treatments should be attempted in infants born prior to a specific gestational age and/or level of organ functioning. This related to routine resuscitation at birth.
- iatrogenic effects of therapy (encompassing considerations of pain and suffering) and
- cost

Various philosophical and theological approaches used to examine neonatal problems, were accepted or rejected based on:

- selected ethical theory (e.g., deontology, utilitarianism, social contract),[dd]
- ethical principle (e.g., autonomy, beneficence, nonmaleficence, justice), or
- ethical device (e.g., personhood and the moral status of the fetus→newborn, *slippery slope*, sanctity of life, best interest standard, quality of life) (Arras, Asch et al. 1987; Dunn 1993; Novak 1988; Walters 1988; Weir 1992).

These concerns and the concomitant questioning continued to push through the 1990s and undoubtedly spill over into the new millennium. In more recent years, the ethical interest in neonates took on an international flavor. Scholars compared U.S. experiences with their own or simply reported the state of the art in various countries lending an ever broader perspective to consider in the ethical dimension

(Brinchmann 1999; Brinchmann & Nortvedt 2001; Herman & Mehes 1996; Levin 1990; McHaffie et al. 1999; Sauer 1992; Szawarski 1990).

Collective Approaches to the Neonate Dilemma

Publicized focus groups and conferences were held to debate issues related to bioethics and neonatal care. In 1974, the Health Policy Program and the Department of Pediatrics at the School of Medicine, University of California, San Francisco organized a conference to explore the ethical issues and policy implications of neonatal intensive care. The results of this interdisciplinary symposium were published in 1976 (Jonsen & Garland). The incentive for this event came from the escalating use of science and technology for infant care, sometimes labeled the *rescue phase* of the first two decades of neonatal care. Now that a variety of highly sophisticated treatments could be applied to premature infants and other compromised newborns, the question arose whether such treatment *should* be used. The California conference also addressed the policy implications related to research and other clinical activities in the NICU.

Another group effort resulting in a major project and report began in 1984 at the Hastings Center. The group, directed by Arthur Caplan, addressed "issues of substance, procedure, and vision related to the ethics of neonatal care" (Caplan & Cohen 1987; Murray & Caplan 1985) The group proposed eight summary points from their deliberations including a need to consider the neonate life after discharge, quality of life for the infant, and education of both professionals and the public about the whole perinatal period (Caplan 1987).

These recommendations appeared to support a stronger focus on the examination of the parental role when decisions are made in the NICU. They also recognized the need to follow these parents after the infant's discharge from the NICU. The suggestions not only seemed to acknowledge the effect of compromised infants on parents during hospitalization, but also indicated a clear need to begin support for parents before birth and continue this support long into the future.

In an advocacy effort, Harrison was instrumental in organizing a 1992 conference of parent and physician representatives to develop a set of principles for family-centered neonatal care. The resulting document was published in *Pediatrics* (1993) so that the principles might be implemented in the NICU setting and form the basis for ongoing dialogue among the parents and health care professionals.

Contemporary Concerns

More recent years in the NICU have seen such issues as newborns with HIV infection and "crack" babies introduced into the ethical dimension of neonatal care. Two major anthologies addressed the continuing challenges of ethics in the NICU (Caplan, Blank et al. 1992; Goldworth et al. 1994). *Compelled compassion: Government, intervention in the treatment of critically ill newborns* particularly targeted the public policy aspect of treatment decision-making for compromised newborns. The other, *Ethics and perinatology*, attempted to analyze the impact of technology on perinatology from a multidisciplinary perspective.

Additionally, as infertility treatments mushroom, the likelihood of multiple births, early labor and/or delivery, and compromised newborn life all increase (Francis & Nosek 1988).[ee] Treatment for high-risk pregnancies can also escalate the need for high-risk newborn care as the newborn is more likely to reach viability even if that viability is marginal. Media coverage of these advanced reproductive technologies and their consequences have not received a balanced approach. Emphasis on the positive outcomes is an unrealistic portrayal of the situation for many families. Another issue, the effects of the environmental pollution and exposure to toxic elements, certainly has implications for fetal development and possible newborn compromise. These specific problems and others as yet unimaginable may seem, but they represent basically the same continuing challenges.

We know the prenatal period is important for the newborn's initiation into physiologically independent life. The effects of cocaine or alcohol use are particularly devastating, but the woman's health status, actions, and behaviors have always had an impact on fetal development and subsequent need for newborn interventions. The needs of compromised newborns and premature infants represent various health care challenges. After all, HIV is an infection, and the risk for infection was an early hurdle to surmount in premature care. Although the devices themselves change, technology and its use or nonuse will continue to be an option for decades.

Woven throughout the medical problems and treatment decisions are confrontations with the ethical implications of these decisions. Although each individual discussion takes on its own particular orientation, Weir concludes the leading ethical position in the 1990s was the best interest standard (1994, 1995). Ethicists were attempting to suggest guidelines for ethical decision-making in the NICU as a result of the tendency to overtreat that stemmed from the Baby Doe cases, while also seeking to eliminate the unwarranted influence of decision-makers who come to the process with vested interests. Regardless of the volume of scientific and objective data, "No one who is intimately involved can be totally objective or completely free of any conflict of interest" (Hammerman et al. 1998).

The currently prevalent best interest standard affirms to some degree the moral status of the infant and requires decisions to be based on considerations related only to the infant itself and its medical condition (Dunn 1993). Certainly this ethical position has profound implications for the parents or other caregivers who will ultimately take responsibility for the infant.

The Parents' Role in Ethical Decision-Making

Over the course of these decades, ethical debate has targeted various aspects of treatment decision-making (Arras, Coulter et al. 1987; Aumann 1988; Avery 1998; Bailey 1986; Carr 1989; Engelhardt 1978; Klitsch 1983; Kuhse & Singer 1987; Marchwinski 1988; Probert & Carson 1984; Sims-Jones 1986; Smith 1986):

- when to treat,
- when not to treat,
- what is obligatory (morally required) and what is extraordinary (not morally required),
- passive and active euthanasia (actively ending life or allowing death to occur),
- medical uncertainty,
- quality of life,
- role of infant care review committees or pediatric ethics committees,
- social responsibility,
- use of resources,
- futility,
- and related public policy

Numerous individuals from a variety of disciplines were represented in these published discussions: physicians, nurses, philosophers, theologians, ethicists, lawyers, social workers, hospital administrators, social scientists, political scientists, chaplains, and journalists (Duff & Campbell 1976; Fleischman 1990; Miya 1989). A number of empirical studies specifically centered on the perspectives of health care professionals when faced with ethical dilemmas for the neonate

(Berseth et al. 1984; Chally 1992; Martin 1989; Miya, Boardman et al. 1991). While certainly the topics were focused in particular ways and contributors had a variety of goals, parents were notably under-represented in this body of literature (Ellis 1984; Gortner 1985; Ketefian 1988).

Germane to the project described in this book was an initial awareness that some authors simply chose not to address the parental aspect. For example, Jonsen and Lister (1978) framed a discussion of ethical issues in the NICU around three issues: iatrogenicity, the experimental enigma, and prognostic perplexity. Parents were never mentioned. Sparks (1988), a theologian, in an otherwise thorough review and development of a typology of the moral basis of decisions to forgo or cease treatment elected not to address who should decide. He acknowledged that parents are among the primary arbiters, but a precise decision on the *who* question was set aside for another time and place. This is noted not to indicate that his book should be dismissed, but rather to document the missing parental perspective in ethical decision-making.

Second, although various authors claimed to represent the parental perspective, parents rarely spoke for themselves in this body of professional literature.[ff] Demands to represent parental perspectives were made in some sources, but the majority of authors wrote *about* the parents' experiences as they (the authors) perceived that experience rather than directly seeking the parents' viewpoint.[gg] Few systematic accounts prior to 1985 endeavored to simply ask parents and subsequently report what they thought and believed. Those persons who would be most affected by the decision-making were actually least represented in the professional discussion of all disciplines.

A few sources devoted their discussion to advocacy for parents of neonates (Blustein 1989; Cerase 1988; Penticuff 1987, 1988). Klaus (1986), responding to a plea from Harrison (1986) for more parental involvement, emphasized the need to selectively communicate with parents (not *to* or *at* them). Physicians needed to assess parents but only provide them with information about the infant's status that they can handle. Others argued for more complete disclosure in order for parents to understand the complex nature of decision-making in the NICU (Brody 1989; King 1992). Scully and Scully's chapter (1987) on the Baby Doe dilemma was written as a directive for parents of high-risk neonates. Shared responsibility was a decision-making concept proposed by Bartholome (1988). This approach focused on decision-makers as a circle of individuals who were all loyal to the child. He rejected a rights orientation, best interests standards, and reasonable person perspective for settings like the NICU. The goal of the interaction was to "fuse, not shatter human relationships."

A few very important contributions from research studies included a parental perspective and add to our understanding of that perspective. In these studies, mostly sociological, the investigator(s) used a participant observation approach to describe the environment of the NICU and the behavior of all of the participants (Anspach 1993; Barber et al. 1992; Bodgan et al. 1982; Frohock 1986; Guillemin & Holmstrom 1986; Gustaitis & Young 1986; Jennings 1988; Levin 1986; Rostain 1986; Rottman 1986). These articles are excellent sources, but the parents' perspective is weakened by being embedded within all of the other material included by the author(s). Numerous perspectives were discussed. The parents' perspective can then be minimized or even lost. Additionally when seeing the action and behavior of all participants, the reader is tempted to rationalize, trivialize, or dismiss parental responses in light of other, especially professional, commentary.

The actual role of parents in decision making shifted over the years. Prior to the Baby Doe cases in the 1980s, NICU personnel discussed withdrawing or withholding treatment without the threat of legal retaliation (Harrison 1996). Then Baby Doe regulations reinforced a hard-line position employed by some professionals that parents were not capable of making decisions for their child (Chaney 1986). Professional observation of the parents' crisis as a result of the infant's hospitalization justified side-stepping parental involvement. Professionals assumed a paternalistic approach to decision-making with parents (Kottow 1998; Paris & Schreiber 1996; Stewart 1998). They perceived parents as unable to absorb sufficient information to understand the baby's situation or to follow a logical, rational process required for appropriate treatment decisions. Not just the present situation but anxiety for the future was shown to affect some mothers (Pinelli 1981). Mothers of infants with congenital heart disease in one study were shown to be intimidated by the anticipated level of care that the infant would require. These findings supported the removal of parents from active roles in decision-making.

Norms of society generally confer decision-making authority on parents for their children (Peabody & Martin 1996). Despite the more-or-less guarantee of parental autonomy by society, decision-making is compromised in the NICU although some professionals advocate for family involvement and autonomy (Jellinek et al. 1992; Luckner &

Weinfeld 1995; Moore & Day 1993). In the present application of the *best interest* principle, who determines the precise best interest for a particular infant is not clear (Hammerman et al. 1998). In some cases it is argued that parents' desires are in conflict with the infant's best interests when they refuse life saving treatment. In other cases, the opposite situation can occur; parents can demand more treatment than professionals recommend which can also be judged to not be in the best interest of the infant. In other words, in some cases, unless parents agree with the professional recommendation for treatment, their decisions can be ethically ignored as not in the best interest of the newborn.

Another area of debate related to parental involvement focuses on the role of emotions and feelings in ethical decision-making (Callahan 1988). On the one hand, many professionals believe parents need to become attached and emotionally invested in the neonate for optimal outcomes (Klaus & Kennel 1982; Lau & Morse 1998). Blustein (1989) argues for the acknowledgment of the intimate nature of family relationships--not just as a psychological consideration but because of its moral implications. On the other hand, some ethicists argue that emotions, especially emotional burdens as well as financial considerations do not belong in the debate. The child should be central to decision-making with family implications considered second or not at all (Pierce 1998). If emotional elements do not have a role in initial decision-making for the infant, the question could be raised as to when and where they do have a role. Certainly emotions, feelings, and finances (also often named as irrelevant for ethical decision-making) have serious post-discharge affects on everyone including the infant. When do they become relevant in decision-making?

The same theme of marginalization of parental decision making holds somewhat true for professional films related to neonatal care. In *Code Gray,* one of the four vignettes focuses on ethical decision-making in the NICU, although the infant is a ward of the state so no parent was involved. Professionals and ethics committee members discussed the various approaches to interventions for the infant (Achtenberg & Sawyer 1983). Given the strong and opposing viewpoints of the nurses in the film, the addition of a parental perspective would have been interesting. Who would advocate for the parents? *Dreams and Dilemmas* follows one couple and the premature twins for 6 months in the NICU. There is no narrative, but the experience includes nurses, physicians, a social worker, and hospital chaplain as well as the parents (Kahn 1998). In the film the nurses and the physicians often stood while the parents sat. Some would interpret this as a clear message of power and authority, an example of talking *to* not *with*. *Born Dying* probes a multitude of viewpoints related to decision-making for a dying newborn. The story is scripted to present several individuals talking to the viewer of the film, who represents the baby's mother. No decision is suggested, but neither is it clear that the parents will eventually make the decision about the newborn (Baxley & Associates 1983). A more recent documentary focuses on families after the discharge of their multiply handicapped, medically fragile children. Parents reminisce about the NICU aspect of their experience with these children and some note an absence of involvement in decision-making (Blaustein & Kasell 1999).

The Public View

A review of the lay literature provides insight regarding the general population's view of the neonate's plight. Of course, these revelations focus on selected, usually individual, parental stories. The personal experiences of several vocal families verify the perception of detachment during hospitalization and abandonment at discharge. Ethical decision-making is not necessarily addressed by name, but in reading these accounts one can envision the ethical dilemmas inherent in the stories these parents tell. Both fathers and mothers want to be good parents and act in the best possible way for their infant, which certainly shows value-based motivation. A number of these parents believed they were disenfranchised from responsibility in decision-making.

One of the earliest personal reports was from the Stinson parents (1979, 1981), who described their son's six-month hospitalization in the NICU as a time of great frustration for them. The Stinsons were unable to make any significant decisions and believed that their son did not really belong to them until all treatment failed. A letter to the hospital administration led to the later construction of their experiences in book form (1983).

Another author, Helen Harrison has long been a contributor from the parents' perspective (1983, 1984a, 1984b, 1986, 1992, 1993, 1997, 2001; Harrison & Kositsky 1983). Her son resided in a NICU about 1975 and was subsequently diagnosed with cerebral palsy, hydrocephalus, near blindness, and severe retardation. Ms. Harrison has expressed a deep commitment in favor of informing parents, involving them in ethical decision-making, and providing on-going support after discharge. She has been a very active advocate for other parents.

Other parents publicized their neonatal intensive care experiences from time to time (Adler 1987, 1988; Alecson 1995; Anderson & Hall 1995; Barthel 1985; Bridge & Bridge 1981; Cuming 1988; Curry 1995; De Pree 1996; Gordon 2001; Isham 1992; Jacobs 1990; Kantrowitz et al. 1988; Kupfer 1982;[hh] Layne 1996; Loizeaux 1993; Stein 1994; Watson 1996; Wingert 1988). Many of these stories make a special plea for readers to understand their plight. Families ask others to sympathize with the difficult circumstances they confronted in the NICU and the challenges they face as parents who daily care for their seriously ill child. The acute emotion parents feel is undeniable. Some are angry about the resulting outcomes, while others celebrate their survival of the experience and the *miracle* of the child's outcome. However, the long-term outcome and adjustment for these families is often unpublicized.[ii] An exception was a more recent contribution (Curry). This mother of a premature son used 16 years' worth of her own handwritten journals to chronicle life with her physically disabled child. Another unique report was at once the story of a personal journey and a scholarly (anthropological) investigation of narratives or first-person accounts of the NICU experience (Layne). Again, although ethics and morals may not be specifically noted in these stories, the descriptions make it obvious that such dilemmas existed for the parents.[jj] It is difficult to say whether these reports are balanced ones--over-representing negative or positive outcomes. Either is possible and all should be read with such an admonition in mind.

In addition to parental contributions to popular literature, media accounts also drew the public's attention to the plight of the premature or handicapped newborn. Some of these were news broadcasts, while others were longer programs. Helen Harrison, the parent advocate, was featured on *60 Minutes* during the news reporters' investigation of the economic implications of NICU. *Born Too Soon* (1991), the story of Elizabeth Mehren's experience with a premature, became a movie released on a cable network in 1993. Even a novel about a family's experience with a pre-term infant has been published (McHaffie 1994). Newspapers and news magazines occasionally run special features on prematurity, neonatal care, or an especially interesting birth experience which entails NICU care (Adler 1987; Born too soon 2000; Kantrowitz et al. 1988; Knief 1998; Rosenthal 1991; Stein 1994).

Scholarly Approaches to Parental Perceptions

Although few systematic, formal investigations that included the parents' perspective existed in 1985 when this project was conceived, several were located or conducted in the interim. Most of these studies did not focus on ethics.

The Baby Doe issue of the 1980s seems to have stimulated interest in ethical decision-making and neonates as well as other topics related to parental experiences in the NICU. The research topics that included the parental perspective were:

- preparation for the NICU experience (Griffin et al. 1997)
- the parents' perspective of ethical decision-making (Barber et al 1992; Belkin 1993; Evans 1989; Rottman 1986; Rushton 1994; Schlomann & Fister 1995)
- parental perspectives of communication in the NICU (Able-Boone et al. 1989)
- the informed consent process (King 1992)
- values of mothers of low birth weight infants (Raines 1998)
- parents' responses to premature death (Palmer & Noble 1986; Wretmark 1993)
- caregiving by parents in a NICU (Scharer & Brooks 1994; Swanson 1990)
- need for and source of support for parents during infant hospitalization in the NICU (Fleishman 1984; Miles, Carlson et al. 1996)
- parental stress in the NICU (Affleck et al. 1990; Bass 1991; McHaffie 1992; Miles, Funk et al. 1991, 1992; Padden & Glenn 1997; Shields-Poë & Pinelli 1997)
- psychological response to infant hospitalization in the NICU with follow-up data (Hummel & Eastman 1991)
- life support decisions from the parents' perspective (Kirschbaum 1994, 1996; Walwork & Ellison 1985)
- transition to parenthood (McCluskey-Fawcett et al. 1992; Miles et al. 1998)
- satisfaction with NICU care (Blackington & McLauchlan 1995; Satariano et al. 1987)
- parents' view of the parent-child relationship 8 years postdischarge (Kratochvil et al. 1991)
- mothers' experiences of caring for severely compromised infants after discharge from the NICU (Catlin 1997)

Several meta-analyses were conducted as well. One identified aspects of the NICU experience that negatively impacted the parents' ability to successfully parent their child after discharge (Rikli 1995). Another summarized the research relating to parenting the premature infant (Holditch-Davis & Miles 1997). Two reviews targeted the studies related to parental stress (Boardman 1995; Lau & Morse 1998). These synopses all emphasized the need to develop interventions to minimize the negative effects of the NICU experience and improve the outcome for both parents and children.

A consistent theme among the studies investigating parental perspectives of ethical decision-making was a lack of involvement in decision-making by parents. Many potential decisions were presented as medically oriented circumstances, or in some cases the parents themselves failed to recognize the presence of ethical events in the course of the NICU experience. Parents discussed both physical and emotional inadequacies. Accompanying any exploration of decision-making was commentary on many other aspects of the parents' experience addressed in the non-ethics focused research: stress, coping, satisfaction/complaint, communication, parental role, and expectations for the future.

Summary

The ethical debate continues, of course. The NICU remains a rather insular environment in the health care scene. Aggressive care persists, however, as physicians practice defensive medicine in our litigious society. Additionally, the idea of conquering medical problems motivates physicians to treat rather than withdraw in order to discharge a live baby from the NICU. Cost containment is yet to become a serious issue, as child protection regulations hold such considerations at bay even in this period of managed care.

For parents with a high-risk newborn, experiences in the NICU and ethical decision-making are only the beginning. In some discussions, the ethical decision-making in the nursery was treated as an isolated event in family's lives (Fost 1981; Sparks 1988; Watchko 1983). Not only do they need to grapple with the crisis of a newborn hospitalization, but also with the life-altering events which follow the closing of the NICU doors at discharge. The seamless connection between the infant in the NICU and family life in the community should ever be kept in mind. Both health professionals and bioethicists for whom the high-risk infant is central to their interest, interventions, and deliberations, bear a distinctive burden to remain alert to the far-reaching effects of their roles in these families' lives. Decision-making may be viewed as strictly medical or objectively ethical, but it has a real life, day-to-day bearing on the subsequent life of the neonate, its family, and the entire community.

Notes

[a] Carol is not the real name of the woman in this study. In fact, all of the participants' names in the entire book have been changed to protect confidentiality. Name changes include direct, individual quotes although the reader will not be reminded at each pseudonym. Additionally, some stories were revised to protect confidentiality. However, all of the material comes from one interview or another, or from a combination of interviews as necessary. Only first names are used for these assumed names which should not be taken as a sign of disrespect for these parents. Most parents asked to be addressed by their first names during the interview.

[b] A premature or preterm infant is one who is born before the end of the 37th week (Korones 1976). Even more specifically "any neonate whose birth occurs through the end of the last day of the 37th week (259th day), following onset of the last menstrual period" (Frigoletto & Little 1988 p. 310).

[c] University of Nebraska Medical Center successfully discharged (1995) a newborn with a birthweight of 320 grams (11.3 ounces). Personal communication.

[d] Specific criteria define the high-risk infant which can be term ("through the end of the last day of the 42nd week...following onset of the last menstrual period") or preterm, or post-term as well (Frigoletto & Little 1988 p. 310). Although many newborns admitted to the NICU are premature, other reasons for admission are discussed in the Appendix, The Research Enterprise, when infant criteria for parents' invitation to participate in this study are described. Briefly, the presence of congenital anomalies, respiratory problems, babies whose mothers experienced a high-risk pregnancy are several reasons for designating the need for NICU admission. A few newborns may be inappropriately admitted to the NICU, that is the condition was not as serious as anticipated and discharge may be rapid.

[e] ECMO is a heart-lung by-pass procedure which mechanically supplies oxygen to the newborn. In the 1970s, the combination of pulmonary hypertension and inadequate intake of oxygen was invariably fatal. ECMO was the solution to such a clinical problem. The procedure was first used without a clinical trial and nine of the first thirteen patients died. Clinical trials ensued but in the meantime more conservative measures were implemented as well.

Results were comparative so the ultimate value of ECMO was not clear (Bunker 1995).

[f] Iatrogenic means a condition of the patient caused by therapeutic treatment. Sometimes such effects are labeled *side effects* as in symptoms which occur as a result of taking medications. Usually iatrogenic is reserved for more complicated outcomes. In iatrogenic situations, the result of using a particular treatment may actually make a patient worse. For example, the provision of excessive levels of oxygen for respiratory problems can result in blindness.

[g] In addition to blindness (retrolental fibroplasia) resulting from the use of oxygen as mentioned above are other examples: intraventricular hemorrhage, bronchopulmonary dysplasia (a respiratory condition in which the lung tissue becomes thick and fibrous), and tissue trauma from the pressure and friction of tubes and other devices used in or on the infant.

[h] C-PAP and PEEP are both used to prevent alveolar (air sacs) collapse. Oxygen is exchanged for the waste product of carbon dioxide in these tiny parts of the lungs.

[i] Bovine-based surfactant was the natural type replacement product generally used to treat premature infants at birth, those at risk for respiratory collapse. A synthetic version has also been tested (Robertson 1983; Tanka et. al. 1986). A more recent alternative currently under clinical investigation for newborns is the use of perflurocarbon. An interesting summary which includes references to scientific publications can be located at "www.med.umich.edu/liquid/whatislv. html"

[j] A fine plastic tube can be inserted into the blood vessel with a needle that is then withdrawn, leaving the tube behind for access to the blood vessel. The tube in the blood vessel can then be connected to a longer tube which in turn leads to a bag or bottle of fluid. The fluid usually contains medications or other substances like sugar in a water base. Since the types of materials required as substitutes for complete nourishment (breast milk in the case of newborns) are *strong* liquids, they need to be immediately mixed with a relatively large amount of blood when they enter the blood vessel. To accomplish this, the tubing is threaded into a large vessel close to the heart. Such a placement of an intravenous (into the vein) tube is called a central line.

[k] The longer survival for lower weight infants needs to be especially considered when evaluating any long-term outcomes research. A 20-year follow-up of very-low-birth-weight infants by Hack and associates (2002) was reported. These infants were born between 1977 and 1979. Treatment today is vastly different and the survival rate for these very small infants is higher now. Therefore the needs of larger numbers of these infants, especially those with serious sequelae need to be considered within the health care arena.

[l] The figures for 2001 equivalents were reached using a conversion formula provided on the internet site "http://newsengin.com."

[m] Although many reactions to the different factors in the blood of pregnant woman and fetus are possible, a common untoward development occurs in the fetus with Rh positive blood (inherited from the father) whose mother has Rh negative blood. During fetal development the woman's body produces anti-Rh agglutinins. These substances act to destroy the red blood cells of the fetus after they have diffused through the placental membrane. The hemoglobin from the red blood cells is converted to bilirubin which causes the yellow (jaundice) appearance of the baby's skin. The post-birth treatment is blood transfusion: immediate provision of Rh negative blood while removing the Rh positive. Transfusion prior to birth is possible. The woman's anti-Rh agglutinin level is monitored and the fetus can be infused with the appropriate blood type as indicated during the pregnancy through a laproscopic procedure. The use of Rho (D) immune globulin (RhoGAM) during pregnancy has significantly reduced the need for infant intervention (Pillitteri 1985).

[n] Congenital hydronephrosis is the dilation of the kidneys from the accumulation of urine, which is prevented from flowing into the fetus's bladder. One possible cause of this condition is a malformation or twisting of the tube (ureter) that leads from the kidney to the bladder. Surgery is implemented to restore the flow of urine from the kidney to the bladder.

Obstructive hydrocephalus is the excessive accumulation of spinal fluid in the brain. The spaces of the brain (ventricles) expand and prevent the development of brain tissue in the fetus. The surgical procedure involves the insertion of a tube into this space allowing the fluid to drain off.

[o] Spina bifida is a defect in the spinal column. A number of different types of defect can exist from mild to quite severe. A portion of the bone of the spinal column is missing and the spinal membranes and sometimes the spinal cord itself can protrude. Infection is a risk if surgery is not performed, and permanent injury to the cord can result in loss of bladder control, paralysis, and/or mental retardation. Intrauterine surgery may limit the damage that such a condition can cause although this is not a common approach as yet (Pillitteri 1985).

[p] This now infamous photograph of Bruner is taken to task by Jones in a New York Times article on fetal surgery (2001). Apparently the photograph of the fetus "reaching" out of the womb and "hanging on for life" as used by anti-abortion activists, is a misrepresentation of the reality of such an event. Bruner admits that he *lifted* the fetal hand out of the incision to hold it in his hand rather than the fetus purposively reaching out and grasping Bruner's finger. Two rationale are provided for the misinterpretation by various groups as the fetus is not developmentally capable of reaching and grabbing plus the pharmacological effects of anesthesia would prevent such a purposeful or even reflexive action.

[q] When regionalization occurred, levels of neonatal intensive care were created to differentiate among the services hospitals were equipped to offer. The most complex care is offered in Level III nurseries while Level II nurseries have some sophisticated services but are not as comprehensive as Level III nurseries. Level I hospitals only care for normal newborns (Frigoletto & Little 1988).

[r] Some examples are listed below. These were available as the book was written. Given the transitory nature of material on the internet, their current status is unknown. Key words to use with any general search engine might include: premature, newborn, parenting, high-risk infant, and support groups.

www.fathersnetwork.org [targets fathers' needs]
www.rhsnet.org/support/groups.htm [sources for support groups]
www.fcsn.org [parenting information]
www.2.com/issue03/wiz_do6.html [Pediatric medicine at the University of Alabama]
rainforest.parentsplace.com/dialog/get/npremature/47.htm/ [specializes in premature issues]
www.cleft.com/brocpar.htm [parents of newborns with cleft lip and cleft palate]

[s] A guide for evaluating internet sources can be located at: http://libweb. sonoma.edu/web/eval.html

[t] For purposes of this project, Merenstein and Gardner's (1985) criteria were used to identify high-risk. In that edition they included <2500 grams at birth, <37 weeks gestational age, Apgar <5, bilirubin >15 ml/dl., presence of congenital anomalies, and/or need for surgical intervention. Although these may appear to be liberal criteria at the present time, these were timely criteria at the time this project commenced.

[u] This genetic defect is commonly called Down Syndrome or less appropriately, mongolism. The syndrome consists of a set of congenital anomalies associated with an extra 21st chromosome. Normally a person has two such chromosomes, one from each parent. The *tri-* designates the presence of three in this abnormality.

[v] Duodenal atresia is an intestinal constriction that prevents the passage of food through the diseased section of the gastrointestinal tract. Death ensues if the constriction is not surgically corrected. The operation carries relatively low risk and is usually performed within 48 hours.

[w] Esophageal atresia is a condition in which the tube to the stomach (esophagus) does not develop normally.

[x] According to Jeff Lyon (1985) in *Playing God in the nursery*, shortly after the death of the Bloomington Baby Doe case, another Baby Doe case ensued in Robinson, Illinois. After an informant disclosed the parent's refusal for surgery to treat myelomeningocele, an investigation resulted but the baby was treated and later adopted. A Baby Jane Doe was born in Port Jefferson, Long Island, New

York, in 1983. She was diagnosed with meningomyelocele, microcephaly, and hydrocephaly. Although her parents initially refused to allow surgery, they later agreed to have a shunt placed, and she finally became sufficiently healthy to go home. See Lyon's book for details about these and other related but less publicized cases.

[y] Conjoined twins is the term for the common expression *Siamese twins*. From the one original egg, two individuals begin to form but the separation is incomplete. There can be varying degrees of union involving the head, chest, or abdomen. Some internal organs may be duplicated while in other cases the two share certain organs.

[z] There is a whole set of debates, about the morality of active versus passive behavior, in bioethics. Some argue that there is no difference, while others claim that actively engaging in activity that brings about harm or death may be ethically wrong but simply allowing a disease to progress or tolerating the compromise that side effects of a drug induce is passive behavior, but not wrong behavior. This debate appears to have a long history dating at least from the Middle Ages perspective on infanticide and continuing to the present (Hopkins 1997).

[aa] This is a cultural or social standard meaning marriage bonds or other legal arrangement existed between the infant's parents.

[bb] Fletcher is one moral philosopher who supported infanticide as a justifiable and honorable practice. He is known for his discussion of personhood and characteristics that define such personhood in order to quantify humanness (1972). Cortical functioning was a key characteristic in his analysis but all traits were selected to help determine what constituted a life with a particular minimal quality. However, he did not specifically invoke his list of traits to determine who should live and who should die. He claimed to have devised his list to stimulate and engage others in discussions about the cardinal essence of humanness in order to reach some resolution about the concept of quality of life.

[cc] An oft cited use of the principle of extraordinary versus ordinary means of medical treatment is from the response of Pope Pius XII (1977) in 1958 to Dr. Bruno Haid, an anesthesiologist, of the University of Innsbruck as he addressed the moral quandary of whether or not a patient had to accept treatment. Dr. Haid's particular challenge related to the physician's obligation to always resuscitate a patient.

[dd] Definitions of these terms and similar ones used in bioethical writing can be located in the glossary.

[ee] "Making babies" was the focus of a 1999(a) *Frontline* television presentation, which clearly linked reproductive technologies, the booming infertility business, and intensive neonatal care. The 60-minute program is available on video tape from PBS Home Video, 1-800-PLAYPBS (1999b).

[ff] In addition to these specific examples (Callahan 1979; Cohen 1976; Duff & Campbell 1973; Penticuff 1988; Rue 1985; Strong 1983a, 1983b, 1984), an

analysis of the literature between 1966-1985 by Davis reached a similar conclusion. Although parents were named as decision-makers in 75.75% of the sample articles, Davis notes that this assessment was made by the authors of the articles rather than the parents themselves. The authors were professionals for the most part, and Davis' personal interviews (1994) with parents did not support a parental understanding of involvement in decision-making.

gg A recent example comes from a study in the Netherlands. Neonatologists and general pediatricians were interviewed. The study showed parents were involved in making 79% of the decisions. However, **NO** parents were consulted in the study. Only the physicians were interviewed. The question is raised as to whether or not the parents would have had the same perception (van der Heide et al. 1997).

hh There are at least two editions of this book. The first was published in 1982 and then a later edition in 1988 which does have some additional material.

ii Two attempts were made to contact these parents. A letter was sent to the Stinsons in care of the publishing firm requesting some follow-up information given the longitudinal nature of this project. The second involved a letter to Jerry Adler at *Newsweek* requesting permission to use a poem he wrote and published as part of his story in the 1987 issue cited in the text. Someone simply wrote **refuse** in a black marker across the request without any rationale for the decision. Realizing the trauma parents experience during and sometimes for years after the NICU hospitalization, we as investigators believed that the stories the parents published had a cathartic effect. They confronted the issue and were now moving on. They apparently did not want to continue to discuss the matter with anyone. We respected that possible position after posing our requests and accepted their lack of response or refusal.

jj As the final steps for this book were being completed, *Reader's Digest* (October 2000) published a special excerpt from *Baby E.R.: The heroic doctors & nurses who perform medicine's tiniest miracles*, a book by Edward Humes, published later in 2000 by Simon and Schuster. The excerpt included the stories of several families' experiences in the NICU. The exact scope of this book was not explored but the content in *Reader's Digest* had the clear ring of familiarity as Humes' stories unfolded after hearing the stories of parents in this project.

CHAPTER 2

A View From The NICU

Asked to look back over the neonatal intensive care experience, one mother began her story:

> I woke up in the middle of the night and my water broke. I thought to myself--well, this is the end of the pregnancy. I'm, you know, not even six months pregnant. Nothing hurt. All I could remember was another family who had a baby that was three months early. But I was *more* than three months early so I thought, well, this is the end. I immediately called a nurse friend and she told me that the sac could seal over but I needed to get to the local hospital. They would transfer me to [town] where there was a level two, intensive care nursery for the baby if it didn't seal. Well, from then on, it was just chaos.

Beginning a discussion of the NICU experiences with an earlier event was not unique among families in the project described here. Whether one talked to these parents at predischarge, six months postdischarge, or four years postdischarge, all of them persisted in describing their experiences in the NICU within the broader context of their lives.[a]

The goal of this project was to examine the parents' perspective of ethical decision-making in the NICU. We gave the parents the informed consent document that included this information, and this goal was verbally described again as informed consent was obtained. However, it would appear from the parental perspective that the NICU experience cannot and will not be separated from the parents' more expansive family history and their total current situation including events outside the hospital. Our expectation that parents would target some aspect of the infant's care or the traditional focus of bioethics on treatment decision-making initially was not met in the anticipated manner.

Several women in the predischarge phase began their descriptions with their joy, satisfaction, happiness, excitement, and optimism about the pregnancy. One of these women responded:

> Actually being pregnant stands out for me. I enjoyed being pregnant. I thought the pregnancy was really good. I was always happy. When Dr. [name] put me on bedrest the last three weeks before I delivered was when I started to feel heavy. I knew then it was time for me to start to take it easy. I had been going to the spa for swimming, you know. I thought it was really good for the pregnancy and everything was going well. My check-ups were just, you know, regular. I was pretty good except, of course, toward the end. It was twins and that was a real problem.

Another woman had the following perspective:

> I've been trying since I was 16...or really pretty much close to 17 and I just couldn't get pregnant. No matter what I tried. One doctor goes, "Oh, I'll put you on the pill, that'll make you more fertile. I'll put you on the pill for a while and then take you off." Well, that didn't work. So the joy of actually finally having a baby meant a lot to me, and my husband. The way my husband reacted to the pregnancy--that is what stands out. It was very exciting and very interesting because he started to do little things around the house...helping me out. Or saying little jokes. Looking back, I see more of the joy and thrill of having a baby than the pains, and the problems of delivery and everything.

The grandmother of one infant described her daughter's situation this way:

> Well, she is a little baby still herself, you know. I let her spend the summer with my sister. At one point she came and told me she hadn't been having her periods. It was just little spots here and there. I took her to the doctors and they kept telling me she wasn't pregnant and she was too young to be on birth control pills. So I finally bought a test myself and made her take a urine test--at seven o'clock in the morning. Well, she was three and one-half months pregnant! I cried like a big baby. I wanted to know, I couldn't understand why blood tests and urine tests they gave her couldn't tell a three and one-half month pregnancy. I figured that I would, jus...you know, I'd take the baby. I wouldn't make her feel embarrassed because I do think it is kind of shameful at her age [her daughter was twelve when she became

> pregnant]. And believe me, I do not talk to my sister because of it either. She let my daughter become pregnant. That's the way I feel. My daughter wasn't doing that when she was home with me, her mother.

Evidence for the broader parental perspective was widespread throughout the entire interview. The parents' approach in attempting to help others understand their experiences provided a particular, important insight into the NICU experience. Rather than a narrowly focused and simplistic response to only the nursery events, the parents' replies encompassed the totality of circumstances impacting the NICU experience. All of these factors were important to them. One woman began with the question of whether or not she was actually pregnant:

> Well, really...they couldn't figure it out. If I was pregnant, first of all. The pregnancy test kept coming back negative. I finally figured out for myself that I was pregnant, the end of--the last week in May. I had been doctoring since the beginning of April. Then in June I went in for another pregnancy test and that's when they confirmed that it was positive. So it took them like a whole month or more, for them to figure out that I was pregnant. In the meantime they were treating me for other stuff first. I was having severe cramping and stuff so they thought I wasn't ovulating. That I just wasn't ovulating. That's what they thought was happening.
> Interviewer: What were they giving you?
> Oh gosh, I can't even remember. One of them was, some...hormone that they give women. I can't really remember what the pills were that they gave me. But anyway, I also had a shot that was supposed to clean out my system. Then they said that I could start taking Clomid.[b] So I would have a chance to get pregnant.

For parents, it seems events in the NICU *could not* be examined nor understood *without* knowing these other factors, including their identity as individuals, their family life as it existed before the infant was born, and then events subsequent to its birth. This emphasis on context and relationships while responding to the request to describe their NICU experience, is a very important reminder to anyone concerned about parental coping or adaptation to the crisis of a high-risk perinatal event as well as any decision-making in which parents are required to participate. Hospitalization of a newborn in the NICU is not an isolated event for families or even the main event, try as some may to make it so.

Before Conception: One Approach to the Parents' Stories

Some of the family history, as noted above, that parents believed led to the NICU experience began years before conception. The most distant events that parents now relate directly to the current infant hospitalization were those focused on infertility. Some families sought assistance for conception many years prior to the birth of this child (or children). Medical assistance for infertility involved tests and procedures, monitoring of bodily functioning, timing of intercourse, and, as several women indicated, the use of Clomid, a fertility-enhancing medication. Physically and emotionally challenging incidents were faced before encountering the NICU, overtaxing families prior to any stress that the neonatal status or hospitalization might provoke. Facing conflict was not new to some of these parents. To have finally conceived just might be considered a miracle for parents with fertility problems. Both parents in the following situation were so eager to describe their excitement that they kept talking over one another:

> Father (F): We had problems, she had problems becoming pregnant so they kept pretty good tabs on her during the pregnancy...
> Mother (M): ...I was just so happy being pregnant. Just finding out I was pregnant and really, the whole pregnancy...
> F: ...then there was the shock of, my wife coming home and saying, we're going to have twins, possibly triplets. We found that out about a month after she found out she was pregnant, I think...
> M: ...I had an ultrasound...
> F: ...well at first, the first couple of weeks, I didn't really know how to take the idea of having twins, pos...possibly triplets. It was kinda a shock at first but then we got a little more excited as time went on. I felt so fortunate that she was pregnant, you know. We, we're in a lot better position than other folks 'cause a lot of other folks can't even get pregnant...
> M: ...and I felt real good too. Except, you know, that I started having contractions...
> F: ...in your fourth month.

At the other end of the continuum, a few had unplanned pregnancies that were their entrée into the story. At least one woman believed her contraceptive pills failed because they were too old or not strong enough, "It [the pregnancy] wasn't planned. I was taking my pills and the next thing you know, I was pregnant." One couple did not agree about this aspect of the pregnancy. The woman claimed that the pregnancy was unplanned while her husband believed it was anticipated. He went on to discuss their apprehension at waiting so long to try getting pregnant again, "...'cause it's, you know, the, the longer you wait, the more...supposedly the risks. The risks are a little greater when you get a little older."[c] Several couples did not take any precautions to prevent pregnancy, including those individuals in their teens.

Some prenatal conditions of the women warranted close monitoring, creating concern for the pregnancy. One couple carefully considered conception before attempting to become pregnant because of the women's preexisting health problems. They received conflicting advice. One of her physicians recommended not allowing an inoperable tumor to stop them from considering conception while another was not sure pregnancy was a good idea. But they decided to attempt this second pregnancy and be as careful as possible without letting the woman's condition rule their lives.

One woman said she was terrified when she became pregnant with her intrauterine device (IUD) in place.[d] This apparatus was imbedded in the placenta at the time of delivery:

> *The forgotten IUD.* Ethyl admitted irresponsibility in monitoring the IUD because, after having it inserted, she never had it checked again. The IUD was inserted after the birth of her daughter and now, six years later, she suddenly found herself pregnant. The ultrasound showed the IUD right up against the fetus and removing it was considered dangerous. Ethyl said that she "couldn't risk losing the pregnancy. I had to give it at least a chance. At least try." Ethyl had a difficult pregnancy which the physician predicted, with intermittent labor pains and bleeding throughout the time she carried the baby. She was told there was a 99% chance the pregnancy would not make it to term. The pregnancy was imminently threatened when Ethyl experienced a sudden, huge gush that was the loss of amniotic fluid. Ethyl thought she would go into labor and deliver immediately but she was placed on bedrest and given magnesium sulfate and terbutaline which averted the delivery for another four weeks. Ethyl also contracted a kidney infection. She thought she would "mentally lose it" during this time, which she attributed to the effects of the medications. Ethyl described the result of this pharmacological prevention of preterm labor as simultaneously, intensely relaxing the body while also causing another acute sensation, like a powerful urge to speed up and move. This dual action was accompanied by headaches and a perception that her eyes

would pop out. Additionally, she had pain from the kidney infection. Ethyl finally requested some adjustment in the medication, either a lower dose or a discontinuing of one or the other medication so that she could tolerate the situation. The magnesium sulfate was discontinued but, two hours later, the baby's heartbeat became critical and a caesarian section was performed. According to the infant's hospital medical record, her weight was 735 grams at birth and she was discharged after three months residence in the NICU.

The Ordeal of a Difficult Pregnancy

Far more parents reviewed a difficult pregnancy as the precipitating event for their story than any other circumstance. More prenatal difficulties might certainly be anticipated in such families given the infants' need for the NICU. After all, some sort of crisis precipitated the woman's or baby's distress. In general, women discussed their perception that once they were pregnant, many of the negative psychological symptoms and feelings they reported were summarily dismissed during prenatal obstetrical visits. Some postpartum guilt about the infant's compromised status could be attributed to these perceptions and the women's hindsight in which they chastised themselves for not being more assertive about their own impressions. Some of these women's symptoms were rather nebulous and might have provided only a weak rationale upon which to base any significant intervention: feeling depressed, scared, anxious, frustrated, tired, generally sick, or unusually uncomfortable. Admittedly the women had vague feelings that the pregnancy "didn't feel right," but they had more specific concerns as well that they felt were ignored.

Women recalled their frustration with obstetricians who failed to attend to even the more tangible symptoms, such as pain. Parents wondered if infant problems could have been avoided if doctors had paid more attention to the woman's perceived status. Pregnancy is a natural event, but many women believed that they were expected to tolerate almost anything that resulted from this state and not question deviations from a previous healthy condition or recollections of a previous healthy pregnancy.

Indeed, several women had been pregnant previously and they compared this experience to their past ones:

> This was different from my first pregnancy. We didn't really expect that we would have to do all this. All of a sudden he [the doctor] told me that the baby would need a transfusion or he'd be in trouble. I was

> having amniocentesis tests done every three weeks. It was getting too risky to do any more transfusions. We understood. We felt confident we were doing the right thing.

Two women believed this pregnancy was easier than their first and, for one of these, no problems developed for the fetus until after birth. A few women had earlier unfortunate pregnancies in which fetuses were lost; therefore they had quite a high investment in seeing this pregnancy to a successful conclusion.

Three women discussed their surprise that their pregnancies might be difficult and the baby end up in a NICU after fertility treatment. One of these women quoted her physician: "He was as shocked as we were about preterm labor with Clomid!" Two couples related that they were fully informed about the possible outcomes for the pregnancy with Clomid. One of these couples with a multiple gestation was clear that they had been told the woman was at "high-risk for having preterm labor" but did not subsequently realize the kind of treatment in store for a small baby like theirs. The other couple made a remark about their awareness of the possible need immediately after birth for the baby to get surfactant.[e]

This woman described her response to a difficult pregnancy:

> It was a miracle that I was pregnant. I really wanted to have a baby but it was real uncomfortable. The baby was real active. And from about the second month on, I was really uncomfortable. There was a lot of pressure in my pelvic area. I was real disappointed in my doctor. I had been told that with my first daughter I had an incompetent cervix. When I went in for my prenatal checkup, I told my doctor from the very beginning. But he just blew me off. And I'd had contractions with this baby from about, I'd say from the fourth month, they started. And he kept saying, "Oh, it's just Braxton Hicks.[f] It's nothing to worry about." So I called the office (the day I came to the hospital) and they said, "Well, it's probably nothing but go get it checked out." I came to the emergency room and I was all the way dilated! The baby was on the way. It was breech and it was pretty traumatic.

The father added, "She was sure miserable the whole time. It was back pain, pressure, and just...everything. At least he was born whole. (pause) But he was fourteen weeks early."

Concurrent medical conditions and/or problems in the woman, such as asthma, excessive weight gain, diabetes, infections, bleeding, elevated blood pressure, and edema could potentially compromise her health and affect the infant's outcome. One couple believed that the physician's initial inability to determine whether or not the woman was pregnant, and then delaying aggressive intervention to maintain the pregnancy, was their worst nightmare.

The development of an incompetent cervix led to the use of cerclage[g] in one case. This pregnancy was the woman's fourth and, hopefully for her, the second live birth. As soon as the physician detected the incompetent cervix, a cerclage was performed. The woman explained, "It wasn't just whether I was going to make it to term or not but whether or not the *baby* would make it whenever it was born."

In three cases there was a failure to place the cerclage. One woman was scheduled for the cerclage but went into labor the day before the appointment. In two cases the physicians neglected to place the cerclage despite both women's knowledge of the incompetent cervix from a previous pregnancy. In one situation there was first a polite request by the patient and her husband and later more assertive insistence that a cerclage be performed:

> *Failure to act.* Crystal told of her and her husband's frustration with their obstetrician. During an earlier pregnancy, Crystal had gone in for a regular check-up at about the 19th week to discover the sac had begun to come down so the obstetrician attempted to place a cerclage. This induced premature labor and Crystal eventually lost the baby. After the loss, the obstetrician told Crystal and her husband that the problem was an incompetent cervix. Should she become pregnant again, she was to be sure and tell her physician about this earlier problem and insist upon a cerclage. If it was done early, this stitch in the cervix would prevent it from opening and avert a loss of the pregnancy. Early in the current pregnancy, Crystal made an appointment with the obstetrician because she was "thrilled" with the possibility of being pregnant again and she wanted to avoid a loss like the previous experience. The obstetrician confirmed her suspicions about the pregnancy but indicated that a cerclage was not necessary, certainly not at this point in the pregnancy. Crystal's pregnancy proceeded without any difficulties for a short time until she really became worried about the incompetent cervix condition. When the couple renewed their suggestion, the physician dismissed it with his admonition that they, as parents, were not in a position to practice medicine. He, the obstetrician, would make all of the decisions. Crystal finally decided to see another obstetrician at the 15-week point. As she surmised, the same difficulty had surfaced and she again was in danger of losing the pregnancy. Much to her and her husband's dismay, the

> second obstetrician admitted that a cerclage should have been done but now it was too late to attempt to place one. It might stimulate uterine contractions and he wanted to minimize such an outcome. Additionally, there was a danger of puncturing the sac at this point. Crystal delivered vaginally at 24 weeks and the boy weighed only 620 grams. After 235 days in the NICU, he was finally discharged only to be readmitted later for complications, which resulted in his death six weeks after the initial NICU discharge.

Both legal and illegal drug use worried some of these women in terms of its effect on the fetus. For example, one woman discussed her shock at becoming pregnant while taking asthma medication and her preference for discontinuing it before conception or at least lowering the required dose had it been a planned pregnancy:

> I don't know if it was the right thing to do to get pregnant. I should have gotten my tubes tied, a long time ago. [I] always put it off. But I knew I was on a lot of medications and I just made up my mind. I'm not going to get pregnant.

The woman who admitted a substance abuse problem (crack cocaine) during the first two and one-half months of the pregnancy did not connect it to any fetal developmental difficulty or the current condition of the infant, which she described as a viral infection. Based on experience with a previous pregnancy, she complacently said that she would have known if anything she was doing would adversely affect the pregnancy. In fact she assured us during the interview that the hospital staff told her that her drug abuse had "nothing to do with her [infant's] condition whatsoever." The only problem during pregnancy that she could attribute to a possible dire outcome for the baby was her "feeling always on edge" because of the child's father. At predischarge she avoided going into this aspect any further but she was living at a shelter for abused women at the time of the interview. In the postdischarge interview (six months later), she was more explicit about the extent of her husband's abuse and her situation during her pregnancy.

Early Labor: A Shocking Turn of Events

Early labor was another outstanding circumstance for some women who had an otherwise normal pregnancy. Seven women failed to recognize initial signs or symptoms of labor, partly because of their early arrival. Several women mentioned enforced bedrest and tocolytic medications to stop premature labor.[h] One couple began their story with their excitement at the prospect of having twins and then their dismay at subsequent need for treatment. The woman starts:

> I will never forget the day we found out we were going to have twins. I was about five months pregnant. They then told us that I would have a difficult pregnancy for the remaining time. I got this really strange feeling. They said that they can keep the babies in [by giving me special drugs]. But I always had, always had the feeling that we weren't going to keep these babies in there very long anyway. That was my major concern. I was twenty-six weeks when I delivered.

What seemed interesting under these various high-risk circumstances was some parents' incredulity that accompanied resulting problems, including preterm labor. Few seemed to have expected the preterm labor as a risk of their pregnancies even when the pregnancies themselves were high-risk. In this group of parents there were eight multiple gestations (six sets of twins, two sets of triplets). Most of the women on fertility medications did not seem to realize that a multiple conception was possible and this in turn would lead to a high-risk pregnancy. Some women had very specific and/or invasive procedures to monitor a high-risk pregnancy: amniocentesis,[i] tocodynamonometry,[j] more than the routine number of ultrasonographies,[k] and in one case intrauterine transfusions for the fetus.[l] Most of these women assumed that, with these treatments, all would turn out well for the infants. Or perhaps it was hope that created such a mind-set.

One woman, who was pregnant with twins, told about her obstetrician's prediction that she might deliver in June, rather than in July when she would be full-term:

> I thought I was gonna have perfectly normal healthy babies in June. I didn't realize that even having them a month or six weeks early meant having a premature baby with possible problems and something like this [admission to the NICU]. I mean, this was never expected. I was never warned. They didn't seem concerned about any premature labor or anything. It was never mentioned that I maybe would have to come to [distant hospital] and have my baby. They shoulda' went into it a little more extensively.

For several women, early contractions, premature rupture of the amniotic sac, and hemorrhage led to frenzied trips to the hospital in the middle of the night. Helicopter transport to a tertiary care center from rural areas and emergency caesarian sections all contributed to these individuals feeling out of control and emotionally torn. Husbands were concerned for the health and safety of both wife and baby. The women's descriptions about the preterm labor ranged from simply surprised and anxious to more intense reactions such as depressed, confused, terrified, stressed, and shocked, but mostly the women were scared.

One woman called the hospital with her report of early contractions (two weeks prior to her due date) but was told to wait until the contractions were five minutes apart before she came in. When she began to complain of severe pain, her own mother made her go to the hospital. Another woman who was surprised by the premature labor went into this state fifteen minutes after an amniocentesis. It was obvious during the discussion that she did not know or remember that initiation of labor was a possible risk of the amniocentesis.

Some women were placed on bedrest in order to control preterm labor. Although the effectiveness of this intervention varied, bedrest was a negative experience for most. But the requirement was one willingly accepted for the health and safety of the baby, ensuring further growth and development of the fetus and a delayed delivery. Simply doing next to nothing was a challenging ordeal, and of course bedrest did lead to generalized weakness:

> I guess the hardest part for me was having to spend two weeks in bed. And, I really appreciated watching out the window...and seeing people walk around and thinking how wonderful just to be able to walk around again. It's amazing how much you take for granted. It's extremely depressing to just lay there. And not be able to move, not to be able to get up and go to the bathroom, wash your hair. I don't know that I would have the stamina to lay there for three months.

Those who were hospitalized for the bedrest and medicated for early labor had an even greater overall negative effect, as symbolized by one woman who contemplated jumping out the window. She quietly remarked at the end of her interview:

> During my pregnancy while I was laying in bed on all that medicine, and feeling guilty about whether or not I could stand it any longer. Or, if I just wanted them to be born so it would be over...(pause)...I had a lot of mixed feelings. And, and at one time I did look at the window seriously and wonder how far down it was.

The women on these preterm labor medications all brought attention to their potent side effects. Tocolytic drugs caused headaches, blurred or distorted vision, difficulty in breathing and an inability to urinate (both due to retention of fluids the women believed), loss of appetite, and mental instability, including hallucinations. These side effects were more or less uniform in all the women regardless of the length of time on the drugs, four days, for example, or several weeks (one woman for 14 weeks). Especially disconcerting were mental aberrations or "feeling like you are going out of your mind," as one woman exclaimed. Buying time for the fetus to continue to develop motivated these women to tolerate the treatment--"...there was no question though that I would do this for my children"--so bedrest and prenatal treatments did not present a conflict for most women.

One woman described her situation as she went into premature labor at work (32 weeks gestation). She did not note any problems with the pregnancy until that moment. Later she was told that an abruptio placenta which she called an "abruption," caused her early labor.[m] She recounted her shock at having sudden contractions and bleeding both within 15 minutes of her first noticing that "something did not feel right." She was taken to the labor and delivery room immediately upon arrival at the hospital. With the administration of magnesium sulfate and terbutaline, the staff was able to stop the contractions by three o'clock in the morning, according to her recollection. She was flat in bed for about a week when it was decided to let her out of bed and monitor her closely. The contractions started immediately so she was returned to bed and the dosage of the medications increased. This time there was no bleeding. After the contractions were under control, she was told that she was on the maximum dosage. If labor began again, there was nothing to do to stop it.

She discussed her assessment of the situation at this point. She felt very, very scared and was not adjusting well to the effects of the medications. She did not like how she felt while she was getting them: "...if one more needle came at me, I was going to attack somebody!" She was afraid that something bad was happening to the baby because she had gone into labor so many times and gotten so many drugs. However, on the positive side, the physician had been able to begin steroid therapy[n] and was preparing to give the baby surfactant at birth.

Several of the men addressed the effect on them of the women's bedrest. One of the more common observations was the recognition of the woman's contributions to the household and its functioning that she could no longer complete:

> Her bedrest made me realize a lot...a lot of the things I took for granted. I had to be home more and take on a lot of things. I just assumed all this was being done by her but when I had to do it, it was so hard.

One father underscored his understanding of the importance of the medications and bedrest to prevent a bad outcome for the baby, which he did not think the doctors emphasized sufficiently for his wife:

> I pretty much was going along with the idea that whatever it took to, for, whatever was best for that baby--for her to stay pregnant as long as she could. I was perceiving from them that they really were not wanting to paint any gloomy pictures about the baby so not to traumatize her. It was really important for her to stay pregnant. For a while she was a little tired of it--lungs filling up, and the medications and stuff. She wanted to get it over with...and I'm thinking. I think maybe they should start painting some other picture so that she could see the dark side of this. So she can see...what she's doing [importance of bedrest to prevent labor and premature birth] for the baby.

He believed that such an explanation would create a reserve of strength and courage for his wife that she might draw upon as she endured the restrictions and the effects of the medications.

Some of the participants questioned whether or not a justification for the treatment would be meaningful for the woman at this point. A number of descriptions by the women led to their conclusion that, although information may be shared or limited choices offered to individuals during labor, a compromise in mental status, especially when on tocolytic medications, kept these women from believing they could adequately participate in discussions or decision-making. Some women acknowledged their inability to concentrate, which made them question their own capacity to make rational choices.

The fathers, of course, did not share these limitations although there were different anxieties and stresses for them. Getting to the hospital for the labor was not possible for some men and several even missed the birth of their child(ren). This absence also meant the lack of any opportunity to participate in any decisions about labor, birth, or initial infant treatment had they been proposed.

In a few cases, women discussed the connection between the preterm treatment and their own later recovery. One woman described how she was so disoriented and weak that, despite her strong desire to comply, standing beside the bed for a brief moment was arduous. Two weeks after her own discharge from the hospital, she continued to have trouble walking. There were other instances of prolonged recovery from physiological insult. Three women were admitted to an Adult Intensive Care Unit after delivery. For one of these women, it was a seven-day stay followed by 11 more days in a step-down unit before she was discharged from the hospital. One woman did not remember her delivery until six days after it was over, and another remained so sick she was unable to get to the NICU to see the baby for two weeks:

> I had no clotting factor in my blood and I started bleeding. And I had kidney failure. I was in intensive care for seven days [post C-section]. I have absolutely no recollection of any of it. I wasn't even aware I had a baby 'til probably five or six days afterward!

All women worried about the effects of these drugs on the baby; they did not want to add to the baby's stress. Whether actually due to these prenatal treatments or not, these women attributed their own immediate, subsequent status to the prenatal treatments. Interestingly enough, only one woman wondered about any permanent effects on her own long-term health and expressed concern about this possibility. Despite the critical condition of three mothers postpartum, no one initially addressed this in the interview. It only came to light later in the discussion as all circumstances surrounding the infant's admission to the NICU were probed.

Birth: A New Life Emerges

The birth experience itself was not mentioned first as often as the pregnancy. One woman initially shared her horror when she thought the caesarian incision would start before she was anesthetized (about half of the women in the study had caesarian sections). Two other families characterized the delivery as chaotic or filled with confusion. As one woman stated, "His premature birth--it really surprised me. It was a normal pregnancy, and then rush, rush, rush." The other woman had one twin vaginally and the second by caesarian section, which was also an eye-opening experience for her. In no case, however, among these 32 families, was the baby's circumstance in the NICU cited first as the most outstanding event no matter how compromised its condition.

Across the interviews, parents raised occasional questions about the delivery, whether or not they noted it as the most outstanding event.

Some women worried about anesthesia and caesarian section surgery. One woman adamantly refused a caesarian section. She took an interesting perspective in refusing the surgery. At this point in her labor, she remarked, she did not think there would be a live birth. If she wasn't going to deliver a live baby, then she wanted to be able to have something from the experience and that something was delivering the fetus herself. "We were going to let nature take its course," she asserted.

Two fathers questioned the decision-making related to the delivery, but only within themselves. They never raised these doubts with health professionals prior to the delivery. One father discussed hearing the physicians debate about "when to take the baby." The physicians' indecisiveness made him very uncomfortable. In the meantime, all he could focus on was his perception of the pain and agony experienced by his wife. He wanted action, quick. He wanted the problem-filled labor to end.

Another man had a somewhat different dilemma. He had already been asked about the caesarian section for which he gave permission, but he perceived that "certain people were trying to buy time" for the fetus's benefit rather than his wife's. Given the couple's experience with toxemia in an earlier pregnancy, he did not want to wait for anything. He reported:

> I told them that I was tired of waiting. It was a four-day ordeal. The doctors told me that all we could do is...pray. By this time she was not in very good shape. I was...feeling that the doctors had made the wrong decision. That will be my feelings for the rest of my life. Keeping my wife alive, that's what I wanted most...but certain people did not agree.

For him, physicians seemed to be favoring benefits for the fetus over a healthy outcome for his wife. Such a conflict is hotly debated within the bioethical literature resulting in a lack of consensus in many discussions and varying institutional policies depending upon where one delivers (Sise 1988). All of these events were grounds for debate in the parents' minds even it not in open conversation with each other (when a spouse or significant other was present) or with health professionals.

For the relatively few parents who did include comments about the infant in the early portion of the interview, only two parents' recital included events from the NICU. For one family, the parents briefly mentioned that the baby was originally admitted to the regular newborn nursery immediately after delivery, then transferred to the NICU when the infant's condition deteriorated. The other parents noted that the baby was currently "just hanging on at the edge," then switched topics and more intently discussed pre-admission circumstances.

Although parents believed or hoped that successful completion of prenatal treatment would result in a good outcome for the infant, once things began to go wrong parents also had pervasive thoughts about losing the baby. Some realized that, whatever the present fetal status, given the mother's condition during pregnancy and labor the baby's chances were better the longer the pregnancy was maintained. Additionally, parents spoke of their concern, once labor began, that babies (especially cases of multiple gestation) could not survive the stress of delivery. For those parents who experienced a very early delivery, the size of the infant(s) at birth produced disbelief that anything so small could actually survive.

Encountering the NICU

The NICU experience gradually became part of the discussion as parents completed their descriptions of pre-admission events. We directed the parents to think about the NICU and to reflect upon the outstanding events. Ultimately, if parents did not address decision-making, possible conflict, or "a time when they weren't sure what was the right thing to do," we led them to think about such issues with the use of various probes.

For some parents, seeing the baby for the first time was a shock, but, as this story shows, parents could differ in their observations:

> *Contrasting perceptions: The Barbie Doll.* Alice had given birth to a 680-gram baby boy at 27 weeks gestation. Alice had a cesarean section and did not see the infant at birth. Bob, the father, was the first parent to see the child in the NICU after he was stabilized. The father says, "I had a confidence inside that God gave me, that no matter what I saw, that was my son...whether he had all of his fingers or toes, or blind or whatever. He was my son and I would take my faith in God's promise in His word...he would be a normal person. There's never been a doubt inside of me about his, about him making it, being a normal person."
>
> Alice continues: "I doubt[ed] it though. The first night I saw him, when I first saw him [long pause]. Bob had come to my room and told me what a beautiful, perfect...little boy we had. And his [Bob's] face was this big, you know [gesturing widely]. And he was just on cloud nine, you know. And when I went in to see the baby, I just...oh my, my

> heart went to my stomach and I just could not believe that this tiny, little kid...that this *tiny*, little kid...[voice trails off]. His body was as big as a Barbie doll and his head was as big as a plum. He just...his limbs were skinnier than my little fingers. He was so, so tiny. *I* just didn't see how he could live."

Parents were afraid to touch such a fragile baby but a few who were brave enough to try, felt chastised. Touching the baby was generally prohibited, according to these parents, especially when newly admitted and for a long time thereafter in cases of very sick infants. Not only did parents not get to hold their newborn as expected, but other anticipated caring and tending activities were carried out by professionals: bathing, diapering, and feeding. Parents had not simply a feeling of uselessness but a deeper sense of incompetence as they realized their child truly needed someone else as a caregiver.

Those parents who could not comprehend the gravity of the baby's situation (and this was the majority), or whose babies appeared less delicate, failed to understand why they could not touch the child or provide the care. The statement below captures some of this dilemma as well as the barrier that the environment created.° The NICU was not a place where most parents felt comfortable, as one woman explains:

> I had a real hard time going in the nursery there so I would stand outside the window. She [the mother of another neonate] came out and talked to me one day. We never really discussed much of her baby. Her baby was doing well. I mean he's the same term as my baby and he weighed a lot less. It was just real hard for me to understand why my baby had so many problems. But that was just how it was supposed to be, I guess.

A question about the infant's status was part of the demographic information collected from parents before the interview about neonatal care was opened. Parents were directly asked the rationale for the baby's admission to the NICU, the present diagnosis of their infant, and how it was doing. One question led to another when they hesitated, grappling for a response. The most common response of parents was that the baby "just needs to grow a little." Generally parents had a simplistic perspective of the baby's condition. It seemed remarkable that parents would merely say that the infant simply needed to grow a little, gain weight, or was as yet unable to take nourishment normally when it was living in an intensive care unit.

The status of *little*, in terms of a diagnosis of premature, and the relevant, potential problems of an early birth were not articulated. Most parents were without a basic understanding of the associated medical problems or pathology accompanying this precarious condition. Bodgan and associates (1982) discussed this as mis-communication between health care professionals and parents. For them the term was "all they need to do is feed and grow." But these researchers noted that...among professionals, this remark had quite different meanings. Even when the medical terms spilled forth in an explanation of a diagnosis or procedure for the infant, few parents in our study were able to expound upon the information. The outstanding exception to the more common inability to describe the infant's health status was the knowledge and understanding related to surfactant. This was the one treatment they were able to discuss in some detail.

Decisions about the use of surfactant were mostly made in the labor phase of the delivery process, although one father discussed learning about surfactant during his wife's pregnancy. Participants were generally correct and clear about this medication. They knew the source of the drug--that is, how it was manufactured. They also knew the rationale for the drug's projected use and what would occur if the newborn did not get it. Given the parents' understanding of the newborn's need and the action of this drug, no one had even the slightest hesitation in giving permission for its use.[p]

The distinct difference between parents' knowledge and understanding about surfactant and their knowledge and understanding related to other procedures or medications led us to conclude that it was not necessarily the mental status of the woman, nor the context of decision-making that explicitly determined the degree of comprehension. The surfactant was proposed for the newborn within a research protocol in effect concurrently with this project. Forms for surfactant use were different from routine informed consent documents. More explanations seem to have been provided and apparently parents more precisely remembered the importance of understanding this choice. The effort expended on the surfactant research protocol seems to be an important variable in parental recall and understanding. Given the informed consent process, the staff was obligated to provide detail and answer all questions. Whether or not any professional wanted to withhold information even for altruistic reasons such as preventing discomfort or fear in the parents, they could not evade communicating detail in the case of surfactant.

Parents specifically discussed the terminology health professionals in the NICU used and complained that words were not always defined. One woman related her conversation outside the nursery window with another mother who asked her how her baby was doing. The woman described her infant's condition:

> She has an enlarged liver and her heart is growing smaller. She is retaining fluid and she is very, very sick. But I don't know what that means. But that is what they have been telling me...all that they have been telling me.

One set of parents related that the physician said the baby was depressed. Although they knew the general meaning of depressed, they had no idea what this meant for a premature newborn. Some parents recognized the incomplete status of the information they received and readily admitted that they knew the child was given X, Y, and Z, but they did not know what X, Y, or Z did. Although neither of us had the background to evaluate detailed information about high-risk pregnancy, birth, or neonatal care, it was obvious on occasion that a few individuals had erroneous perceptions. Incorrect terms were used to describe common treatments or procedures; *normal* ranges for laboratory tests were misunderstood; goals or outcomes for interventions or examinations were simply wrong. Not knowing or understanding the baby's experiences worried some parents. This lack of information most often caused parents to fear that the situation was worse than they imagined while simultaneously allowing them to hold on to their belief that all would work out in the end.

Given many parents' lack of comprehension of the infant's serious status or its fragile grip on life, they had many questions about the need for the infant to remain in the nursery. They were impatient for discharge and in many cases sincerely believed the baby would improve more quickly "if only we could take it home." Parents often observed that the *other* babies in the NICU were the *sick* ones. They mentioned the use of complex machinery and sophisticated treatments in the NICU, but most distinguished between the more critical needs of other children and their own baby's needs. They discussed their wonder at other families' ability to cope with such desperate situations or minimally viable babies. One couple embellished this view. The mother was an experienced NICU nurse and so both she and her husband knew that all high-risk babies did not go home as normal newborns. She said of her husband, "But of course, he was sure ours would!"

When describing their infant's residence in the NICU, the parents mostly focused on the usual domains of parental responsibility for those infant needs they had expected to monitor and fulfill before their circumstances led to hospitalization of the infant: feeding, cleanliness, and sleep. Parents preferred to discuss these concerns and possible decisions related to them rather than the more technical aspects of their infant's care or areas usually identified with bioethical decision-making.[q]

Nutritional needs were a common point of discussion as some mothers were faced with a decision regarding breast-feeding. Women had to decide whether or not they were going to invest in pumping their breasts now, and perhaps for some extended period of time, in order to breast-feed the child when nippling and sucking began. Many factors had to be weighed to determine if it was reasonable to consider breast-feeding: a) distance from the hospital and the frequency of visits, b) length of time until the baby could suckle the breast itself, c) demands of family, and d) other children (nineteen of the thirty-two families had other children at home). Breast-feeding was the only decisional aspect of feeding about which parents felt they had a legitimate opinion. Parents were interested in how and what babies in the nursery were fed. They assumed feeding their child was a relatively simple task and the means to provide nutrition was available. Waking babies to feed them and using a nasogastric tube--"force feeding," several named this, disturbed some parents.[r] Parents particularly noted their dismay when formula was put in the tube and then seemed to immediately run out the baby's mouth. Was the baby really getting adequate nourishment?

Bathing and diaper changes were other areas of infant need about which parents could address their concerns. One father was upset that the nursery did not have "preemie" diapers and he wanted his son to have them, so he purchased them himself. He was also concerned about the exposure of his son in the isolette to what he perceived as a hot, dry environment--too hot and too dry. He explained his discussion with the nurse about his observations of the baby, the fast heart beat and rapid respirations:

> But I asked them. I know he's hot. It's ninety degrees in there--he's hot. And they said, "Oh no, oh no, no, no, no, no. It's normal. It is normal." And then I went home and I called later. I asked, "Is the kid hot? Just put your hand inside that hood. It's ninety degrees in there." I know

> what it's like to try and breathe when you're hot. And he's... Well, I bitched and bitched and just kept on it, you know. "Can't you just turn down the heat?" But they said they couldn't do it. Well, I come back the next day. I looked and they had it turned down four degrees. So instead of ninety degrees it was eighty-six. And--*he was resting easier!!* I knew he was hot, why couldn't they listen to me?

In the context of possible life-and-death issues in a NICU, one might question the father's resulting hostility (his term in the conversation) toward the nurses about a mere temperature issue. But it is more important to note his frustration, which apparently led to the hostility. It was obvious in his comments that he may not have the knowledge to question a laboratory test, a drug, or a medical procedure but he did believe he knew about babies and comfort. He noted that he himself knew what it was like to be so hot that it was difficult to breathe. If his assessment was erroneous or his conclusions mistaken, then the NICU staff should have explained why he was wrong in order to give him peace of mind.

Parents drew from their experiences with other children or those experiences they anticipated for their firstborn, as a standard for what was normal functioning. The baby's general comfort was a concern. Sleep in a cozy bassinet or crib, placed in a darkened, quiet room was one of these standards. The NICU was a far cry from this vision. Parents discussed the ever-present lights, noises from machines and personnel, and procedures (including the provision of medications and nourishment) that interrupted their baby's rest. Parents also noted the "uncomfortable" position of the baby. Some infants were sprawled in frog-like positions with arms and legs askew rather than curled in a fetal-like position. Parents were concerned about the ability of the infant to rest or sleep well under such circumstances.

Parents also addressed the experience of pain for their infant.[5] As one father responded, "You wonder how much pain they're in. If they're suffering or what." They questioned how many of these procedures and treatments were not simply uncomfortable but in fact caused pain. One common example they cited was the withdrawal of the infant's limb during heel sticks for blood tests. Parents felt they had valid points when they raised their concern about infant comfort. But they surmised that they would have little impact on the plan of care by discussing possible changes with health professions. Parents felt impotent in their attempts to make any modifications in their infant's life at this moment in the NICU.

Despite parents' basic familiarity with these areas of infant care, in the NICU even the most common task of infant care such as a diaper change, was framed within caregiving of such a sophisticated and technical nature that parents were quite intimidated. Parents felt they had little control over any related decisions and, moreover, they could not easily question caregivers or refuse treatment. Parents capitulated to the professional's expertise. Any decisions they might have wanted to make simply slipped through their fingers as they saw caregivers functioning so effectively and efficiently in what was to them, a foreign environment:

> Interviewer: Did you feel you were a part of the decision making?
> Mother: No, not really. Well, yeah, I guess, I suppose I could have said no, but it wouldn't have done the baby any good. I mean, I could see the benefits and why they did it. I suppose I had the choice. But I only thought about what they said about the baby.

Parents recalled that possibilities or alternatives were seldom offered to them. They were simply told what the professionals were required to do, what the baby needed, or what was suggested as the best treatment. A few parents cited kidney failure, jaundice (hyperbilirubinemia[t]), lung problems (bronchopulmonary dysplasia[u]), ventricular bleeds, sepsis, and seizures as especially serious cause for alarm and worry, but not decision-making. Parents noted the use of selected treatments or procedures such as complex eye examinations, various medications (lasix, caffeine, insulin, antibiotics), oxygen and ventilators, placement of intravenous and central lines[v], chest tubes, transfusions, and assorted surgeries. They characterized discussions about these treatments not in relation to decision-making, only in terms of agreement with what was necessary for the baby's recovery. As one parent said, reflecting the position of most parents, " No, [there was no conflict]...the right thing to do was to give him every possible option for success, for life."

One father shared his experience with his daughter. He and his wife were in the nursery on a Sunday and noted how large the baby's "stomach" had become. The parents were able to talk to the doctor and, when they expressed their concern the father recalled this response:

> ...'yeah, we're concerned but sometimes they get that way when they don't have a bowel movement.' Then we get this call the next Friday. She was bleeding. She had been doing real good up until that point.

> They were getting ready to put her in an isolette, which you know is kind of a big step for a premature baby. I just felt like maybe they ignored, ignored her stomach, her internal bleeding. I felt at the time that something could have, should have been done a little sooner than what it was.
>
> Interviewer: What did you do?
>
> Father: I, no, nothing. I just...lived with their decision.

Generally, the informed consent process necessary for many of these procedures was not an instance of conflict nor did it pose a dilemma. Parents could remember little of the content of those informed consent documents. They only knew there were many forms they had to sign: "I've signed so many papers I don't know anymore what I signed." Informed consent was discussed as a perfunctory activity. Step one: the baby needed something; step two: parents had to sign. Sometimes health professionals had to telephone for the informed consent. Telephone requests required witnesses for this verbal informed consent, that is at least one person in addition to the one requesting the consent, who would legally verify the telephone exchange. This was an especially anxiety producing situation because it usually related to emergency requests. Parents had vivid memories of these random calls. Still, parents posed few questions about any of these situations. They believed that a baby who needed something should have it. Besides, parents expected that the treatments and procedures would be implemented even without their permission:

> Most of the time I never thought anything went on in there [the nursery]. They just kind of, you know, they went ahead and did it. They didn't really need our approval to do it.

The informed consent document itself was required, from their position, for the baby's record. Some parents noted that the consent might also be used to protect the hospital in case of legal action.

Few negative responses were articulated about this state of affairs in the predischarge phase. A majority of parents merely expressed gratitude and appreciation for all that health professionals were doing. Most parents verbalized genuine positive impressions. A positive view of the situation could have a significant effect on the parents' convictions that decision-making was not needed. On this positive side, one father shared his experience:

> They really go out of their way to make you feel a part of everything that goes on in there. Almost like a surrogate mother and father for every baby in the unit...like...my own family.

Another parent, a mother, observed a resident physician by her baby's isolette as she came to visit one evening:

> I'd walk up and there'd be a doctor by her crib and he'll be strokin' her foot and tellin' her, "Come on baby, you gotta' hang in there." They're not cold and heartless you know.

Professionals were informative and caregivers kept parents up to date, but parents did not have to make decisions. It was quite clear that professionals were in charge, there were no choices, there were no decisions, and there was little conflict related to newborns because parents were not part of decision-making. Parents were accepting and comfortable with their role. One parent supplied a rationale for this perspective:

> It's obvious that we have not been a part of the decision-making as far as the medical treatment that he gets, simply because we are not the ones trained for it. To a large degree you have to trust the doctors and the nurses that they're gonna do, that they're gonna make the right decisions. But, first of all we trust the Lord, have faith that the Lord is directing those nurses and doctors.

Other examples of specific statements representing thoughts about decision-making for about half of the participants are displayed in Table 2.1.

A singular example where a number of parents felt they actually made a decision relative to a procedure was their choice to have a circumcision for male infants. In fact, one family noted the decisional aspect of the circumcision and contrasted it with the fact that the child *had* to have a respirator.[w] No decision was involved in the respirator's use, since it was necessary for breathing which in turn was necessary for life. Parents believed that these treatments would result in a normal baby.

Families felt disconnected from their newborn and expressed feelings of emptiness and a lack of fulfillment as they confronted the reality of an empty nursery at home. These feelings originated in emergency measures at delivery or the immediate whisking of the baby to the NICU. Parents described a lack of interactions with the infant

Table 2.1 *Summary of comments from parents about decision-making in the NICU*

- ...we left decisions in the hands of the professionals. I accepted that they knew what they were doing, everything was under control. I worried about an infection, but I just took one day at a time.
  - You just don't know what...if it's right or wrong. They can tell you something that is not even close to being right and you'll never know."
- I just wanted him to be OK.
  - They told us everything. The baby is doing OK. We need to wait until she comes home to make decisions.
- Most of the time nothing went on. They went ahead and just did things.
  - I just kind of left it up to them to do whatever was best. Whatever was best for the baby. They've got their rules and they're the professionals. We really feel left out of this whole experience.
- It wasn't so much asking. It was more just doing and then they'd tell you. We didn't know what should be done. We thought the one might have to have surgery and we wondered about that decision, but it never came to that.
  - None [decisions] really. We weren't offered choices and we are confident of what they do and why they do it.
- They [professionals] make the decisions. They got to get your permission to do anything to him before they do it...the surgery on him. But I really haven't made too many decisions because they make them all. I just come and see him every day.
  - We didn't have much of a choice, the doctors told us. We are comfortable with decision-making--the professional's decisions. We didn't really question it. That was just the way it was.
- They more or less do what needs to be done. They have always been right on top of everything. They check 'em and they find the problem right away and try and correct [it].
  - Making decisions was not a problem. I just talked to the doctors. They explain. I asked questions and if I thought it was gonna' help, help him being so little, I was willing to go along. Just as long as they can explain it.

Table 2.1 *Summary of comments* (Continued)

- We have made no decisions since the baby was born. We just did what had to be done. The things they were doing were logical. There was no choice about the respirator. He needed it so they put him on it. [Later, on the same topic] However, they weren't telling us anything, how sick he really was. I felt the child wasn't ours. He belonged to them and they just seemed like they didn't care if they told us anything or not. We finally went down there and demanded--what is going on? Then one of the doctors sat down and talked to us about him. We wanted him home so bad. I guess that is what made us finally demand to know what was going on.
    - Whatever happens, happens. We already thought we lost him once. Everything [since then] has been pretty easy to take. I've had this time with him and it has helped me to accept whatever happens.
- So when you're making a decision, it doesn't really involve the parents all that much. It's among the doctors.
    - They [health professionals] got to follow the rules. And you got to pretty much go along with what they know is best for them [neonates]. They'd say, "It's best that we [fill in the procedure]..." And of course we wanted the best for [boy's name] so we agreed to whatever they suggested was best.
- It sounded like they had made the decision in the morning and just hadn't told us yet.
    - I look at a child [in the nursery] that died, that had multiple anomalies as well as respiratory failure and wondered if I would have wanted them to continue [treatment] for him. And so, I ponder this, I think about it from time to time. That wasn't a decision we had to make. And based on my own personal values, I don't know if I could have called it [treatment] off. They thought that there was a reasonable chance that he could live. What if he were going to be retarded as a result of his treatment? Is that reason to stop? There are some pretty frightening things to think about.

---

itself which they had expected to begin at delivery. Some of this disconnected feeling was attributed to the environment in the nursery. Otherwise, the distancing of parents could be explained as an extension of maladaptation observed during high-risk pregnancies, which of course, some families experienced (Penticuff 1982). When the outcome of the pregnancy is threatened or harmed, ambivalence toward the infant results until the condition is resolved.

Most parents were not familiar with a NICU; they had not seen such a unit before, although a few were able to recall television programs that featured such a setting. Parents emphasized their timidity about coming to the NICU based on their lack of comfort with the unit, the busy atmosphere, and their own feelings of inadequacy related to the infant's care. The amount and complexity of the machinery housed in the NICU made parents wary of their surroundings when they came to visit their child. They were fearful that they would inadvertently disconnect some tubing or damage some device. They felt clumsy and ill at ease. Most were not accustomed to situations where death could occur on an hourly or even a minute-by-minute basis, if not for their child certainly for most others in the nursery. Parents' sensitivity to their visitor status in the NICU may even originate from an other-wise well-meaning comment from professionals such as those encouraging parents to "take a break" or "go get a cup of coffee" (Sudia-Robinson & Freeman 2000). Rather than taking such suggestions at face value, parents can interpret these as the staff's perception that they are in the way or visiting too much.

Sophisticated medical technology and highly invasive procedures represent a scientific paradigm that promotes separation, objectivity, and a valence of individuation (Sandelowski 1988). This is in opposition to concepts of attachment, subjectivity, and interaction with others that parents anticipated for their role with this baby. Although the procedures and devices may be beneficial, they also produce estrangement. They have the potential to fracture the human meaning of these events in people's lives. It is not simply because the parent or practitioner (physician or nurse) is often removed from immediate connection with the patient. But in this case the patients themselves are individuals who are unable to express their awareness of or regret for any dissociation. Parents and family can be threatened by the technology that is a necessary life force for their child but prevents them from enjoying the physical closeness they anticipated with a newborn.

Those families, whose babies had extended stays in the NICU of course, were challenged even more by the difficulty of maintaining a relationship with the infant over a long period of time. One mother lamented that it just "doesn't seem right to leave the baby here [in the NICU]." Normally a baby goes home soon after birth and she was concerned that eventually she would feel like she adopted this child. Actually, in some adoption cases, parents take babies home much earlier than the more seriously ill NICU infants. The average length of stay for these infants was 55 days--almost two months. Parents were concerned about being able to generate feelings of attachment.

In the early 1900s. Dr. Martin A. Couney had an interesting comment about parents of the babies he sent home after they had been treated in his incubators at side shows or fairs (Silverman 1979).[x] Couney felt parents were unappreciative of his care and showed little affinity for their infants. Silverman (1992) found a parallel experience in dramatic neonatal intensive care where "superb technical experts make an all-out effort to support [the] life" of the newborn. He had his own professional experience of parental rejection in 1945 when he was a senior resident. His joyous feelings of success as he managed to keep a 620-gram baby alive for three and one-half months were in tension with the numbness of the overwhelmed parents. Silverman was proud of his miracle and was annoyed that the parents were only thinking of the uncertain future. He was a hero at rounds for setting a hospital record for longevity while the parents focused on disability, social consequences, and financial drain. Those parents resented his enthusiasm.

When parents examined their pregnancy, birth, and NICU experiences, they included perceptions of the care providers. Professionals were part of the NICU environment. Parents viewed the health professionals as experts equipped to make decisions and in an authoritarian position to carry out these decisions. Both positive and negative comments were predictably scattered throughout parents' conversations. Most remarks were affirmative and more frequently addressed the relationship of the parents with the nurses. Trust and faith in professionals were terms customarily used to describe parental perceptions of the relationship. Parents were grateful for the presence of nurses for their infants, the communications that they had with them, and their professionalism. They "explained everything," parents regularly remarked and one mother added, "in English!"

> She [the baby] wasn't a reality yet. I don't remember going through the delivery. I don't remember the time they said I had a baby, so it was all just really strange. Then when they brought down the videotape, it was, it was nice! There she was. Of course at that time she was hooked up to just about everything imaginable. But the nurse explained everything...

Nurses encouraged parents to call and check on the baby's status when they were not able to visit.

Communication, however, can also be misinterpreted. The best of intentions can go awry, as indicated by one mother. Nurses told her to "...not worry. We'll take care of him" when suggesting that she go get something to eat or go home and rest. Instead of being reassured that her son would do all right and she did not have to be there so much, she felt shut out by this comment. It made her think her presence in the nursery was totally superfluous. Yet visiting the infant was an important, useful activity for parents. Scharer and Brooks (1994) noted the struggle over control perceived by some mothers in their relationship with nurses. Mothers were left feeling dissatisfied with NICU care when they could not trust nurses while nurses were unable to acknowledge their competitive feelings relative to mothers while caring for the infant.

By the parents' descriptions, most conversations with the staff occurred by the infant's isolette as parents maintained their vigil over the newborn. Parents mentioned that this situation could be troublesome for them. The "bedside" was not private. Not only were parents physically on display during these visits, but conversations were not confidential. Anyone standing within a few feet could hear the discussion. In fact, parents recited parent-staff consultations involving other families with whom they had no long-term relationship or for whom they had no responsibility. On the occasions when nurses were simply conveying the status of the infant or relating positive events of the previous day, there was little parental concern. But when setbacks, failures to improve, or negative results from tests were shared, then it became a challenge to maintain one's composure.

Parents consistently indicated the need of a private place for discussions about the infant's status or potential treatments. They were not sure they could or should ask for a different setting, yet they acknowledged that they were not able to concentrate or retain information when they were worried about appearances and others' evaluation of their actions and behaviors in the public space around the isolette.

A desire to sit down for at least some conversations was an important element of the parental request for communication. Sitting down to talk had quite a different meaning for parents than standing around the isolette or chatting in the NICU entrance or a hospital hallway. As might well be predicted, sitting down meant that the professional was not going to quickly relate some information and then scurry away. Sitting down provided parents with permission to ask questions or more thoroughly pursue information they did not understand. Sitting down symbolized the parents' importance and their responsibility for the future health and well being of the infant in the NICU. Someone who sat down was perceived as willing to listen to the parents' verbal stumbling as they often struggled to express their perspective. The professional who sat was more likely to help them articulate their fears, anxieties, and doubts and help them to request what they did not yet know how to express.

Parents thought the nurses were mostly caring, honest, and doing a good job. Several parents phrased their relationship with the nurses in terms of the nurses' willingness to "put up with them," as if they did not have a right to visit their infants in the nursery. A few timed their visits with the infant after they comprehended the routine schedule of events, to avoid those periods when physicians were busy making rounds or the unit was bustling with activity. They felt that they were in the way and might contribute to less than adequate care in the course of their infant's treatment. One father, taking this perception to the extreme, believed that

> ...the perfect parent of a premature baby that's in that intensive care nursery is the parent that comes up ten minutes on Sunday and calls once a day. That way you're not in their way. You just come get the baby when he's ready to go home. And...they give you a big slap on the back and say what a great job they've done.

One father mentioned that he thought nurses were not paid enough given the kind of work required for these neonates. Another father noted that the unit was understaffed at times but he also pointed out that the hospital probably never lacked a billing clerk!

Parents indicated that they could discriminate between "regular" NICU nurses and substitutes. Several concluded that a few nurses were not comfortable taking care of these infants compared to normal newborns. They noted that occasionally nurses were transferred from the newborn nursery because of staff shortage or nurses were "just temps" in the NICU. One mother described her distress when the regular nurses were not assigned to her infant. She then decided to simply stay in the NICU herself those days to observe the care and make sure that a regular nurse would respond if her infant had a crisis.

The videotapes of the babies taken by the nursing staff were treasured. Parents who lived at a distance and were unable to visit as often as they liked were especially appreciative. Additionally, the videotapes were for the most part, a record of progress. They documented growth and development, which in turn meant potential wellness and discharge.

Parents differentiated between physician professionals and nurse professionals in certain instances. Some parents criticized their physicians. Comments extended back to the pre-admission period when parents had not been prepared for the NICU experience. They believed the obstetrician should have warned them during the woman's pregnancy about the possibility of early birth or neonate problems. One father wanted to visit the NICU before his child's birth so that he would not be going into the unit for the first time to see his own baby, but he said he was discouraged from this strategy. Parents whose children were in the NICU for a long time observed the regular change of physicians and medical residents. They needed assurance that new house staff would rapidly become familiar with the current status of their child.

A frequent comment was the unavailability of physicians or the lack of direct information about the baby's progress and status from physicians themselves. In fact, several parents were quick to tell us that physicians did not like to talk with them, or avoided them, or did not stay in the nursery long enough to contact for discussion. Parents appreciated information from nurses but perceived that the ultimate authority resided in the physician's camp. Some parents did not realize they had a right to ask for an appointment with the physician or they would have initiated this action earlier. As one father said, "Professional people are to listen to you first before healing can take place." However, if parents do not have an opportunity to sit down and talk with physicians, no listening takes place.

Two couples felt quite strongly about their lack of information. One couple thought their questions were not answered from the beginning (after her amniotic sac ruptured and they went to the hospital). The couple relayed conflicting stories received from the staff about the women's condition during labor, the possibilities for the baby at birth, and his subsequent course of treatment.

They had also observed the same problem with another couple in the nursery. They felt sorry for this other couple because a physician kept telling them their baby was very, very sick. While the physician kept repeating "sick, very sick," the father of this sick baby was getting angry. The first couple looking at this other child and tuning into the tone in the physician's voice believed the infant was in fact going to die. "Why not just tell the parents the child might not pull through?" this father wanted to know. Why was it so necessary to hedge? To have another professional come along and put the truth more bluntly or yet another to say it even more tentatively was confusing to parents. This father indicated that, though bad news is hard to take, parents are adults (or they should learn how to be adults) and they will find a way to deal with the unsuccessful outcome as well as the successful one. Bodgan and associates also noted this communication gap (1992). Whereas professionals may use "very sick" to mean "going to die," for parents this description may simply mean a few extra days of hospitalization.

As might be foreseen, parents differed in their preference for good news versus bad news. For some, any bad news or negative comments were unwelcome, while others wanted regular reality checks. One father remarked that "the staff treat us like idiots--I'm a college graduate!" On the other hand he also disliked the "black picture" the staff always painted. He went on, "It never turned out that way--why did they always have to be so negative?" Thorne and Robinson (1989) identified a similar response in their research of the provider-family relationship. Although trust is the first stage, this is a naive type of relationship. Disliking staff remarks would come under their second stage of disenchantment when families discovered the discrepancies between their perspectives and the health professionals' perspectives. The last stage is one of guarded alliance wherein families attempted to balance passivity and assertiveness.

The father quoted above was not alone on this issue. Some parents did express their desire *not* to hear any bad news and in fact perceived objective negative descriptions of the infant's status as information they did not want. A number of parents did not seem to believe the infant's status was as seriously imperiled as described to them but they failed to verbalize their outright disagreement with the physician's judgment.

One father remarked that the nurses were always telling them their child was going to die and yet he had no doubt that he would live. He respected the professionalism of the staff but believed they were continually stressing the negative. He told of a very strong sign he had received that gave him the strength to believe his son would make it:

The Red dog. Ken is the father of David, one of the smallest babies represented in the project. There were dire predictions for David as he began his life at only 680 grams. Ken was one father who did not like to receive any bad news about his baby. He did not want to be prepared for any negative events. In this he was rather unique among parents in the study--he did not want an objective prediction for the future of his child. Ken felt strongly that thinking positive thoughts and believing everything would be OK was a philosophy that would help his baby through any obstacle and effect a positive outcome.

One of the signs Ken received that convinced him he was correct relates to a dream he had. One night Ken dreamed that he was in his backyard on a hot, summer day. As he came out the door and walked down the steps, he saw a three- or four-year-old boy playing in the yard, laughing and throwing sticks for a red dog to retrieve. The playful, happy scene made him feel good even when he woke up the next morning and went off to work. Several days later he was sitting at his desk at work when a colleague came up to him and said, "Say, I heard that you just had a son and I was wondering if you might like to get a dog for that boy?" Ken thought for a minute. He and his wife did not have a dog and he had not thought about a dog for their boy, but it was worth considering. The colleague quickly added, "Our dog recently had puppies and we have one left. Why don't I have my wife bring the puppy over here after work and you can take a look?" Ken agreed. After work, the two men went outside to the waiting car. Ken looked inside the blanket-lined box on the back seat. There was the red dog! He was only a puppy now but, in a couple of years, he could be the dog in his dream, playing with his *normal* son right in his own backyard!

A few parents indicated their disappointment in specialists. One family had a particularly trying situation with the urologist called in for a consultation. Another family wanted to have a neurology consult and felt that they were inappropriately talked out of this action.

A common sentiment expressed about the nursery and the staff related to evaluations of the parents themselves by the staff. Parents definitely felt that they had to present themselves as mature, responsible, and capable adults. Parents should be people with confidence, and confident people did not have to ask questions nor did they express anger and fear. Such perceptions led to a number of different behaviors enacted by parents because their own reputation and subsequent status were on the line. Many parents felt, for example, that they had to contain their emotions while visiting the infant. Crying was not an acceptable response nor was an inability to receive whatever news staff had to impart. The possibility of being evaluated also affected parental visiting. One mother explains:

> I spent as much time in the car as at home during the first two months of [the baby]'s life. I felt as if I had to be there daily or they'd think his Mommy didn't care. What *good* mother would leave her new baby in such a frightening place?

The sensitivity of parents to their potential evaluation by the staff and the importance of the staff's opinion of them are related in the following story. It shows how vulnerable parents felt in that they realized the staff had to provide the care for their infant. The baby was in their hands and parents did not want their own behavior to be the grounds for any compromise in the infant's care. Parents did not want to upset the health professionals or the system in which they worked. Although this story describes a predischarge incident, it was not mentioned until the six-month postdischarge interview. This timing raises the question of researchers as sources of intimidation for parents although neither one of us worked in the NICU. How much are participants in a study willing to share when a family member continues to require health care services?

> *The case of the disappearing formula.* One mother, Alma, tells the story of her interaction with another mom, Pam, in the NICU. Alma's baby was progressing and in order to prepare for discharge, Alma was coming in to feed the baby several times a day. Pam's baby had been in the NICU for some time and she was more comfortable than most mothers were in this environment. Pam had apparently been observing Alma one evening as she tried to get her baby to take a bottle. Alma said that she was having a difficult time as the baby kept falling asleep and did not seem to be hungry or interested in sucking on the nipple. She was getting very frustrated and worried about what the nurses would think of her if she couldn't get this baby to take the bottle. She feared discharge would be delayed, which was the last circumstance she wanted to face. As she stroked the baby's lips with the nipple, the bottle was suddenly whisked out of her hand. Alma looked up, startled, to see Pam take the bottle over to the sink, remove the nipple, pour the formula down the drain, replace the nipple, and thrust the empty bottle back into Alma's hand while moving quickly back to her own baby's isolette. Before Alma could speak or even think of any response, a nurse passed by and noted the empty bottle. The nurse was full of praise for Alma at her successful feeding. Alma saw Pam wink at her.

> The nurse immediately removed the sleeping baby from Alma's arms and put it back in the isolette. Alma felt in a quandary. Should she tell the nurse the baby did not take *any* formula? If she told the nurse what really happened, what might happen to Pam? If Alma didn't tell the nurse, could any harm come to her baby who was not fed? Would the missed feeding prevent a timely discharge for the baby? Alma felt like a coward and knew she was not a good liar, so she quietly left the nursery and went home.
>
> That night Alma did not sleep well, fighting nightmares that showed her baby shrinking to skin and bones and nurses yelling at her for being a terrible mother. Alma hurried back to the hospital early the next morning only to be greeted excitedly by the charge nurse. "I don't know what you did last night when you fed the baby but she had the best night ever, she really drank her next feeding hungrily, and she's gained a little more weight. She's even closer to a stable discharge status!" Alma nearly collapsed from relief. As she sat in the rocking chair holding and feeding her baby again, she began to laugh to herself. What a joke! One of her worst nights since the baby's hospitalization had been transformed into a turning point toward an imminent discharge.

One parent described what he called "the rules of behavior for parents." After he had ascertained them, he was tempted to write them up and post them outside the NICU door so that other parents would not have to waste their time figuring them out. To document this parental belief that their visits were evaluated based on some vague set of rules, one parent affirmed that he found notes on the infant's chart hanging by the isolette that infuriated him. He read a whole page of notes about his wife and her behavior and only two lines about the infant. He wanted to know just who was the patient and who was the most important object of professional care?

Parents who lived out of town felt particularly vulnerable to judgments about infant visiting. Others held full-time jobs and were exhausted at the end of the workday; they felt unable to add a hospital visit to their already overwhelming schedule. Women with limited maternity leave went back to work immediately after delivery in order to save their time off to coincide with the infant's discharge. Of course, some families had commitments to other children and activities for which they had obligations. It was not that the hospitalized infant was not important. Mostly a realistic limitation of time and energy led to decisions not to visit. Sometimes visits were replaced by telephone calls, and parents were grateful that nurses encouraged these calls and in fact spontaneously called parents as well. Except for the emergency calls for informed consent, the telephone was a welcome connection to the infant through the nurse. Such communication was an important element of support. Telephone calls also allowed the parent to change the setting as well as enjoy the privacy afforded by the lack of visual interaction. Neither person had to maintain a facade for the other person's benefit.[y]

This group of parents seldom mentioned other forms of support at this point in the project. One family did make note of how their community responded to their circumstances and "people we hardly know have come out to help us. Just...been amazed." A couple of families referred to the importance of communicating and visiting with other parents of babies currently in the NICU. Several mothers were disappointed not to be able to locate a more formal parent support group. One woman discussed talking with a mother from a group called "Parent-to-Parent." She called other nurseries in the region and beyond until she finally found a group in Texas from which she was able to find strength. Religious beliefs, faith, or spirituality were not absent, but rather the target of less frequent remarks at this time by these parents.

A few parents emphasized the importance of their own spouse for them during this crisis. One woman noticed that other couples came to visit their infant together and she lamented that her husband was unable to come with her. She missed his support on these occasions. Her husband had already lost two children in a previous marriage and did not want to deal with the possible loss of this child. She said:

> I miss the support some other parents have when they are here with their wife or husband. That bothered me at first. I'm trying to do it on my own...it'd be nice to have somebody to lean on.

Perception of Decision-making

Although these events were all described as examples of experiences that stood out because parents "weren't sure what was the right thing to do," few felt they had to actually make decisions. They were in conflict or had doubts, but for most issues others made the decision. This was especially true for the situations involving neonatal medical care. One exception prior to the NICU admission included several teenage mothers and a decision they considered throughout the pregnancy as to whether or not they should keep the baby. They actually had to resolve this issue themselves. Permission to use surfactant upon the baby's birth was perceived as a definite request for permission to treat that parents technically could refuse. Ten families were involved with this issue. However, in the parents' initial discussion of a possible conflict, they most often named, or first named events that occurred prior to the NICU experience.[z] One woman's adamant response to her absence in decision-making represents the status quo among these parents:

> We are not in charge. We are not in control of *our* baby. A lot of the times, I don't agree with the way they are doing something, but I have no choice. They are in charge of my son and I am *just* the mother.

Frader discussed the control aspect of neonatal care as chairperson of the American Academy of Pediatrics Committee on Bioethics (G. Clark 1996). He characterizes pediatricians as more likely to form a partnership in decision-making with parents than neonatologists. This difference is quite likely in that pediatricians cannot force decisions as easily on parents who have a history with the child and who can more readily take a child home after an office visit or switch physicians during a hospitalization. Parents of neonates are more or less a captive audience for the neonatologist.

Although we had anticipated that parents would recite lists of treatment dilemmas and other conflicts they encountered in their experience while the infant was hospitalized, this did not generally transpire. We sought assurance for the lack of moral conflict through several probes before the conversational thread was shifted. Although parental perception of conflict or doubt might have existed previous to the birth of the child, conflict related to traditional bioethical decisions for the infant in the NICU rarely existed for these parents (see Note "q"). Part of the parental perception may stem from viewing a calmly functioning staff who went about their work in a skillful, routine manner. How could there be serious ethical concerns or moral imperatives in an atmosphere without panic, with so few apparent emergencies?

Only two examples emerged in this predischarge discussion that did reflect traditional bioethical discourse. One family noted a "bleed" in one of their twins and discussed its effect on the quality of life for both children.[aa] The father prefaced his remarks with this conviction:

> [We will] do everything we can to save these children. Because they are the only children that we'll probably have. We went through a lot to have these babies.

The female twin went from a Grade III to a Grade IV bleed. The parents were informed that there was a chance that the baby would be severely handicapped and possibly develop cerebral palsy. The mother expressed her concern about the baby's future quality of life. There was apprehension on the part of both parents, shown by their question not just about this child but both children: "How were they going to come out?"

In light of this concern, the mother said that they requested a consultation with another physician, a specialist. "I mean, how long do you go on making a baby live?" she asked. They had sought counsel from a friend, a nurse, who indicated that if her baby was in a similar situation, she would want a consult. "[It] seems like they can keep 'em alive...for as long as they want [deep sigh]. Where do you draw the line?" the father implored. Ultimately they felt they were talked out of the request for a consultation and led to accept the recommendations for aggressive therapy. They were told that a consultation would simply be an added expense they did not need to incur since the physician in charge was very experienced and another opinion was not necessary. This, they said, was the hardest time of the baby's hospitalization thus far for them.

Not all parents were enamored of technology and the interventions available for pregnancy and birth. A few questioned just how many treatments should be administered, "Modern technologies get a little carried away with bringing babies into the world...you just gotta draw that moral decision somewhere." The second example, then, revolves around the status of the baby at birth. This was the only couple who recounted an ordeal about whether or not extraordinary means should be used. The situation originated at the time of delivery. These parents emphasized their request to refrain from extraordinary measures if the baby was only marginal at birth. Labor began quite early (25½ weeks gestation by ultrasound) and the couple understood that the fetus was extremely small and marginally viable. They were led to expect that the fetus might be born dead or die shortly thereafter. "I didn't want a baby that wasn't really strong. We didn't want them to take extraordinary measures," the mother said. The father agreed using almost those exact words.

> They told us that it would be our choice as to how much we tried to...how much life saving measures were taken on our baby. We called a nurse friend in the middle of the night when I was in labor. She is a very strong Catholic, so she is against abortion. Very--so prolife. She thought we made the right choice.
>
> The father continued: [W]e asked the doctor about legal ramifications if the baby should live and what measures could be taken. He said, "The law doesn't enter into this." He did say that if the baby ended up in good condition, specifically if he weighed more than they predicted, then they would ventilate him. Of course, then when we saw him, we were really excited and there was no question [about saving his life].

In discussing this further, the ventilator was the only special measure used in NICU medical care that fit this man's definition of extraordinary means. It was acceptable although he was unable to discuss its long-term effects or the implications of ventilator use for future decision-making.

This couple was unique in this particular group of parents. They discussed decision-making relative to their other children as an example of their problem-solving processes. They indicated that when they were dissatisfied with answers, they sought more information. They operated from the premise that "doctors weren't God." They believed they had a responsibility to educate themselves and ask people's advice, and not to do something because a physician said so. Few other parents demonstrated such assertiveness and comfort in stating their beliefs and desires, and then acting upon them with the professionals.

One other couple vacillated about their role in decision-making related to discontinuing the use of the ventilator. They initially stated that they were not involved in decision-making, then after some reflection decided that they may have been included in the decision related to the ventilator. Mixed with their descriptions of the information about the ventilator were comments about "living with decisions the health professionals made." "We raised few concerns," one parent remarked, recalling that they mostly just listened. They emphasized the professionals' focus on the baby's suffering while she remained on the ventilator, including counsel from their own priest. The parents clearly understood that she could not live if the ventilator was turned off. So in effect, their final decision was simply agreement with what was most strongly recommended. When we examined the decision-making process with the parents in depth, whether or not the decision was really a choice among viable options was questionable.

Finally, one family discussed a moral dilemma in the nursery but not one for which they had decision-making responsibility. There were no struggles between right and wrong decisions for their own child but they knew of a woman whose newborn was going to need a liver transplant. The parents tried to comprehend how someone could make that decision. They had asked the woman how she decided and she told them that she knew of another baby who was not offered a transplant. She believed all possible treatments should be extended to children. The father went on:

> I've often wondered about that myself...just how do these people decide. What if one of our girls needed a liver transplant or something like that. Something really serious like that. We wouldn't know what to decide. We could say one thing now, but if it came down to the final decision it could be totally different than what we think right now. What is right and what is wrong? It's a personal decision. I don't think there is a right or wrong answer. Should you just let things take their course? [The baby] might not survive. But is it right to put the child through months of misery and not have them survive? Right now we can only accept things for our baby as they come.

One father presented an interesting perspective on morality which did relate to the couple's situation and the birth of high-risk infants. During the interview this man selected the implantation of multiple fertilized eggs and the possible option of abortion to reduce the pregnancy as a moral dilemma for some individuals (but not one he and his wife encountered). He posited a very prolife position and was concerned about the over-zealous actions of some physicians in implanting several embryos. The multiple gestation increased the risk of an early delivery for the woman resulting in premature fetuses. This man's wife had been on Clomid[bb] for the treatment of her infertility. He lacked sufficient knowledge about the pharmacological action of Clomid in increasing the maturing and release of multiple ova, which had the same potential for multiple gestation and risk that he abhorred in IVF (*in vitro* fertilization[cc]). He obviously did not recognize the similarity between IVF and the use of fertility medications, or that his own situation involved the same moral dilemma.

The complete discussion and examples of parental perceptions of moral or ethical decisions will be presented later in the section on moral orientation. Most of their responses were not directly related to their predischarge circumstances or neonatal care.

More parents did discuss areas for possible decision-making prior to the baby's admission to the NICU rather than NICU care as already described. Parents were more confident that they possessed some authority in pre-birth decision-making situations, especially prior to hospitalization of the woman, but not always. However, outside of the hospital, parents could seek alternative physicians and consultations, which they sometimes did. Medical advice such as the decision to place a cerclage, could be followed, ignored, or altered. Parents had some flexibility in determining the exact time of admission to the acute care setting for pre-birth care and monitoring. Most of the decisions for these babies would be made after the parents took them home, the respondents concluded. Then they would really become parents and could take on the roles they had originally expected to fulfill.

From interviews with parents in later phases, they acknowledged at least two additional bioethical dilemmas and decisions they made. One was a combination about a No Code and removing a child from the ventilator. The other decision was about who to save if the choice was between mother and child during the birth. However, for whatever reason, those particular situations were not included by the parents at the predischarge interview. The ventilator decision could have occurred before discharge but after the interview for this phase.

One brief mention of the allocation of scarce resources needs to be included here. Justice related to the financial requirements of health care is an important issue in bioethics. Myriad discussions and numerous essays address monetary problems. The NICU is no exception to this concern. Only two parents expressed their concern about the cost of this hospitalization at predischarge. One, already noted above, criticized staffing shortages and their financial implications. The other parent more directly targeted his concern for his own hospital bills:

> They [physicians] were concerned again about something and they had another doctor look so that was *three* exams. Now they want to do yet another exam. But you know, the baby is OK. One doctor says he is going to go blind and another observes that it will heal over by itself. It's just something they watch. How are we to know? But it is just sometimes you feel that they're running up the bill 'cause I've got good insurance. And this [hospital] is a business! And it's a profitable business, hospitals are, you know. I'm sure every q-tip and cotton ball is costing me a fortune.

Medicalization of Parenting

Overall, prior to the discharge of the infant from the NICU, parents described their role as passive, waiting, expectant. Hence the label for this phase, the medicalization of parenting, meaning that parental responsibilities were appropriated by health professionals who provided medical care. Whether duties were physical or psychological, and because the infant's life depended on skilled, sophisticated interventions encompassing complex technology, most parents willingly abdicated their expected roles. From the parents' perspective, health care professionals, including physicians, nurses, social workers, and others, were in complete charge of the newborn and responsible for both its care and associated decision-making. These staff people were there 24 hours a day, while parents could be present only a few hours a day. One mother said:

> No, they make [the decisions] mostly. The only time they call me about him is if, like they gave him his surgery on his hernia...and I had to sign the papers for them to do it. I really haven't made too many decisions because...they make them all. I just come and see him every day.

This decision-making encompassed all aspects of care for the infant, some of it medical or nursing care but some of it not. Although parents generally felt they made few decisions, most parents were quite comfortable with these arrangements--at least as they described their situations in the interviews prior to the discharge of the infant from the NICU, "I thought it was just great. Whatever can be done. We want it done...anything that the doctors felt would be good to do, we were just more than willing."

Other scholars have also labeled similar parental experiences as medicalization.[dd] Steinfels (1978) used this term in a theoretical sense for the imposition of the medical model on pregnancy and childbirth milestones, which changed them from family events to medical events with health professionals in control. Mitchell (1986) observed this phenomenon in her neonatal clinical practice as nurses monitored the hospital centered crisis instead of a mother supervising a normal family's developmental task. Arras and associates (1987) cited the physician *wait for certainty* philosophy as a rationale for usurping decision-making. Certainty can only be determined by expert personnel making every decision a medical one rather than an ethical one.

Jennings (1988) in his examination of the connection between ethics and the description of NICUs in ten selected ethnographic studies, claims that "NICUs seem, as cultural systems, to avoid using an explicitly ethical vocabulary when decisions are made; the 'medicalization' of ethical questions is widespread." La Puma (1999) makes an even more harsh interpretation as he observed *both* physicians and ethicists engaging in *double talk* using a language only those in the discipline would understand. Earlier Figlio (1977) differentiated technological medicine of the 20th century from earlier practices. Both social and ethical problems in medicine were transformed into a *biomedical format* for which the physician provided the answer.

Why might parents be generally complacent with this surrogate arrangement? According to the parents' own testimony, at least three factors, as described above, could contribute to this passive stance:

- the parents' compromised emotional and/or physical state,
- the parents' estrangement from the newborn who required care they could not provide, and
- the environment in which the infant was hospitalized, including the authority and control exercised by health care professionals.

Our additional observations affirmed the parents' naiveté, first, when we reviewed the infants' charts and second, during the secondary analysis of the interview data. We finally comprehended the error of the parents' simple understanding of their circumstances when we examined the babies' medical records subsequent to the completion of all interviews. Although we had just finished talking with parents for hours, we were not prepared for the sheer volume of documentation resulting from the hospitalization of any one child yet alone the quantity of paper generated by the records for 42 infants. It was a perfect moment of revelation. The interviews with the parents had given us little understanding of the generally serious nature of most infants' conditions, therefore we had not anticipated the meaning of days and even weeks of hospitalization and the accompanying mountain of records it created. Intellectually we understood the possibility of a stray infant or two inappropriately admitted to the NICU for critical care when its needs may have been marginal. But we realized this outcome was not possible for 42 infants. However, parental discussion did not support the professional assessment of the infants' circumstances as documented in the charts. Our goal to clearly identify and accurately describe an uncontaminated parental perspective was impeccably met given the difference between the infants' data in the charts and the parents' descriptions.

We had set project admission criteria based on the infant's status and we trusted the intermediary personnel to follow the protocol. Yet, as already discussed, most parents could not fully articulate their child's major problems and/or the rationale for admission to the NICU. The parents had little understanding of the seriousness of a NICU hospitalization, or treatments and procedures in particular.

One interview in particular illustrated this phenomenon. During the interview, the baby was in the conference room with the mother and me. Initially the television was at an extremely high volume but the baby was asleep in an isolette right next to the set. It was impossible to hear anyone speak so the television was turned off. I was concerned that as the session proceeded, the baby might wake as a result of the conversation and other noises, including the grandmother coming in and out of the room and other distractions heard from the hallway. Yet he was totally undisturbed by any sound at any time. Later when we read his chart, his discharge summary revealed the fact that he had been extremely premature and was at risk for developmental learning problems secondary to major visual, auditory, and motor perception deficits. Now his lack of response made sense. There was some doubt that he could even hear all of the clamor that surrounded him. In addition to his lack of response was the other fact that the mother, when describing his status, did not mention any of these conditions. She had merely said that he was admitted to the NICU because he had to gain weight (his birth weight was 1278 grams).

There was an element of cognitive dissonance for us as researchers during the interviews of the parents prior to reading the medical records of the infants. On the one hand was the staff's assurances that parents invited to participate in the project had neonates who met the high-risk criteria for admission. On the other hand, we found it difficult to believe there was no voice given to ethical problems as parents described their infants and their experiences in the NICU. Other than a gentle, periodic reminder to our NICU liaison about meeting the infant admission criteria for the project, we were too busy to press the issue and seek any more detailed information from the staff about the infants' courses of treatment. Procedurally we wanted to know the infants' status solely from the parents' perspective, so we did not schedule a chart review until the post-interview stage, after the analysis of the data had been completed.

As we finally realized, this particular group did *not* represent a cohort of infants who were marginally ill. Their high-risk status was verified by the chart review (see Table A.4 for a summary of infant status at birth). Most infants had some degree of prematurity and presented the expected comorbidity issues. Others were initially admitted to the NICU for birth trauma or precipitous changes in status shortly after birth; some required transport from community hospitals when this crisis occurred. There were no cases of extreme congenital anomalies although several infants had hydrocephalus; others had orthopedic problems, and one baby had hydronephrosis. Eleven newborns had hyaline membrane disease and ten infants had intraventricular hemorrhage. Most infants had a central intravenous line at one point in their hospitalization and about one-fourth were on a ventilator for various lengths of time.

Many of the comorbidities, treatments, and procedures were common occurrences in a NICU but not within the domain of the parents' usual experiences with children. Many problems were actually iatrogenic effects from treatments which parents did not discuss.[ee] Some infants were scheduled for extensive interventions after discharge and will require considerable medical care for years in the future. Blindness, deafness, compromised physical functioning, and/or various degrees of mental retardation among the infants in this group were present. However, parents could not envision or discuss these potential outcomes.

Another way to categorize the seriousness of the status of this group of infants can be based on Merenstein and Gardner's criteria (1985), which were used to screen potential families for admission to this project. Basically there are six criteria: birth weight, Apgar score, gestational age, bilirubin level, presence of birth anomalies, and need for surgical intervention. Ten percent of the infants in this group met one criterion to gain admission, 41% of the infants met two criteria, and 37% met three criteria. The remaining 12% met four or more criteria. It appears then that this group of infants represented a broad range of conditions:

- a few with only minimal problems
- the majority with serious but not necessarily life- threatening circumstances resulting in a recovery which might evolve in either direction and
- some with sequelae that were likely to lead to significant compromises in future years.

The long-term outcomes were as yet undetermined for many of these children and their status at four years postdischarge will be discussed later (see Table 4.1).

Given the infants' health status and the many complex procedures implemented during their care, the potential for ethical issues existed. However, these parents did not identify such issues nor were they involved in ethical decision making for the most part. One example provides a dynamic contrast between the parent's discussion of a decision and the status of the infant. The most outstanding decision for this couple was whether or not to breast-feed. Yet these are the parents of a child with profound problems that will be challenging issues for him the rest of his life. One consult with a specialist alone is several pages long, spelling out many difficulties and future prospects related to the status of only one body system. The dissonance between the parents' description and the chart data was overwhelming.

The parents' inability to articulate more than a superficial understanding of the rationale for admission to the NICU and for continuing care at this level does not imply that parents were not informed. When discussing these issues with us, a little over half of the parents indicated that "they always explained things" or "they kept us informed." Parents were both informed and desirous of *more* information. Some blamed themselves for this lack of knowledge, "I was real confused about some of the things they were talking about. I guess it's my own fault. I should ask more questions, but..." Additionally, parents wanted to better understand and retain what they were told:

> Well, you know, it's kind of tough to say. Because, being so small, you really, you really just don't know what. You don't know if it's right or wrong. They can tell you something that is not even close to being right and you'd never know. There's so many different things that they can do for an infant.

A minority of families perceived an inconsistency in information provided to them. For example, one parent indicated that what you learned depended upon the resident who was on duty. Later, when the resident changed, so did the information. Another parent responded that, even within a few days, different nurses gave them different answers to the same question. This situation was true for other personnel as well: one physician versus nurse, a resident versus the neonatologist, the social worker versus the nurse. Parents were unable to connect the disparate responses to any significant change in their infants' status or treatment so information was puzzling rather than helpful. Deborah Alecson (1995), the author of *Lost Lullaby*, also noted differing information as a source of great confusion for parents. She claimed that based on her and her husband's experience with NICU, objective treatment is not what occurs. Rather treatment depends upon the neonatologist on duty (G. Clark 1996).

During the post-interview chart review and analysis, we located extensive documentation in the medical and nursing notes regarding discussions and teaching sessions. However, in the course of their interview, parents appeared not to remember sufficient information from those meetings, denied the existence of knowledge that had been shared with them, or chose not to discuss what they were told. It must be noted that being informed, retaining information, comprehending it, and explaining it to someone else require different cognitive skills, all of which may not have been used.

In ethical decision-making, information and understanding are prerequisites for completing the informed consent process. We had anticipated that parents would possess a wealth of information about the infant since the child was the central feature in decision-making. However, this was generally not true. Some parents did recognize the precise gravity of the situation. Since parental understanding of the infant's status is such a pivotal element in discussing ethical decision-making in neonatal care, these parents' lack of understanding may have led to their failure to recognize a need for serious decisions.

The second observation documenting parental passivity requires an important but more complex explanation and will be reserved for later. It requires jumping ahead several years past completion of the three phases of the project and so, at that appropriate point, the observation will be described. This particular insight into the parents' situation was not possible until the later two interviews were completed. However, it is important to note here that there is additional documentation for the medicalization of parenting within this project.

When we look for evidence of participation in ethical decision-making and fail to find it, it is disappointing. These people are, after all, the parents of children for whom they will be responsible on a long-term, ongoing basis. Considering the growing emphasis on bioethics and health care, the lack of parental in ethical decision making absence seems somehow unethical. Many explanations might be offered for the parents' responses: lack of recall due to stress and other personal characteristics or failure to understand the processes in which they were actually involved, among others. Parents could have been in denial or perhaps they did not want to discuss certain aspects of their infant's care with us. Evidence from the infants' charts documented educational sessions with parents and a different perspective of the situation from the professionals' positions. However, that does not change parental perceptions. Contrary to discussions in the literature, most of these individuals left the NICU experience believing not just that they did not make significant decisions, but that there were no bioethical decisions to make.

Initial Suggestions for Other Parents

The interview concluded with a request for parents to add anything that they wanted to relay about their experience, which had not been addressed during the discussion, or to provide us with any advice for other parents undergoing this same experience. Parents said to get support as the NICU events were encountered:

> I been worrying a lot...a stillbirth, a miscarriage, now this. It's hard. I think you need to have lots of support. If you got somebody, that helps. Somebody to talk to, not if they understand but just willing to listen and try to understand. I talk to my parents, my mother mostly. Me and the baby's father doesn't stay together but we do talk. So that's a big help; he understands me. But he has his own worries. He is one of those types of people where actually going to see him [the baby] all hooked up to tubes and everything...[sound trails off] He can't really deal with that.

Parents need to be prepared for the possible lack of family support and understanding, some families advised. One father noted that most people who asked how he and his family were doing really did not want to know, or did not care about his response. Most parents did not expect neighbors and other more distant friends to necessarily become a support system but they did expect families to jump right in. These parents warned others that disappointment could ensue when support did not materialize. Parents were genuinely pleased to have participated in the interview because it was important for someone to pay attention to them and what they said.

Some parents suggested that making friends with the parents of other infants in the nursery would help especially when formal support groups were not available. The opportunity depended upon how often and how long parents themselves visited. Seeing the same individuals coming in and out, standing in the hall outside the NICU, or taking a break in the cafeteria could eventually lead the way to contact and mutual support. Similar crises draw certain parents toward one other.

One mother stressed interacting with other parents as soon as opportunities arose and gave a specific example. She overheard another couple discussing the possibility of putting a shunt into their newborn. She was able to tell these parents, recognizing situations vary of course, that she herself had a shunt for almost two decades and was doing fine.

The professional staff could be a vital support, parents noted. Most parents crave information about the infant but do not always know what or how to ask them. Parents simply have to overcome this reticence. One parent admonished...

> Parents have to ask lots and lots of questions. They have to learn the terminology. It is scary but you will get used to it. Once you are educated then you can pretty well determine for yourself how things are going. It is a struggle at first. They [health care professionals] aren't used to people being educated or asking questions. You [parents] need to stand up for yourself. They don't expect it but they will respond if you let them know.

One mother suggested another strategy for other parents...

> If you want a feel for how your baby's really doing, go in the NICU and sit next to his nurse and talk to her and observe *her* anxiety! They realize where your baby's at. We appreciate what they, the physicians say. They give it to you on the line, because I don't want anyone glossing over things and suddenly finding your baby is *really* sick. But talk to the nurses to get to know your baby.

Technology and the progress medicine has made will amaze you, parents cautioned. Initially NICU or special nursery will have no meaning. How the staff and equipment overwhelm the tiny infants in their isolettes will be a surprise or even a shock. Numerous parents said that more people should know that these nurseries exist and the kind of care that can be provided for infants like theirs.[ff] Generally, however, the full meaning of this experience, the future impact of this special infant upon each of these individuals and their families had yet to be realized.

Discharge: The Next Milestone

General contentment seemed to characterize the parents' predischarge perspective, but none of these parents had yet experienced total care for the infant. Parents of newly discharged, recovered high-risk neonates as well as those who require chronic care even when long-term needs are predicted, often cannot imagine how much a tiny baby can impact family life. Many mothers observed that these babies who had been hospitalized seemed different from their other children especially when they had significant experience with children from routine deliveries and discharge.

Therefore, what exactly did parents say they were expecting for the future? At the conclusion of the predischarge interview, a little over half of the babies would be coming home soon--"things have worked out," as one parent said. "Soon" varied among the parents' definitions from the very day of the interview to as much as six weeks later. As one mother remarked, "It's a bit scary but they [health professionals] are real positive about them." Some acknowledged that this time frame was a "guess-timate." They admitted that weight gain was not always steady or predictable but they had a target discharge date in mind.

The remainder of the parents related a more complicated time frame. A few infants were scheduled for surgery (eye procedures and reconstructive surgery on a ureter) or remained on a ventilator and still required weaning. These parents believed their child needed to gain weight but reaching this goal required an unspecified amount of time before the child could be discharged. Uncertainty best describes their situation, through for a few parents it was unclear why their future was uncertain. Waiting was the name of the game for them and the term often selected to describe their perception of the neonate's immediate prospects. In these cases, the description reflected the uncertainty of the staff as communicated to the parents and remembered by them. For example, one parent described waiting for cultures. Lung problems had developed and the infant had to be put back on the ventilator. The staff was investigating the possible cause of these problems and cultures were thought to provide the necessary clue about the setback. Another parent noted an increased heart rate and the fact that the infant's organs were not working right, in addition to its weight problems. Regardless of these variations, all of the children except those who died, were eventually discharged and parents were next interviewed six months after discharge.

What are parents' experiences after discharge? What differences, if any, do child-care and the integration of this baby into the family make as the parents look back at their NICU experience in light of their present circumstances?

Notes

[a] See Table P.2 for previous publications relating to these phases.
[b] Clomiphene citrate (Trade name Clomid) is one of several possible pharamacological agents available for the treatment of infertility in females after male fertility has been established. Mentropins (pergonal) is another choice. These drugs stimulate ovulation and therefore increase the possibility of becoming pregnant. Overstimulation of the ovaries is a risk and fertilization of multiple ova is possible (20%). Pregnancy with multiples is in and of itself is a high-risk process. The greater the number of fetuses, the greater the risk (Lobel & Spratto 1983).
[c] This conflict would not have been likely to be detected with most couples in this phase of the project. As opposed to the usual procedure for this set of interviews, the parents in this case were interviewed separately due to scheduling complications.
[d] An intrauterine device (IDU) is a contraceptive apparatus that is inserted into the uterus (Pillitteri 1985). One or two strings attached to the devise extend into the upper vagina and can be felt, thereby allowing the woman to regularly check if the device is still in place. It is generally believed that it prevents pregnancy by causing a local inflammatory process in the uterus that interferes with the implantation of the fertilized egg.
[e] Surfactant is a naturally occurring substance secreted by the alveolar membrane (lining) into the fluids that coat the sacs (alveoli) of the lungs. These alveoli are the final destination for the air (with oxygen) we breathe. Surfactant is necessary to prevent collapse of the alveoli with a subsequent inability to receive air and allow the blood which surrounds the alveoli to absorb the oxygen. Fetuses delivered earlier in gestation may not as yet have the capacity to produce surfactant or, for other reasons, this production may be decreased even in full-term infants. Surfactant is now produced artificially and can be introduced into a newborn's lungs, preventing this collapse. It must be injected before the newborn takes its first breath.
[f] Technically Braxton Hicks are described as intermittent contractions of the uterus; however, they are usually painless, palpable contractions occurring at irregular intervals (Thomas 1977).
[g] During a cerclage, a stitch of nonabsorbable suture is placed around the cervix to prevent it from dilating. The timing for this procedure is critical as

manipulation of the cervix during the placement of this stitch may induce labor.

[h] Magnesium sulfate and terbutaline sulfate are tocolytics, a classification of of drugs employed to halt uterine contractions of premature labor. They relax or suppress uterine muscle. They are used after 20 weeks gestation and prior to 36 weeks. Another drug that suppresses contractions is retrodine hydrochloride. Bedrest, a more conservative approach, is often employed first but later combined with a pharmacological technique should bedrest alone be ineffective.

[i] An amniocentesis is a procedure wherein a sample of the fluid surrounding the fetus and cells floating in that fluid are removed through a needle inserted into the uterus. The fluid can be tested for chromosomal abnormalities and neural tub defects (anencephaly, encephalocele, spina bifida, myelomeningocele) as well as estimate fetal age, well-being, and pulmonary maturity (Fischbach 1984).

[j] Tocodynamonometry is monitoring for premature uterine contractions. One woman in this study who described her experience wore the monitor around her abdomen for an hour in the morning and an hour in the evening while she remained at home. The device recorded and taped uterine contractions. She then called the center where the tapes were read once a day and excessive activity could be detected. If at any time she felt that she was not doing well, she could record and telephone it in, 24 hours a day.

[k] An ultrasonography of the fetus uses ultrasonic waves, similar to energy waves but of higher frequency, to measure and delineate deep tissue structures. Waves are created and directed toward the object of measurement; in this case the procedure focuses on the uterine cavity and the fetus. As the waves strike various thickness of tissues they are reflected differently. A pattern of reflections is created and an image of this pattern is produced on a screen. Often abbreviated as "ultrasounds."

[l] An intrauterine transfusion is a procedure designed to treat maternal-fetal blood incompatibilities which could result in the destruction of the fetus's red blood cells. Through an amniocentesis technique or fetoscope, 75-150 ml. of washed red blood cells are injected into the fetal abdomen. The transfusion may be instituted only once during pregnancy or repeated every 2 weeks for 5 or 6 times (Pillitteri 1992).

[m] An abruptio placenta is a premature (early) detachment of the placenta (Thomas 1979).

[n] Steroid therapy is initiated during preterm labor to facilitate lung maturity in the infant while still in the uterus. These infants are then targeted for the instillation of surfactant at delivery. These treatments enable the alveoli (air sacs) of the lung to expand when the baby takes its first breath rather than sticking together and thus resulting in asphyxia.

[o] The design of the NICU is changing. In the past features of the NICU were based on concepts from emergency rooms and operating rooms. See "New concepts, science, experiences drive innovative designs? The changing face of the newborn ICU" and "Innovations in newborn intensive care design: A photo tour" both of which are in the Summer 2001 edition of *Advances in Family-centered Care,* 7(1).

[p] During this first phase of the research, the use of surfactant was experimental. Obtaining informed consent from one of the parents was required. The informed consent document was more detailed than consents that were used for other procedures and surgeries, given the experimental nature of the drug use. Surfactant is no longer an experimental drug.

[q] That is, bioethical decision-making as commonly and frequently described in the bioethics literature and addressed in Chapter 1. Very briefly, these bioethical issues might be treatment related: to decide to start or stop a particular intervention such as a ventilator, a feeding tube, or surgery. Whether or not to institute a "Do Not Resuscitate" order is another common ethical issue. An ethical issue might be related to who ultimately makes the decision: parent, physician, or a judge within the court system. An ethical issue can also develop when various parties involved (parents, health care professionals, hospital administrators, social workers, pastoral care personnel) do not agree.

[r] Prematures and other infants in the NICU may have problems with normal feeding. Some cannot suck or swallow. Additionally, there is the potential problem that the gag reflex may not adequately function, creating the danger of aspiration of oral fluids. Sometimes sucking causes excessive fatigue or cyanosis occurs. Feeding through a nasogastric tube, or gavage feeding, as it is sometimes called, is a means of providing nutrition for the infant by a tube inserted through the nostrils, past the pharynx, down the esophagus, and into the stomach slightly beyond the muscle that surrounds the opening to the stomach.

[s] Professionals' beliefs about pain in newborns have varied. One early theory posited the lack of pain reception in newborns, especially prematures, due to the immaturity of the neurological system. Anesthesia therefore, was not used during circumcisions. Other procedures, including more complex surgeries, were also implemented without anesthesia. The toxic effects of medications to alleviate pain were believed to be a greater risk than the effect of pain itself in later philosophies of treatment. More recent research supports the need for anesthesia and some changes have been made in practice. For an excellent overview, see Franck (1992). Also see Butler (1989).

[t] Jaundice or icterus is a yellow appearance of the skin, white of the eye, or deeper tissue. Hyperbilirubinemia is the presence of bilirubin in the blood to an excessive degree, which usually indicates an abnormal destruction of erythrocytes or red blood cells. When this concentration is sufficiently high, it

can be clinically viewed as jaundice (Thomas 1977).

[u] Bronchopulmonary dysplasia (BPD) is a dysfunction of the lungs which is believed to result from prolonged dependence on the ventilator (breathing machine).

[v] A central venous line is essentially a tube of inert material inserted into a major vein and threaded through the superior vena cava (one of the large veins that returns blood to the heart) to the right atrium (cavity or section) of the heart. Fluids and medications can be infused through this tubing as well as nutritional substitutes for normal oral feeding.

[w] The terms respirator and ventilator are used interchangeably for mechanical devices employed in cases of respiratory failure. The machine assists or controls the respiration of the individual. Various machines operate on differing principles so the type of device is specific to the individual case, or the usual need in a particular critical care area. Ventilation is a complex therapy that poses many risks for the patient.

[x] See Chapter 1 for a more detailed explanation of the history of the side shows.

[y] See the Appendix for additional information and discussion of telephone interviewing versus person-to-person dialogue which can be applied to parent-staff communication as well.

[z] Specifically, for most parents the discussion focused on the pregnancy [*n*=22]. Next in importance was the birth experience [*n*=20]. Of equal but of relatively less relevance were the issues of conception [*n*=13] and the status of the baby but not necessarily its treatment [*n*=12]. Obviously some parents included more than one issue.

[aa] This particular "bleed" is a condition medically labeled an intracranial hemorrhage or more specifically, if appropriate, an intraventricular hemorrhage. In the premature infant, capillaries are more fragile than in the full-term infant, which makes it more likely for vessels to break and allow blood to leak from them, or hemorrhage. This can further assault brain tissue and cause various dysfunctions or mental retardation in the child depending upon the area of hemorrhage. Hemorrhages are graded according to the severity, I the least severe and IV the more severe.

[bb] We failed to ask the women how long they had been on Clomid or other fertility enhancing pharmacological agents. When considering financial implications, drug therapy is of less significance than other more invasive techniques if one only considers the treatment costs. However, the high-risk outcomes would be similar.

[cc] *In vitro* fertilization (IVF) is a process whereby a female's ovaries are stimulated with fertility drugs to produce multiple mature eggs. Another drug is given to promote their release at maturity. These eggs are retrieved with a hollow needle inserted through the abdomen with a laparoscope or directly

through the vagina. The eggs are fertilized with sperm in some sort of laboratory container (i.e. test tube, petri dish). This mixture is then provided with nourishment and warmth: incubation. A limited amount of growth ensues before the resulting embryos are then placed in the uterus of the woman who has sought the pregnancy or the embryos can be frozen. Eggs can be her own or donor eggs; sperm can be her partner's or donor sperm. It has been the practice in some cases to place more, rather than fewer embryos in the uterus to offset the possibility that all embryos will not implant themselves and develop. However, the higher the number of resulting viable, implanted embryos, and therefore developing fetuses, the greater the risks in the pregnancy--both to the woman and the fetuses.

[dd] Although Steinfels' article (1978) was published prior to this study, our use of "medicalization" for this first phase was not consciously based on her work. If any work should be cited here I would have to say that Ivan Illich's *Medical nemesis: The expropriation of health* (1975) was the first place I saw the term medicalization. Illich specifically used the "medicalization of life" as a descriptor for his observations of the process wherein physicians and their medical practices have become central to one's entire life in many countries of the world. I was unable to locate previous uses of the term. Myra van Zwietan of the Department of Ethics, Philosophy, and History of Medicine, Catholic University of Nijmegen in the Netherlands, who is investigating the concept of geneticalization and using medicalization as a comparison concept, was also unable to provide any earlier references to medicalization.

[ee] Several dictionaries define "iatrogenic" as physician-induced, describing a patient response that occurs as a result of autosuggestion based on a discussion with the physician, an examination by the physician, or other suggestion made in the course of the medical visit. Illich traces the history of iatrogenic in *Medical nemesis* (1975). Literally this term describes an action that produces physicians, "something that only medical schools or parents of future physicians do. But for 80 years the term has been commonly used for health-damage induced by doctors" (p. 17). More recently "iatrogenic" has been used to refer to those outcomes, usually undesirable, caused by the treatment itself. In most cases, however, physicians order these treatments but the common approach in various texts is to discuss these effects as caused by a procedure or device rather than target the person ordering or implementing them.

[ff] At one time when I was working on this section, "Supertwins: triplets, quads and more" a 2-hour program was broadcast on The Learning Channel (aired January 22, 2000). Although the program was generally an informative one, there were serious limitations given my experience with the families in this study. Such limitations underscore the lack of understanding and parental preparation for the NICU experience. The program's focus was the increasing number of multiple births given the current surge in treatments for infertility

and the prevalent feeling conveyed throughout the program was an overwhelmingly positive one. No data was provided about the number of cycles necessary for pregnancy to ensue or a resulting live birth. The program provided the correct statistics about live births in cases of multiples, but never included representative families in the show. A quad pregnancy spontaneously reduced to three survivors, who were all eventually discharged from the NICU, was one specific example of a multiple fetal pregnancy. The problems of a high-risk pregnancy were noted including both prematurity and other sequelae in the resulting infants but only one couple whose children had cerebral palsy was shown. Even when negative material was presented, the video portion did not show the negative side visually. Finally, no financial information was reported. The volume of supplies and paid assistance necessary for multiple births was noted. However, all families appeared to be in good financial standing--based on their houses, neighborhoods, appearance, and activities. Given the slanted view offered by such a presentation, a lack of knowledge and preparation for a high-risk perinatal experience is understandable.

CHAPTER 3

The Infant at Home

Finally the baby comes home. The joy, the ecstasy, the thrill--the happiness in taking that first step toward normal family life. The chores, the sleepless nights, the erratic schedule--all of those elements contribute to a disrupted family life as parents struggle to adapt to the newborn's needs. But the baby that was brought home was not a normal newborn. Parents vacillate between attempts to make life as normal as possible and grappling with unexpected duties as a result of life with their special baby.

One mother begins a review of her experiences since the discharge of her twins with this discussion:

> It's a lot of work and it's a lot of fun. It's, it's rewarding. But I don't think anything has prepared us for what was involved with them. Like a full-term baby would eat and go back to sleep. But we might mess around for an hour feeding *one* infant, and...you know, they'd...they'd drink a little bit here and drink a little bit there. It would take two hours to feed two babies and pretty soon you're ready to start all over again.
>
> There have been times when we didn't know whether we should be worried about something or not, and maybe took them to the doctor unnecessarily. But, we would rather be safe than sorry later on. So when she [one of the twins] ended up with something on her lungs, we'd go and have her checked out. 'Cause she was the weaker of the two. Instead of waiting, usually it would happen on a Friday, so instead of waiting until Monday, we'd go and have her checked. Her lungs were worse [than the other twin's] and it was always hard to tell whether she was coming down with something or not.
>
> And we do have a tendency to spoil 'em more because they were in the hospital so long, you know. We hold 'em more and rock 'em more and...we don't do it intentionally. But, we just felt they needed a lot of more tender loving care because they were so tiny.

She also adds:

> Talking to mothers of twins is important. They can relate their experiences with each other, you know. People [later identified as other extended family members] that...people just don't understand that having twins is not like having one baby. They just think, you know... We don't go much and they want to know why, why we don't bring the girls to town and stuff. Well, it's just not that simple. Not by yourself anyway. And, when we first brought them home, the doctors advised us to keep 'em in, you know. Keep them home because...from germs, colds and all that kind of stuff. I think that is how we got through the winter the way we did. We kept them away. But people don't understand, understand why we don't take them to church.

Integrating the Newborn into Family Life

The child, or children, was definitely the focus of the parents' current stories at six months postdischarge. And this focus was particularly on the physical changes in the baby. They also described the tension between the joy and happiness of getting the baby out of the hospital and their own fears and hesitation in taking a special baby home. Parents perceived the baby to be special when medications were ordered, follow-up tests and/or clinic visits were scheduled, particular formulas were prescribed, apnea monitors accompanied by CPR training were necessary, and other specific discharge instructions were relayed to parents.

Secondly, the parents emphasized the baby's effect on them. The demands of this baby, whether it was the first or a later child in the family, required modifications in their lifestyles. Only one woman said things were exactly the way they were before this baby came home. Most parents indicated that the infant necessitated changes in both roles and relationships. Parents' sleep was especially affected, and their use of time. Activities they formerly prized had to be set aside, however temporarily, for childcare. The few parents whose baby died (5 deaths, 4 families), described the effect of a baby's death on their lives and relationships. Sometimes these parents wistfully speculated about what might have been their situation had the infant lived.

A whole range of responses was elicited in the stories of the immediate discharge experience although there tended to be more pessimistic comments than optimistic. The miracle of the baby's birth and survival was noted as well as how fortunate these parents felt.

Parents emphasized the six months of development, the joy, the baby's smile. Their thankfulness was very apparent. Many felt exceptional in that they had survived this challenge of the baby's hospitalization in the NICU and were able to bring the infant home. However, even the most positive descriptions often included a cautious element or downside. For example, parents first responded to probes about the infants' status by indicating they were pretty good, healthy, fine, okay, staying well, or in a couple of cases, excellent. But upon further discussion, parents shared a number of issues and concerns, varying from the common cold to bradycardia episodes, additional surgery, and monumental delays in physical and/or mental growth and development. Additionally, the parental perceptions of infant care were no longer detached or disconnected, in contrast to the predischarge phase. Parents finally felt like parents.

A few individuals immediately encountered what they described as challenging issues. One parent interpreted an infant who never stopped crying on the way home from the hospital as an ominous sign; no usual comfort strategy was effective. Identifying the most suitable formula, taking smaller amounts per feeding, and requiring more numerous feedings were all mentioned in the nutrition dimension. Of particular interest were those parents who finally learned that the usual measures of darkness and quiet at sleep time were not going to work for a former NICU resident. Some learned by trial and error while a few were grateful to the NICU nurses they called who clued them into recreating the light-filled, noisier environment of the hospital nursery. Numerous parents reported more than expected crying, fussing, colic, wakefulness, and discomfort without any particular etiology. Respiratory problems were another common complaint. Responding to apnea alarms was the cause of much anxiety until most parents finally realized that the baby's situation was usually not an emergency--just false alarms. For one mother of twins, however, one alarm going off one afternoon sent her off on a frightening tangent, since she was alone with them. She suddenly thought, what if the other alarm should go off? Then what do I do? She could perform some simple stimulation on both but what if *both* needed CPR? She finally decided that such an emergency was unlikely to occur and she should not dwell on it.

Any new parent could have made the most frequently noted negative remarks--the work that the baby required, the sleepless nights, and how scary this all was. One baby was so fussy and worrisome that his mother attempted to cope by handing him over to sitters as much as possible, even after leaving him at day care while she worked full-time. One mother found life extremely hectic:

> There's just a lot of things going on at home, having him home and everything. It was nice to get him home but I almost missed goin' up to the hospital. It had gotten to be such a comfortable routine. Seeing everyone up there and everybody was so nice.

Parents who brought home more than one baby simply had double or triple the work, which they were quick to address. One mother told us that she finally quit trying to breast-feed her twins so that her husband could help with the feeding. She was overwhelmed by the constant need to have one baby or the other at her breasts.

There was great concern about the baby's health and whether or not the baby was developing normally or even beginning to catch up with babies who had not been in the NICU. It was not that parents did not know generally what normal development entailed, but they wanted to know what was normal for a baby who had been in the NICU. Also they were confused about abnormalities within a range that did not warrant any concern given the hospitalization. They frequently asked themselves how long they should wait when the baby did not seem to be *normal*. If the baby is crying excessively, is something wrong? Or will a baby who was in the NICU be *OK* but just different from full-term infants? Some parents were quite comfortable calling the physician's office, the NICU nurses, or the follow-up clinic personnel, but many others did not want to be a nuisance or bother busy professionals. Beyond the infant's physical status, questions arose about breast-feeding the high-risk infant, the use of pacifiers, and the safety of utilizing other caregivers (family, neighbors, baby-sitters).

Childcare for this infant was definitely an issue for those women who returned to work. Finding suitable, experienced caregivers, especially if the child or children had special needs, was an onerous responsibility, "I think probably the hardest thing for me was hiring people to help take care of them. It's like I run a small business instead of being a parent." People who would have normally volunteered to baby-sit were now hesitant to offer their help for infants who had unusual needs. One woman described her feelings of isolation given the infant's status:

> It was real hard to go anywhere when you have a tube about this arm with a big bag on it and ah, so I was...I felt through all of this whole

> time...I felt like I was a prisoner in my own home. A lot of the times, you couldn't really go anywhere. He was too sick to go somewhere or it was just really difficult. You can't even get him in a car seat. He couldn't wear most of his clothes because of the tubes and stuff.[a]

Most fathers shared some childcare but several did not see infant care as their responsibility in any way:

> I knew he didn't want another child. I mean he really didn't, you know. He's having a hard time, especially with this one. He's scared of him [the baby]. He can't be in the same room with him because he said, he'd just catch himself...listening to how he was breathing and everything. And just worry. So, I do it all.

These men viewed themselves in traditional roles as providers of income for household functioning rather than sharing childcare tasks.

Experienced parents indicated that already having had a child helped them and they felt sorry for parents who were taking home a NICU graduate as a first child. But even experienced parents recounted some features of care for which they were not prepared. It was surprising how many parents in this immediate discharge period identified infant problems after initially stating how well the infant was doing or what progress the baby had made since discharge. We asked ourselves, whether saying the infant was fine, was simply a socially acceptable behavior enacted initially by parents.

In about one-third of these families (11), the parents expected that both the infant's life and their own lives would eventually return to a more normal state, or at least one more commonly experienced by families in their same stage of development. This was a reasonable and realistic expectation. For approximately another one-third, it was quite clear that normal growth and development would never transpire (10). These children were seriously handicapped and would most likely need special interventions for their entire lives. The remaining one-third (13), faced possibly the most difficult circumstance psychologically: their future was the least assured of the group. The final outcome could be fine but then again it might not. Some disabilities and handicaps cannot be determined until the child has developed further, sometimes as late as school age. Parents did not necessarily recognize the status of the infants in these latter two groups. But this question was on every parent's mind -- what did the future hold? Even if our lives are hectic now, should we hold a bright outlook for the future? Will a good future really ensue?

Parents also discussed doubts about their pediatricians but were not sure that they had a right to question the professional's care, to obtain another opinion, or to simply change physicians. One mother recalled her baby's need for further surgery subsequent to the NICU discharge, an experience which led her to reconsider her role relative to hospitalization:

> *A nightmare hospitalization.* Irma's infant was sent home with the understanding that he would need follow-up care related to kidney functioning. Apparently the child's condition changed more rapidly than anticipated for, instead of the needed surgery in six months to one year, the infant was rehospitalized just three weeks after he was sent home. Both parents perceived problems related to the facility during the NICU hospitalization and wanted the next surgery to be scheduled in a different hospital. But this change did not prevent criticism. Irma discussed her disappointment with the postoperative surgical care, the surgeon's decisions, and her observations that the unit appeared to be understaffed. She disagreed with the plan of care relative to feeding, pain medications, and time for discharge. Irma went on to explain how she provided her child with most of his care, which was fine. Although she did not object to providing the care, she worried that any early detection of possible problems might be missed since the professional staff was not in the room very often.
>
> Irma was also critical of the mother of the child in the bed next to her own baby's bed. She found the other mother's behavior and that of the mother's friends who visited the child, unacceptable. She complained that they were smoking in the room. Their appearances were "tough" and she did not always feel safe. The other mother and her friends were quite young, in their teens, and Irma was shocked at their language and topics of conversation. However, she did not take any action relative to these observations at the time of their occurrences.
>
> She now says, "...we could have been very, very angry. A lot of people were saying, well, you should try to file, to sue [the doctor]...but we thought, what's the point? We now have a healthy baby and that's all that matters." On the other hand, she expressed some regret for her inaction: "...if we would have spoken up, asked more questions, and knew that we had more rights...we found out we have a lot more rights than we realized that we did."

The importance of control is undeniable at six months postdischarge. In their own homes with this infant, all parents were now able to make the decisions and do exactly what they wanted to do. Several families did decide to select different physicians after discharge. One family related a more long-term worry about the possible loss of control should they have to institutionalize their severely disabled infant.

A few parents may have made drastic decisions reflecting their backlash against what they had perceived as a total lack of influence while the infant was in the NICU. They discussed their decisions such as discontinuing medications, refusing to use the apnea monitor, varying formulas, and using alternative therapies. Fortunately, the parents' efforts to express control did not seem to have any ill effects in the infants.

One family described pouring all of the infant's medications down the toilet as soon as they got home from the hospital. They did not believe in prescription pharmaceuticals so they instituted their own plan of care based on advice from an herbalist who they believed was key to their family's good health. Following this advice, the mother provides the child with vitamins and other recommended substances. The infant is unable to tolerate formula and is on goat's milk. The mother believes these supplements are helping him to remain healthy and overcome some of his sensitivity. He has never been sick or had any other difficulty since discharge.

Another couple left the apnea monitor in the box in the front hallway, because they believed that their own personal vigilance was more than sufficient for the infant. The "machine" would keep them from close contact with their infant, just as many devices had interfered with their relationship to the infant in the hospital. Apparently there was some mix-up in the delivery of the monitor and a second was sent as well. Then the company wanted to exchange the monitor for a different type. "They said they were going to mail a substitute and would we send the other back," the mother noted. The parents thought this was amusing. The mother kept trying to say, "Don't bother--we're not using any of them. It's never been out of the box."

In a third example, a mother explained how she changed the prescribed formula. She also disagreed with the designated treatment plan about the respiratory interventions. Her approach to respiratory care included a self-devised plan to wean the infant off oxygen and to discontinue the theophylline and apnea monitor. This couple had sought the advice of a pharmacist who gave them the insert for the medication. Basing their decision on the side effects listed for the drug, they believed the treatment and medication were agitating the baby and making him nervous. These plans succeeded. The oxygen and medications were completely eliminated. No monitor was used and the baby was finally calm and peaceful.

Parents emphasized the singular importance of support from their families and the community at large. Participants discussed their relationships with their spouse or partner, their extended families, others in the community, and health professionals. A multiplicity of roles made demands on them. Although parents could envision themselves as more mature, happy, excited, and better able to deal with stress at this point in time compared to the NICU experience, they also confessed to being very upset, scared, terrified, and even bitter at times. One parent made an enlivening attempt at humor in her response, "So I do have a lot more patience. Either that or I'm brain dead!!"

A crisis is undoubtedly a time of relationship testing. The most obvious relationship at risk in this time of vulnerability is the marriage or the affiliation with the partner. Feeling connected with others can provide a measure of security for some individuals and some parents were able to build a closer and stronger relationship as a result of this experience. Unfortunately, not every parent had this support. Some even had major difficulties on this front.

One single mom discussed whether or not she should marry the father of her child. At this point in her life she was not sure that she wanted to share her entire life with this man. Another young, single mother had been abandoned by her boy friend when she found out she was pregnant but she did have her own mother to support her in this experience. A third single woman described the father of her child as a "playboy," not at all interested in marriage to *anyone*. Personal support from this man was intermittent. "I thought, you know, he'd be more responsive to a baby, but he isn't," she relays. So he is generally not a caregiver for the child but he does pay child support. She is very ambivalent about the relationship and his future role with this child. This woman had a subsequent pregnancy within the six-month postdischarge period and she had an abortion. She felt enormous self-imposed pressure to have the abortion:

> Two months ago I found out I was pregnant again. That was, it [abortion] went against the, all my morals. But I just could not see myself with two kids, single. I didn't tell the father until it was all over, because he is very strict. I think, for me, it was...what would people

> say? I mean - here, she's dumb enough, people thought that when I got pregnant. Oh my God, how could that have happened a second time? The first time I had an ear infection and the antibiotics counteracted against the pill and I got pregnant. But how could I explain a second one? The baby's father and I weren't having sex that often. So I messed up on the pills. I was behind and I thought I could catch up but it didn't work.

She went on to discuss the meaning of "what would people say" and its relationship to her support system:

> I was concerned with my family, my mom and dad 'cause they were upset the first time and I could just see me going to them and saying, guess what, I'm going to have another one. I was afraid what my father, and my friends would say. They would think I was out to get the father, you know, to marry me. If he didn't marry me after one child, maybe he'd marry me after two. I just didn't want that.

Of those parents who were married approximately five couples had obvious relationship concerns. One marriage had already dissolved. This was partially associated with the death of the infant but also due to many other factors as well, including domestic abuse and drug use, which were important elements in the woman's story. Several couples discussed the issue of fidelity and the effect of stress on their relationship. As one father noted, "You do things a lot of times when we're tired...that we're not really proud of. But we're still together and so far we're still hanging in there." A mother commented:

> Fidelity. Yeah, now especially, ya know when there is all this stress, and we don't get to talk, be alone together, and stuff like that. This is probably still something that is even more of a concern now. It would be pretty rough goin' if he [her husband] were trying to sneak away.

Finally, three couples did not verbally acknowledge any difficulty during the interviews but, given the observations of the interviewer, the field notes indicated some potential distress in these relationships based on the couples' interactions and other nonverbal signs. At the four-year postdischarge interview, one of these couples was indeed divorced and the second couple continued to struggle with marital adversity. The status of the third couple is unknown, as they did not participate in a four-year postdischarge interview. Regardless of whether or not a couple legally separates or divorces as a result of children with serious sequelae, such a statistic is not necessarily an adequate indicator of marital failure (Sabbeth & Leventhal 1984).

Couples conceded that their partnership required work but that special infant demands, jobs, extended family relationships, and other children all seemed to get priority over the marriage. This is similar to any other parenting situation in which infant care supersedes partnership needs, whether it is the first child or the fifth. However, some parents expressed a nagging worry about the rationale for the increased responsibilities brought about by the needs of the NICU graduate. Interviewees asked:

- Which parent might be blamed for their unique circumstances?
- Was there some factor related to conception wherein either parent might have contributed to the risk for such a crisis developing?
- Or was the high-risk infant's condition due to something the woman did or did not do during the pregnancy?

These quandaries were not a focal point of discussion but in describing their search for some meaning of this event in their lives, a number of individuals certainly expressed this idea. No parent was radical in this pursuit as one father in a study flatly denied his role in conception when faced with his physically and mentally compromised newborn. Instead he accused his wife of conceiving the child with another man (Palmer & Noble 1986)

Families were responsible not only for integrating a newborn into family life but also for easing the adjustment of older children to the demands of a new baby. They realized how hard this whole series of events was on their other children. As one mother indicated, parents needed to be, at one and the same time, special parents to this newborn and a normal family for the older child. Since many of these newborns required more than the anticipated amount of care in a number of cases, parents were often concerned about the focus on the newborn and its potential negative effect on the siblings. The parents' increased awareness of the tenaciousness of life aroused by the newborn's hospitalization extended to their perception of their other children as well, making them think about risks their older children might face such as drug abuse, unplanned pregnancy, coping with chronic illness, and teenage violence and gangs. This crisis also motivated some parents to re-examine their parenting of their other children:

> I think I take my role as a mother more seriously than I did. We're actually working, kind of in and out of some therapy with our oldest

> daughter and her diabetes. It [the high-risk experience] kind of opened up our eyes to things that we could have done differently for her.

Parents were also proud of these older children's responses to the newborn and the assistance that they provided. Some siblings can only complete simple tasks but others are old enough to contribute significantly to the functioning of the household, "We're closer now. I appreciate her [older child] more now. I know that's awful, but...I do."

Generally, as various people served as a source of support, the neonate family benefited. Grandparents could be an especially important element because parents usually trusted them and felt comfortable asking them for assistance. "A crisis shows you who your true friends are," one mother commented, describing how neighbors pitched in to help. Sometimes friends and relatives did not know how to respond to such a crisis and ignored the parents. Misunderstandings occurred as well. Parents described several poignant situations related to support, which emphasized the importance of both extended family help and understanding, and the community acceptance of their special situation. Here are two stories from parents about extended family relationships: Thanksgiving Holiday and The Harvest:

> *Thanksgiving Holiday.* Parents Louise and Frank, who had seriously handicapped twins, tell the powerful story of the first family Thanksgiving after the birth of their children. This family celebration included another relative who had recently had a baby so there were three new babies at this gathering. Frank and Louise were absolutely crushed by their relatives' treatment of the twins. No one actually *did* anything to them--but the twins were virtually ignored during the entire day. All of the attention, praise, compliments, and caring were directed at the third new baby. It was as if the twins were not even present. Louise and Frank perceived that their children, in their handicapped condition, were not welcome in the family. No one looked, cooed, fussed, or wanted to hold the babies. Both parents went home crying after a long, trying day, feeling totally rejected by those from whom they expected and needed lots of love and support in order to face the many hurdles and hardships ahead of them.

> *The Harvest.* Taking home one premature newborn is challenging but taking home twins or even triplets can be overwhelming. Greg and Jane were taking home triplets! Although small--their birth weights were all slightly under 2000 grams--they were born at 33 weeks so developmentally they were quite advantaged. Two of the babies came

home from the NICU in less than one month while one stayed another ten days. There was little time to adjust to the heavy demands of triple baby care. Jane had part-time help to assist her in taking care of the babies and running a household that had more than doubled in size virtually overnight. Greg worked on the family farm but, except for this activity, both parents were constantly busy changing diapers, feeding one baby or another, or comforting a crying infant. By the time of the fall harvest, all three infants were home, but only by a couple of months. Traditionally, all extended family members participated in the harvest. This work had a social dimension to it which served as a renewal of family spirit, but it was also a lot of work and entailed long days in the fields. Jane reminded her husband that her responsibilities this year were in their home, caring for the children. Although Jane had part-time assistance during the day to help with infant care, there was no way to arrange for total care of the children. In addition, Jane was still recovering from the pregnancy and birth. For fourteen weeks she had been on bedrest and medications in order to carry this pregnancy for as long as possible. She continued to have difficulties that she associated with those medications. At the six-month postdischarge interview, she was still unable to walk normally.

As harvest time approached, Greg's family members were planning the work schedule and the target fields as well as the food necessary to feed all of the workers. Greg informed his family that Jane would not be participating. They all found this decision incredible! How could someone *not* participate? No one seemed to understand or acknowledge that triplets could prevent assisting with the harvest--it was simply something that everyone did. Greg was firm and defended their decision, which made it difficult for him to work side by side with his relatives and, later, difficult for Jane as well when she had contact with the extended family. For the family, farm life went on regardless of personal issues or demands, even apparently, triplets and compromised health. Somehow one managed to participate. The decision fractured family relationships and would not be forgotten easily, if ever.

It was not just the parents of the most seriously affected infants who indicated a need for support. When support was lacking, even in cases where infants were responding at a fairly acceptable level and progressing in growth and development, parents did not cope well. One couple explains their circumstances and how trapped the woman feels:

Father: I wished I had known that all that baby-sitting wouldn't of paid off.

Mother: Ah...yes, paid off. That does upset us. We did a lot of baby-sitting for both sisters. And I just...

> Father: No, 'cause they have a two-year-old boy now and it's harder when you have a two-year-old.
> Mother: I do think it's harder for someone when you have a kid of your own. We didn't have kids when we were baby-sitting for them. It was fun to have other people's kids. But now...it is harder for them to baby-sit. They [the twins] are a lot of work. Staying home all the time is a big change. You really don't know until the time comes how big a decision that is. Day care would be $300 every two weeks so returning to work was not financially worth it. They were both on monitors so you really have to have a good baby-sitter. We didn't want to take them out in the cold during the winter...expose them to a lot of extra germs and that sort of thing. It is just hard to be home all the time. [Husband] is trying to get ahead in his job and going to night school, so he isn't here much of the time.

The couple's expectations of help from their family were not met and despite the regular progress of the children, the lack of support disappointed them. The negative attitude permeated a number of their observations about their outcome at six months.

In contrast to this lack of support from families, parents' church communities were particularly helpful through prayer and emotional support as well as their willingness to meet physical needs, "Lots of prayers. There were people as far as Canada praying. There were people we didn't even know until later, hundreds and hundreds of people praying. I think it was just a miracle." Pastors and priests were discussed with high regard and respect. The presence of clergy both in the nursery and outside, for the most part, was helpful during this crisis. Their intervention had been important to parents in a number of situations. For those parents on a quest for meaning, which involves the crisis of an NICU experience, the relevance of religion or spirituality was fundamental. More individuals noted the importance of this dimension in the six-month interview than in the earlier one. Certain individuals were motivated to examine their spiritual life as they had never been led to do before. Religion was a conduit through which they attempted to find the meaning of this experience in the context of their lives. They believed prayer, either their own or that of their spiritual community, was important for the well-being and progress of the infant.

Some community members were so helpful as to have caused a sense of debt in parents, "...because of the positive response that we've had from so many different people...if somebody would ask me to do something, I'd bend over backwards to do it for them." Another positive experience for a few families was their connection with a parental support group. Most parents did not seem to know about these groups while the baby was in the hospital, except for two mothers, the one who located a parents' group in Texas and another who named her contact with the Parent-to-Parent program. But several mothers now mentioned the importance of their current membership in "twin groups." Although not a formal device, some families remained in contact with other parents they met while the infant was hospitalized. Personal socialization was limited but they continued to communicate with one another over the telephone or in writing.

A number of families had less positive experiences in the community, especially when the infant died or was obviously handicapped, or when the parent was attempting to secure additional resources. The following judgmental stance by a community member in the work setting was a rather dramatic response to one parent:

> *"Too nice" for a mom with handicapped children.* One of the mothers, Alice, described an event that took place at work shortly after she and her husband brought their handicapped children home from the hospital. At Alice's place of employment, she meets with the public regularly and one day she was in her office interviewing a couple as part of her job-related responsibilities. The interview began with some social chit-chat and, as the friendly conversation drew to a close, the client expressed what Alice first believed to be a compliment: "How very nice you look, Alice." After Alice said "thank you," the client went on to remark that she couldn't understand how people with handicapped children could dress so nicely. Alice was aghast at such a caustic, personal remark and could barely keep her composure. In some ways the statement was perplexing. What was the connection between her clothes and a child's handicap? But, more than that, Alice found it difficult to understand how people could be so judgmental about her appearance. Both she and her husband really needed support. If this was an example of what was happening in their small community, then their future could be even more bleak than they already anticipated.

Continuing ties with the NICU were informative and supportive for many families, especially those who lived at a distance or who were in such small communities that readily available local resources for advice were not an option. As already indicated, parents sometimes were friendly with other families and the NICU nurses occasionally provided the avenue through which parents maintained ties with those families. When parents talked with the nurses, they were able to get updates on other families as well. Several parents also asked us about these families after the interview was completed. Due to the confidential nature of the project, we were unable to fulfill these requests. By the parents' own admission, the support was also present in infant follow-up care through the high-risk or other clinics. Nurses were available in those settings during clinic visits and ready to respond to parents' questions or the need for advice on the telephone. Communication was important to the parents as they adjusted to the needs of this newborn, and nurses were viewed most positively on this dimension.

Working with the health care system, insurance companies, physicians, social services, or other potential resources was not always pleasant, however. At six months, families were concerned about hospital bills, insurance reimbursement, and other financial assistance to meet the escalating costs of health care for their child. There was no need to ask about finances during this interview as parents spontaneously raised these concerns. Given the length of hospitalization for some children, it would seem likely that bills or insurance reports would have been sent prior to discharge, but almost no parent mentioned cost in the earlier interview.

One mother, attempting to secure funds to supplement the insurance payment for the hospital bill, described being, "...shoved around so much that, the only way to get anything done is to almost be mean, you know, and yell and to really not be very nice." Her assertiveness was not perceived positively by those who had to deal with her. Yet being polite, waiting your turn, and following the chain of command simply did not work, according to her experience. The parental need for funding was pressing. In the course of contacting state senators for some assistance, the father said one senator told them "not to make waves because we didn't want to be known as..." The mother continued, "[We were told] you don't want a reputation as being known as a bitch." The woman persevered in her fight undaunted, however, and succeeded in her efforts to secure additional funding to meet medical expenses.

Parents also had financial complaints. They described their situation as "chronically low on money," "budgeting problems," or needing to even "take out a loan." Extraordinary hospital and physician bills were in addition to the usual expenses of running a household, which some families had difficulty meeting. One father explained:

> I'd say you really gotta put an effort into it, we're just gettin' by. We got a bill after five months that we knew nothing about. We got a bill from a doctor who said he had worked on the baby's feet. They were takin' care of their feet, which is fine. They put the foot in a splint. But this was all takin' place without our knowledge and so we were gettin' doctor bills from people that we never even knew.

Families who lived a distance from the follow-up clinic had the added expense of travel for services unavailable in their hometowns. Two mothers mentioned the father's failure to pay support. A few women felt obligated to continue employment after the baby's birth either because the income was essential to meet family needs or because the insurance benefits were attached to the mother's employment rather than the father's. Some women's inability to return to their job because of infant care demands produced a significant strain on these families. Families were generally prepared for changes in financial status related to pregnancy and postpartum recovery but, when hospitalization of the infant extended from a few days to weeks or even months in some cases, as one mother shared, it "nearly destroyed us."[b]

A major concern was the hospital billing system, which was uniformly judged as unnecessarily complex and unwieldy. Some parents did not appreciate the general format for the bills they sometimes received. These individuals acted as watchdogs over the medical charges. They wanted specifics as they reviewed the bills and tried to determine exactly what comprised their debt for the child. This was especially important when insurance or other sources did not cover the cost of the hospitalization and parents were left to pay the balance privately, "If we could have had insurance, 99.9% of the weight would have been lifted from my shoulders." Simply having an insurance policy was not the whole story for these parents, however. During her pregnancy, one woman added a rider to her policy for high-risk infant care; otherwise there would have been no coverage for the infant's stay in the NICU. In other cases, certain procedures or types of care were not included. Also, the number of days or the dollar amount the policy covered in one calendar year limited hospitalization benefits. It was upsetting for parents to be sued by the institution or to have bill collectors sent to their homes, especially in smaller communities where "everyone knows." At the extreme, one parent could not believe that, on a $185,000 bill, the hospital would sue because he had not as yet paid a balance of $494. This father went on to complain:

> We've had stress over the money situation. They sued us...we're working on it but we ain't got that [much] right now. But, we have a right to know what they're charging you for. They had insulin sent up every day for weeks and he was never on insulin. Now why should my son have to pay for insulin that he never needed? Then they sent up this bag of hyperal and they only gave him 200 ccs. And, they threw the rest away!

A limited number of families had to deal with canceled insurance policies, which was another extreme. One family lost insurance benefits for about three months, which made money tight. The parents had to examine each of their contributions to the family income as well. In this situation the mother did not like living in the town where they were located, but the father's educational commitment required that they at least live there until he finished his degree. She finally decided to leave her husband temporarily and go live with her parents. In this different town she expected to find suitable employment, regain insurance benefits, and have the amenities of community life that were readily available, to her satisfaction. She did not take their children with her; the husband said that she could leave but the children were going to stay. That left total childcare responsibilities for him as well as work and school.

The father and mother were both concerned that their own parents would think that they were having marriage difficulties. Indeed, the woman expressed her feelings of desperation given the infant's status. Although she secured new employment in her parents' hometown, and lived there for some time, the couple finally agreed that a distance marriage was not going to work. She moved back with her husband but not without regret, continuing to lament that "no one understood my point of view." He responded that he planned to be more attentive to her and try to recognize the importance of her perspective in the future. In addition, financial pressures lessened as insurance benefits were reactivated at that point.

The most vivid example of economic problems came from a family dealing with handicapped children and long-term medical expenses. The father explained that the insurance company decided "to cancel out on them." When pursued for further clarification, the father explained that actually, the company had been bought out which necessitated a change in insurance carriers. The new insurance company would not accept the extended medical needs and concomitant payments for care as covered in the original policy for this family's children. The insurance company put a rider in their individual policy eliminating their children from coverage. Loss of insurance created a serious financial bind for this family.

In some cases, as exemplified above, financial stress added to the other stresses of a high-risk birth, led parents to consider possible legal action in retaliation against medical personnel. Although there is no evidence that parents from this study actually sued any of the institutions, four families did discuss the potential for a lawsuit. As one parent remarked:

> I just have the feeling that he [the physician] messed up on some stuff. I really do. We're not the type that's out for any lawsuit or anything like that. But I'm still gonna draw it to their attention, so that he doesn't do it to somebody else.

Another claimed:

> There should have been an x-ray taken and they should have figured out, by her clinical signs, that there was something, other than, just all of a sudden, a turn like that. I just cannot...I still may pursue that some day.

Most infants admitted to the NICU graduate and are sent home with their parents. Most of these cases are considered success stories and indeed are such, judging by the progressive growth and development of the children. However, all families require some degree of adjustment, given their experience with the crisis of a NICU hospitalization and the time necessary for recovery. Some parents continue to face enormous problems within their family and in the community after the infant is discharged. These results confirm the conclusion drawn by Silverman (1992), a pediatrician, who has studied after-care for NICU graduates and their parents. Families themselves, he says, could benefit from an effort comparable to intensive care to assist them with the needs of the infant after discharge. In order to determine fully the extent of family requirements, one needs to re-examine the NICU story.

Looking Back on the NICU Experience

Asking the parents to retell the NICU story during the second interview enabled us to expand upon our understanding of this experience. The recapitulation of the parents' perspective was not sought to affirm or refute earlier findings. Perceptions do change over time. For example, one woman who openly discussed her unplanned pregnancy in the predischarge interview vehemently denied that the pregnancy was unplanned during the current interview. When asked to confirm the earlier understanding in the course of discussing pre-admission information, she went through her denial of the unplanned pregnancy. Out of respect for her perspective the research assistant simply indicated that there must have been some mistake and went on with the conversation. To fully appreciate the parental position on a long-term basis, it is beneficial to examine the construction of these stories at various times, simply to see how individuals are shaping their perceptions--what is important, what is trivial, what is added, what is deleted as the family history is created.

Although parents cooperated with us in sharing their perspectives of the NICU from this six-month postdischarge vantage point, we noted that the six months with the infant at home was undoubtedly a more favored topic. During this set of interviews the parents' spontaneous discussions primarily focused on bringing the infant home, integrating it into family life, and adjusting to any adaptations it required. When responding to the request to describe what stood out for them given the whole set of experiences connected with the infant, they clearly emphasized the initial months at home.

We found this phenomenon quite interesting. When parents had been asked to describe their experiences in the NICU while the infant was housed there, they proceeded to relate the entire set of circumstances that led up to the admission, whereas, after discharge when asked to look back at the NICU experience, they favored a discussion of the present and the events since discharge. We made no attempt to determine a rationale for this preference since it was more patently noticeable during analysis rather than during the intensive interviewing process. The simple fact that the six-month experience was new (and new to us as well) while the NICU experience was now in the background could explain their choices. At any time however, the NICU may have been the least comfortable topic.

Overall, time seemed to have stood still in the NICU as parents reflected back over their experiences from a six-month postdischarge perspective. The NICU experience was perceived as surprising, miserable, decent, hectic, confusing, scary, unreal, "time going on forever," or a total disruption of life. Only six months after discharge, the NICU situation seemed now like something that had occurred very long ago. Some parents described it as a dream they had had; a few said it was a nightmare. One father captured this feeling very vividly:

> You know, it is funny...after she was born there was a commentary on TV about a NICU. We sat and watched it and kind of felt overwhelmed by it, or at least I did. Maybe it was a delayed reaction. At the time it was happening I kind of glossed it over or was just caught up with the everyday mechanics of, well, let's drive over there and scrub up and everything else. But [several months] later or so, watching this program and reliving all that. Watching another family, another couple, scrub up. Watching one kid come home and another who didn't make it and everything. Wow! We really went through a lot! Maybe it didn't or at least I didn't realize it at the time. This show had to bring it all back to me.

Although parents may not now spontaneously recall the impact these events had on them and their lives, when faced with a request to revisit this experience the events and the emotions return. One mother described it well:

> When I look back now after having him home, how I felt as we were about to deliver a premature baby. I thought there's no way in the world I can ever stand, I could ever stand the stress, the financial, the back and forth hassle...just seemed so overwhelming. I look back and think, well, it wasn't that big of a deal. *But*, I read back in my diary, of how I felt those days and it *was* a big deal. I do remember a lot of really hard weeks when I didn't know whether they would have to commit me or not.[c]

Generally, most parents were positive or neutral in their general recollections of the NICU experience. They acknowledged both how difficult and emotionally draining it was for them as well as how much they appreciated the expertise, dedication, and support of the staff. Many of their specific memories were similar to those they had shared during the predischarge interview. Indeed, it was almost uncanny how many of them used exactly the same words and phrases to describe a particular event. A major difference, however, in describing the NICU experience after six months versus predischarge was in the parents' quest for the meaning of this ordeal, both as an isolated entity and also as an element in the whole scope of family life.

Virtually all of the parents in looking back over the pregnancy and subsequent experience in the NICU now sought a rationale of the loss of what should have been a normal course for pregnancy, birth, and newborn nursery events. While some parents assumed responsibility or blame for their circumstances, others eliminated their own behavior as a possible precipitating factor in their situation. In the former category, one parent admitted:

> They told me while I was pregnant I would have to be extra careful because I could have her early. I didn't pay no attention to that and ran around...like I wasn't even pregnant or nothin'.

Another parent said how scary the whole series of events was and added, "I guess we were just so young." In the latter category, parents focused on having done everything they could have done: "I ate right, I exercised, I read everything, I didn't have caffeine--I did everything right." Or, "I can't blame anything I did." Mothers in particular scrutinized the events, their feelings, and their physical status in an attempt to pinpoint something that would explain the crisis. "Perhaps if I would have..." a mother pondered. "Was I being punished for a previous sin?" another mother asked. Parents mentioned that their physicians indicated quite firmly that there was no single good explanation for the course of events in many cases. Bad luck and an unfortunate confluence of factors entered into possible explanations for their predicament and the infant's outcome.

Women are well aware that they are sometimes blamed for the ill health or problems in the newborn, which may have led to the above self-recrimination, either by health professionals or others they contact. Women know that actions and behavior during pregnancy can affect infant outcomes as publicity about the use of drugs including excessive alcohol ingestion and smoking is widespread. Environmental hazards, nutritional status, and even exercise (lack of or excessive) are also touted as potentially effecting the fetus. Whether these factors are significant relative to fetal outcomes is immaterial, women do take on this burden. The contribution to the health of the newborn via sperm and its health status has received little attention. Yet, there is possible damage to the fetus from sperm that is slowly being documented (Nelson 1992).

Parents now lamented this loss of the *normal* in the premature birth or critical newborn events. Mothers specifically noted the loss of a normal pregnancy. One mother related, "I wasn't even big. Most people did not even know I was pregnant yet. That's kind of a letdown." The women felt this loss as a shock, a surprise, a state of confusion, or resentment. Women thought that the early termination of the pregnancy denied them an appropriate transition to the parenting role. It was difficult to adjust to this new role during the infant's hospitalization because of the empty nursery at home and the lack of a pregnant status. Such a loss can extend for a period of time:

> Right now I'm going through, just kinda of a, a bad time. My sister is expecting a baby in a couple of weeks. And you, you know, I don't wish for someone to have a sick baby. But I, I feel like, well she is probably going to have this *well* baby. I feel kind of, some resentment that my baby was so sick.

Had these been normal births, the mother would have spent only a day or two in the hospital and then gone home to immediately bear total responsibility for the baby's care. The baby would have been at her bedside during the entire hospital stay and most of the infant's needs would have been met by her. Instead, precipitous events foreshortened pregnancy or escalated the risk of the birth/newborn phase. Two mothers again emphasized that they were unable to see the infant at delivery or even immediately afterward.

In searching for a meaning, parents included the lack of sufficient information about their infant's circumstances. Whether or not parents were actually told is irrelevant for this discussion. Parents cannot construct a cohesive story, nor can they gain adequate understanding of their experiences and move on to the next milestone, without *retaining* pertinent information. Parents, however, believed they were not satisfactorily informed by health professionals, and this is the element of the NICU experience that they would most like to change. They do acknowledge the difficulties posed by medical terminology and complex infant diagnoses and treatment plans. Additionally they can now especially comprehend how emotionally exacting this period was in their lives.

However, the message parents send is that NICU professionals ought to be sure that they do communicate and that, secondarily, the information is received, processed, understood, and remembered. What parents have learned since discharge only emphasizes their perceived lack of knowledge during hospitalization. They do now acknowledge that some information came from physicians but not necessarily when those physicians talked directly to them. Parents picked up bits and pieces when physicians talked to other parents around the isolette or when parents managed to stay in the unit while the physicians made rounds.[d] A couple of parents acquired the infant's chart after discharge in order to narrow this information gap. In addition parents sought information from other sources, including the medical libraries. On the other hand, parents drew attention to exceptions to the usual lack of communication. One father explained his fruitful discussion with a consultant for his son:

> We were really impressed with [the physician]. He was the one person who would sit down and just listen to us. He said there wasn't much to say about the suggestions, but he let us vent. He said that was real important for us then. It was what we needed.

In expressing a need for information, parents noted the timing of the provision of the information, which for them began prior to the admission of the infant. Most of these individuals believed that they should have seen the NICU during the pregnancy. Infant status in the NICU is a shock to parents but it is a shock to most lay people at any time. At least, if parents see the unit before their own child's admission, they do not have to have the double shock of the physical appearance of the unit as well as the possibly grave condition of their own child. Those with multiple gestations, believed that since the risk of having prematures was greater for them, there was an even more urgent requirement to become knowledgeable about possible outcomes.

Parents continued to emphasize that living at a distance from the nursery was a problem for those whose infants had been transported to the medical center from another facility. Families look back and wonder if being closer would have made a difference in their own feelings and perceptions about the experience. Parents question how this distance affected bonding with the child and how that in turn may have affected the baby's progress. As one mother asked herself, "How do you bond with a baby you can only see twice a week?" Distance certainly affected their own physical availability, and of course parents contemplated the relationship between their availability and status of their infant. When a crisis occurred, parents were not able to be on the scene immediately. Although parents believed their infant's treatment was not compromised, informed consent procedures that transpired over the telephone for the best interests of the infant and to expedite emergency care increased their anxiety. These telephone consents also contributed to the distancing the parents perceived and further accentuated their marginal status.

Families varied in their ability to temporarily move closer to the hospital. When parents needed to care for other children (61% of the families already had other children for whom they were responsible), run a business, or keep a job, then living close to the newborn was next to impossible. Cost was another consideration despite some available assistance for actual living quarters. The parents still needed to figure loss of work time, the actual travel and its expense, possibly childcare, and similar concerns. Parents now asked themselves whether they should have been so frugal or whether they should have completely devoted themselves to the infant. When parents were able to relocate themselves, extended families did not always understand their need to simply put everything else on hold until this infant was secure in its progress. This was especially true when holidays or special family events coincided with the parents' absence from their hometown. One parent discussed how her extended family did not understand her need to spend the Christmas holiday near the NICU rather than in the hometown.

Searching for a suitable explanation of these events was necessary for the processing of the experience and its integration into the family history. However much parents re-examined the time the infant spent in the NICU or considered possible explanations, present-day responsibilities pressed in upon them. Questions were unanswered. Constructing a meaningful story of the ordeal was as yet incomplete as their lives continued in the context of relationships with those around them.

Basically, at six months postdischarge, as most families examined decision-making in the NICU, they were in an ambivalent state. They now questioned the decisions in the NICU and were not positive that the decisions were the best possible. The parents were faced with the reality of the infant's condition and not only had to presently care for it but also consider the meaning of an outcome different from normal or what they had expected, for possibly the rest of their lives. Some parents now believe they had an inherent right to make decisions for their child but were unable to make those decisions when the infant was in the NICU. They look at the significant decisions they make for this child now, at home, and wonder why they were not involved earlier.

On the one hand, from the six-month perspective, parents better understood the child's condition in the NICU, yet they still clung to a belief they previously held. Parents recalled, if only they could get their infant home and resume what they had anticipated as a newborn experience, everything would be all right. This desire mostly reflected a tension between their lack of understanding of the seriousness of the infant's condition and their longing to be in charge of the child's life. Parents continued to acknowledge their lack of sufficient information and the presence of stress, which could have hampered decision-making. However, even considering these factors, they were presently rethinking those conclusions reached by health professionals and their own lack of involvement. Parents were *not* taking the position that the child should not have been treated in the NICU. At this stage, no parent was willing or able to indicate that the child had such a poor quality of life as to warrant omitting treatment or ending its life. Given the child's current needs, however, most parents did believe that they could have been better prepared, particularly for unfortunate outcomes.

A number of families viewed the need for a NICU fatalistically, as a case of bad luck. They expressed the opinion that they were not able to effectively intervene in the nursery and certainly cannot change things now that occurred in the past. These parents viewed themselves as pawns who now accepted their circumstances and lived one day at a time, waiting for the situation to stabilize. For a few, the outcome for their child was God's will and they endured their predicament through faith and prayer. Parents were better able to accept the dire NICU circumstances when the outcome was acceptable: "if the outcome was okay, then the process for getting there was okay as well...we have a fairly healthy baby now and that's all that matters."

In describing their perceptions of the NICU experience from the six-month vantage point, some individuals looked back and saw that they simply had to bide their time until discharge, then they could do as they desired. Not all of these families expressed these intentions prior to the baby's discharge. More parents, after discharge, stressed the importance of control of the infant and an active role in decision-making.

Emerging Ethical Consciousness

Overall, six months after discharge, parents expressed concern in the ethical domain: whether or not the *right* decision had been made about the treatment of their child. The label, *emerging ethical consciousness* represents this phase. Parents communicated their puzzlement as they reviewed the NICU experience and the events that had affected them since discharge. Their expression of doubt or their questioning was only *emerging* because parents seemed hesitant and tenuous in this discussion. No clear, definitive explanation for this parental reticence was apparent. But now more parents could discuss the life-or-death nature of decisions that had been made relative to their child's hospitalization in the NICU. However, prior to discharge, only a few families articulated specific episodes that could be categorized within the traditional ethical dimension of neonatal care. This number increased from the predischarge phase. When we probed for details about this ethical dimension, parents discussed various decision-making events for several medical treatments, including surfactant, which was an experimental pharmacological agent used at their child's delivery, do-not-resuscitate orders, and ventilator use. Whether or not they had had an active role in the decision-making or even whether or not their decision was of substantive value in the treatment regimen were separate issues.

A few parents were anxious to discuss those experiences that occurred prior to discharge. A certain number of individuals mentioned treatments initiated during hospitalization without health professionals either informing them or seeking their permission. When parents came to visit, the baby's nurse simply indicated that *such-and-such* was done today and it went well. Some parents were surprised that the plan had not been discussed with them on their prior visit to the baby or that no one had telephoned them about the treatment. They wondered if they should have asked more questions about the infant's care instead of waiting to be informed.

One couple discussed a *No Code* decision at the six-month interview that had not been addressed earlier.[e] At first they even doubted the legitimacy of their role in this life-or-death issue until they later conferred with their minister. He affirmed the validity of their active participation in this decision. The discussion with the pastor also helped them to understand the exact moral nature of the issues involved in this dilemma and to assuage them of possible guilt for making a *wrong* decision. Exploring alternatives, examining the child's situation from all dimensions, and then reaching a reasonable decision were all part of the support the minister offered during this process.

The couple explained their experience in a very emotional, deeply moving manner. The neonatologist and nurses told them about their daughter's condition and her prognosis, neither of which was very good.[f] The physician thought that a No Code was the best decision under the circumstances. The parents were told that their daughter had been revived several times in the past, and had been taken off and put back on the ventilator. But, as the father stated, "If something would happen now, we'd let God, you know, let nature take its course--either way."

So this couple agreed to the No Code. But when they explored simply discontinuing ventilator support with the doctors rather than waiting for a crisis, the mother said:

> No, we didn't know we had, ah...those options. At first we didn't even know we could put a No Code on her. And we didn't know that we would have to ask to have the respirator taken off.

The father continued:

> The doctors kept telling us that they had a moral code to uphold and that there would be no such thing as that [turning off the ventilator] down there.

The mother proceeded with their story. Sometimes her daughter's condition made the mother so terribly distraught that she went into a nearby room to cry. Something was seriously wrong with her baby and she was not getting better. The mother was in that room one day when a nurse came and talked with her. It was then that she learned there were options, there were choices, and they did not have to sit back and wait for a crisis to occur. The parents asked for a meeting with the doctors but, before the meeting could occur, they were told that the physicians had decided that treatment was futile. According to the parents' understanding, the doctors would remove the baby from the ventilator and then let the No Code order go into effect. If she did not breathe spontaneously, she would be allowed to die.

The parents were prepared for the worst possible scenario--that when the ventilator was discontinued, their daughter would in fact die. Given that possibility, the parents bought a dress for her (they had not yet bought newborn clothes) and planned her funeral. But when the ventilator was removed, her respirations were fine. Breathing was spontaneous and adequate, although the general prognosis did not change.

"The CAT scan[g] showed absolutely no brain matter...only brain stem and fluid," the father related. "There was nothing there," the mother continued. "The potential for any quality of life was nil. There were consultations with doctors in New York and Chicago and San Francisco. They gave us all the reports." "There was very little chance for her," concluded the father, "but she has not died." So, at six months postdischarge, they described their current situation as a nightmare, a hard, never ending battle that they could never have imagined when they set out to finally have a family.

Another mother explained the decision put before her...

> The first time she got really, really sick and her heart rate dropped, they go...well, you know we can give her something to bring her back. Do you want us to bring her back? I said, "yes" because I didn't want my baby to think that I gave up on her. You never know. They could have brought her back if I would've said no. But maybe that's all she needed. That little extra boost to bring her back because she did live for two weeks after that.

Another family whose daughter died thought the "hardest thing in the world" was the last few days of her life. However, they did not believe they had made any critical decisions. The mother stated:

> If I had to do it over again, when it came right down to the end...if I would have had my way, I would've just said, enough is enough. Because even if she would have survived, she would've been severely handicapped. I mean she would've been to the point of never being able to learn anything. And, at that point, I didn't think she deserved to be in a body like that, trapped in there. I still think that it's every parent's right to say when enough is enough...but we had no control whatsoever.

This mother perceived the condition of her daughter to be going downhill for several days and questioned the continuation of any therapy under those circumstances. The baby was on the ventilator; the parents and physician had discussed whether or not to start her heart again if it stopped. The parents had said no but, given her grave condition, they did not think it was really a decision, a choice. The parents believed there were no legitimate options for them to consider. It was obvious to them what ought to be done, and, in fact, from the parents' perspective, something should have been done earlier to prevent aggressive treatment.

Another parent affirmed the positive nature of the decision-making, but continued to support decision-making by a health professional rather than by parents:

> I think I made pretty good decisions. If there was something I could do for him, I'd do it. And if it is something that I don't know anything

about, just involving his health or whatever, that's when the doctor comes in. I'm pretty sure the doctor...they took care of him this long and got him this far. I'm pretty sure they wouldn't do anything that would endanger him. I'm put[ting] my trust in those people up there in the NU [NICU] and the doctor and all those. I love 'em with all my heart.

Looking back over the NICU experience at the six-month postdischarge period, parents viewed decision-making negatively rather than passively, as had been true when the actual experience happened. Most problems revolved around communication and the provision of information. One mother discussed the need to educate people about what to expect. She recalled her admission to the hospital for what she described as "slight cramps and an infection." She thought the doctors could easily stop this development but instead the cramps continued and to her surprise she delivered a 25-week infant. When she was in labor, she and her husband wanted to know exactly what to expect relative to the infant's possible outcome. They felt they were not prepared. Therefore the baby's need to be in the NICU was an unfathomable experience for them. Not all parents would say that and certainly parents could have different opinions during the situation versus looking back to recount it. But these parents believed that health professionals could conduct some sort of reasonable assessment of parents to determine what they needed to know given them as individuals and their particular circumstances. One mother requested a video about preterm labor and the NICU.

Condense the information and put it on a video. If parents choose to watch, they can. If they don't, that's fine too. But you know, a lot of people are not going to sit down and read.

Other parents noted that it was not a matter of being completely uninformed, but rather what the health professionals had elected to say (emphasis is theirs):

In some cases, in one case in particular, we were treated slightly dishonestly. They weren't really being dishonest--they weren't telling us the *whole* story.

This evaluation took place when the parents reviewed the medical record of their infant. After discharge, this couple obtained the baby's chart and were enlightened by the information about the baby's condition as well as the notes about their own behavior and response to the ongoing hospitalization. At the moment health professionals informed them about the baby's condition, the parents felt they were taking part in the care and decisions about the infant's potential outcome. After reading the chart, however, the parents realized exactly how little they had been told and that decision-making had occurred as the health professionals deemed appropriate rather than what they as parents may have wanted had they been fully informed. From reading the chart, the parents believed health professionals had decided and then met with them to convince them to agree with the decision, rather than actually meeting with them to make a decision.

In another situation the parents were able to utilize their pediatrician as an advocate to help them obtain information. They later had verbal verification of a difference between what health professionals said and what was really going on with their infant:

> At first we weren't getting good answers from the neonatologist. But I called our pediatrician and he found out and talked to us. One day he [the baby] looked really sick and I talked to the nurses about holding him if things really got bad. They kept saying that things weren't that bad. But later I ran into one of the nurses and she said, "You know how lucky you are--*he was so sick*!" But they didn't let me know at the time.

The families' struggles with these experiences were indisputable whether the infant was recovering in a reasonable fashion or had extended, special needs. Although the ethical dimension of high-risk neonatal care was not a strong element of their stories, at least not as traditionally addressed in the bioethical literature, it was becoming evident as they now had to grapple with the reality of caring for the infant themselves. They could now look back more calmly over their NICU experience. Few parents, however, endeavored to act on their current observations. Indeed, what could they do now about past events? Questioning appeared to be merely at the intellectual level at six months postdischarge in their family history--it was *emerging*. But their newly gained insight did have the potential to impact their future.

Despite a major concern in the bioethical literature about the allocation of scarce resources, the cost of the NICU and financial considerations were not generally a part of the parents' discussion of their experiences with the high-risk neonate until the six-month postdischarge phase. In fact money was notably absent as a topic of discussion prior to the predischarge set of interviews--except for one family. That father believed useless procedures were done to "run up my bill because I have good insurance." For example, he was critical of the multiple eye exams, which he presumed were worthless because they did not uncover any problem. The other parent who noted understaffing as a problem (with financial implications) continued to complain that his son had to "wait his turn," which he believed incurred additional stress for the infant, delaying his recovery.

The importance of information for decision-making continued at the six-month phase. The parents' level of knowledge compared to the predischarge phase increased but they still needed to grow in this area. As these individuals provided total care for their child, negotiated the health care system, and acquired information about resources, their familiarity with diagnoses and treatment improved. The meaning of their infant's status at discharge and its immediate impact on the family was now much clearer to most of these individuals. During hospitalization, they had expressed their inability to even know what to ask. Now they realized how much they did not know. In particular, they lacked knowledge sufficient to anticipate future development and the need for interventions, whether their own strategies or professional action. Parents had begun this task but, in many ways, adjustment of family life to the infant's discharge was a priority, so the present required their full attention. They were as yet neither ready for nor comfortable with future, detailed planning, particularly long-term planning for the infant and themselves.

Recommendations for Other Parents

Most parents at six months postdischarge, had various suggestions to improve the situation in the NICU. As a rule, parents would say something like, "The NICU is a good place for your premature baby, but..." or "There are some really good people in the NICU, but..." Most of the suggestions for improvement focused on communication and provision of information. Advice to other prospective parents generally could be classified into three areas: parents should be assertive and obtain the information they need, they should insist on a working relationship with *all* health professionals, and they should get the amount and type of support they need. Parents should insist that physicians be available. Harsh retorts from nurses, as noted by few parents, should not be accepted.

Exercising control is one very clear message to other parents in similar circumstances, "I think the one thing I would have done from the very start is ask a lot more questions...not just blindly hand my baby over, you know. Another couple agreed while reiterating a message of both trust and control in this dialog:

> Father: Try to stay calm and let them do their job--they're good. They can do amazing things in there. But just ask all the questions you want and don't feel bad.
> Mother: Even through all of our frustrations and anger we still love everyone in there [in the NICU].
> Father: Trust these people because they know what they are doing. Trust the nurses more than the doctors. Use the nurses as interpreters of the medical jargon.
> Mother: You can go in and look at the nurse's face and determine if your baby's okay or not.
> Father: But if it doesn't feel right in your gut, go with it. Go with your gut feeling. You *do* have control and you *can* help in some of these decisions.
> Mother: It's *your* baby.
> Father: Trust the people in there yet have enough confidence in yourself to take part in the decision-making process.

In general, future parents of NICU infants were encouraged to pursue information about all options and seek the opinions of others, not to necessarily accept what was first told them. Since medical care is not infallible, parents need to be prepared for those treatments and procedures that do not achieve normalcy in the infant. They should try to keep prayer, hope, love, and support alive as they experience the tenuous life of a high-risk newborn and the tragedy of hospitalization. Only a few parents were so completely negative that they were unable to view the experience and explore the possibility of change and improvement. One parent addressed the downside of the experience with some very important advice about the adverse responses engendered by this sort of ordeal, "...confusion, anger, hurt. But these are all normal for parents under arduous circumstances. The point is to not let them destroy you or your relationships with others." As another father noted, those who really care about you will understand and accept your responses, realizing that you need time to adjust to such a disaster.

Two women were pregnant again and parents were prompted to emphasize the need for pregnant women to take very good care of themselves, particularly if anyone was pregnant with multiples. They wanted these women to ask questions and be sure to talk to the doctor.

Offering their suggestions spurred some of the veteran parents to seek advice from the interviewers about their own situations. Additionally, as noted in the Methodology, some conversations continued after the tape recorder was turned off as we made recommendations to families about resources related to our concerns for the infant's status and/or family functioning. We decided that, from an ethical perspective, we could not simply leave those homes without at least attempting to alert the families to our professional concerns and remind them of the selected elements of the discharge plans. One example will illustrate such circumstances:

> *Strong denial.* The interview with Sally did not begin on a very good note. Although she had readily agreed to the session when contacted by telephone, Sally seemed surprised to see the interviewer when she answered her door. Sally invited her in but did not offer to take her coat or indicate where she could sit. During the initial conversation Sally assured the interviewer that she understood the request for the interview and was willing to participate, and that this was as convenient a time as any, so the interview should proceed. The physical position Sally then took, however, belied her previous affirmation of her willingness to be interviewed. Although Sally sat next to the interviewer on the sofa, she turned away from the tape recorder on the cushion between them. Nevertheless the discussion began, but not before the interviewer repositioned herself on the floor with the tape recorder between Sally and herself, in order to adequately capture the dialogue.
>
> Sally warmed to the conversation as the interview continued and was boldly forthcoming in sharing her story about the NICU and her child's initial six months at home. During the discussion, however, the behavior of the infant, Larry, and his interaction with Sally drew the interviewer's attention. Larry was enormous and his size was difficult to comprehend given his discharge weight. He screamed periodically throughout the interview and each time Sally would put a bottle in his mouth. As Sally became absorbed in her responses to The interviewer's, she failed to pay attention to how she was directing the bottle and would jam the nipple in Larry's cheek or stretch his mouth way to the side. Eventually the bottle was empty but Sally continued to thrust it in Larry's direction each time he shrieked.
>
> Although Larry seemed reasonably alert and smiled at times, he did not have the physical movement normally expected for an infant his age. He did not yet turn over. His eyes tracked the bottle as it wavered over his head so he seemed to be without excessive visual problems. Based on the discharge summary for the infant and some additional

assessment by the interviewer, he was thought to be mentally retarded or possibly deaf. He was scheduled for auditory, visual, and motor assessment in the interval since discharge, in order to minimize learning disabilities. When discussing his status, Sally seemed oblivious to his growth and development trajectory and any identifiable problems, despite her education and professional experiences closely related to her own son's possible problems.

At the end of the interview, the interviewer abandoned her research role and urged Sally to get some special help for Larry--for example--an infant stimulation program. There had been recommendations at discharge for follow-up with specialists and involvement in such a program. Sally was not accessing any additional resources in the community but was instead simply dropping the infant off at a private home for routine day care when she went to work. In the evening she was quite tired, she explained. It was all this slender, petite woman could do to complete a task or two around the house, get her own supper, then feed and bathe Larry before she collapsed into bed herself. Sally was amenable to the suggestion for her infant, however, because she truly wanted the best for Larry. She agreed that something additional would probably improve his functioning and she promised to make the necessary telephone calls.[h]

What the Future Might Bring

A variety of parental outlooks were collected as we left parents at six-month postdischarge and they themselves were asked to look forward. On the positive side this father whose children have serious problems, comments on the necessity of:

> ...always being optimistic, always being hopeful for the best thing. You have to think that the future's going to be bright. Just have a positive outlook.

His wife replies:

> I'm still very concerned about her, very concerned. Even if somebody has a slight handicap...you know how mean kids can be. They can make fun of them. But I'm going to try and accept it more and more, I think.

Another woman ponders the effects of her baby's death on herself and her future:

> Right now, even though I am going through changes...I just sat down and watched the videotape [of the baby] the other day for the first time. I know even though I do hurt inside, that she is better off where she is. Especially with the changes that I've been going through. It has affected my two-year-old greatly which affects me. I'm a bit more sure of myself now. I know that maybe in the future I'll be ready for another child...everything's that happened is helping to make me just a little bit stronger.

What might we really encounter in parental responses after several years' hiatus from the NICU experience and additional years of experience with the child? Time certainly has a totally unpredictable effect on people's lives. What specifically will occur in these families? What memories will families continue to harbor about the NICU event? What advice will parents give from a more experienced perspective? In the next chapter we will jump ahead several years to find out.

Notes

[a] Brinchmann (1999) discusses the phenomenon of the home as a "prison" when a child with special needs is cared for by parents. Although the parents in Brinchmann's study were caring for older children, the same themes of less than adequate rest and sleep as well as the problem of feeding the children were present.

[b] Gennaro's findings (1996) support a change in employment for women in families of preterm low birthweight infants during the first six months postdischarge. Fewer women returned to work than those without preterm births and families incurred non-reimbursed expenses (2% to 4% of their income).

[c] This woman spontaneously offered a copy of her diary to us. We gratefully accepted and would like to once again state our appreciation for this gesture. The information was enlightening and added to our understanding. There was nothing in her entries that would have led us to change any of the material we have produced related to this project. It was, rather, further affirmation of our interpretation and conclusions of the results. She began her diary with the initiation of labor at 25-26 weeks gestation and gave us her entries up to and including the date of the six-month postdischarge interview.

[d] Debate continues about whether or not parents should be present during medical rounds. This debate is summarized in "Parents on rounds: The debate." 2001. *Advances in Family-centered Care,* *7*(1), 21-24.

[e] Cardiopulmonary resuscitation (CPR) is one treatment that must be implemented immediately to be effective. CPR is different from the usual treatments in that health professionals operate under the presumption that CPR will be used unless otherwise indicated. A "No Code" or "Do-not-resuscitate" order (DNR), is used to designate a decision whereby CPR will *not* be used on a patient when cardiac or pulmonary arrest occurs. Should the patient stop breathing, or the heart stop beating, the natural processes that follow the crisis will be allowed to occur. No attempt will be made to revive patients by breathing for them, compressing the heart to possibly start it again, or other emergency measures such as the use of stimulants (drugs). A DNR or No Code order is often specified for those patients who have a very poor prognosis and will not recover, or who are unable to withstand the trauma of the resuscitation.

[f] At the moment this couple was describing the No Code decision, this was the only description they gave of the infant's condition. The discharge summary indicated that the developmental potential of this infant was very much at risk considering the degree of her cerebral damage and cortical loss. The overall potential was "guarded." The father went on after the No Code discussion to more specifically describe their daughter's present and potential functioning.

[g] *CAT scan* stands for computerized axial tomography, which is a noninvasive examination of deep body parts. It combines x-ray beams with a computer to create three dimensional representations of these parts.

[h] A follow-up contact with Sally affirmed her pursuit of services to meet Larry's special needs. At the four-year postdischarge interview, she had indeed accessed some limited services for her son. He continued, however, to have very serious problems--mobility, visual, verbal, mental, and behavioral--which will require life long assistance. Sally admitted, however, that her own decreased financial resources and personal relationship problems have prevented her from establishing and maintaining a consistent program of interventions for her son. Her life is a struggle on several levels.

CHAPTER 4

Four Candles on the Birthday Cake

Four years have passed since Herbert's discharge from the NICU. His parents, Kathy and Mike, discussed in their separate interviews how Herbert has been doing since that discharge. Although both are quite positive about Herbert's status in response to the initial question, replying that he is good or fine, when asked to explain this answer each takes a somewhat different approach. Mike immediately downgrades his evaluation and then goes on to explain the speech problems Herbert is experiencing, while Kathy at first skates around the issue and gets more specific only after she is pointedly asked to affirm that there have been no problems since the discharge.

Mike mentions only the problem related to talking and has difficulty explaining Herbert's speech impediment. Finally, he simply defines it as speech that is hard to understand. Herbert is not seeing a therapist, which Mike questions. The pediatrician indicated that Herbert will grow out of this lack of clarity but, although he has improved some, Mike is not happy with the current situation. He compares Herbert to the couple's other son and declares his reservations about the "wait and see" approach to his son's difficulty.

Kathy starts her description of Herbert's problems with the respiratory complications; she calls these asthmatic problems and goes on to explain the continued monitoring of his hearing and vision. Herbert's hearing has been found to be fine but the physicians want to continue to evaluate his vision. Herbert has had a series of allergy tests that have been negative for grasses, pollen, mold, and wheat, but Kathy has noted that cigarette smoke and sudden changes in the weather really bother him. He was hospitalized four times in the first year after discharge for asthma attacks and continues with daily medication for the problem.

As Kathy continues with her explanation, her description of Herbert's health expands to include the apnea episodes that he experienced when he was first discharged. Herbert was discharged on an apnea monitor and remained on it for about nine months. Simple stimulation was sufficient to get Herbert to breathe when the monitor's alarm sounded and CPR was never required. Although she was assured that these episodes were not related to his prematurity at birth and that normal, full-term babies also have apnea, Kathy was not convinced. She also connects the asthma to these episodes.

In general, Kathy believes that Herbert has been slow in growth and development. Although the pediatrician vouches for his placement within a normal range for children his age, Kathy says, "We tend to do that naughty parent thing and compare the first one with the second." She finds his progress slower than his older brother- rolling over, sitting up, walking, talking. She wonders about future development and whether or not Herbert will catch up.

Returning to the hearing evaluation, Kathy expresses her lack of assurance that "everything is OK." She says that she is not at all happy with the way things are. Kathy asked point-blank whether there could be a connection between a possible hearing problem and the fact that Herbert simply does not speak clearly. Kathy then repeatedly presses the interviewer to give her opinion about Herbert's speech. The child is present off and on during the interview and some of the garbled speech is recorded on the tape. Herbert asked several direct questions of the interviewer but on each occasion the interviewer has to look to Kathy for an interpretation--it was impossible for a stranger to understand this four-year-old, even a pediatric nurse. A denial of the problem is neither logical nor ethical.

At the close of the formal portion of the session, the interviewer returns to this issue and works with Kathy on a possible approach that she and her husband might take when they next visit the pediatrician. the interviewer affirms Kathy's uneasiness about Herbert, as a legitimate parental concern that could be pursued with the physician. While respecting the pediatrician's opinion, Kathy could simply express her and her husband's continuing worry and request a referral for further speech and hearing evaluations of their child. Kathy seems satisfied with this suggestion and relieved to have her perception validated.

When describing their current situation, Kathy and Mike are exemplars of the families at four years postdischarge when describing their current situation. All the parents view their circumstances in a somewhat different fashion. For the most part, they are managing family life with the special needs of their child. However, they could use a little assistance in optimizing their level of functioning. The stories of families at four years postdischarge and their recollections of the NICU experience equip us to better understand the challenges of their lives.

Life Goes On

Four years after discharge from the NICU, families had moved into a new phase of their lives. The newborn experience was definitely past although residual effects of that situation may not be far below the surface. Some parents were quick to recall the events which most powerfully impacted them as they faced life with a high-risk infant.

The theme for this phase, life goes on, comes from one father's evaluation of their circumstances. They had twins with serious sequelae. He was headed down a bitter, resentful path when he and his wife turned their mental attitude around. The children were born at 26 weeks at 700 and 840 grams respectively. They were hospitalized for 159 days. Both children remained in conditions requiring total 24-hour-a-day care...

> This has been a very, very difficult experience for my wife and I, but we've learned a lot. We've matured a lot. Back when we first started this we were a couple of snot-nosed kids who thought we knew a lot but we really didn't know anything. We've...ah...it's brought us closer. It really has and basically we're fairly... we're a happy family right now. We've made a commitment. We made a commitment to these children and I'm not going to shirk it now. Down the road, who knows what will happen. As we get older something will happen to these kids but we'll accept it. Live with it...and die with it, you know. We've learned to accept, enjoy the good times and accept the bad. We've been very, very, very bitter. We were blaming it on someone else. We basically lost all of our friends. No one wanted to listen to our crap, no one wanted to hear about it any longer. Sure you've got problems [they said], but let's go on with life. And so, with time, we are making it. You come around or you don't survive. Life goes on.

Parents with young children like these do not have the time to dwell on the past. Child-care for normal children is very demanding so anyone with a special-needs child has few moments for concentrated reflection, although parents shared some of this type of musing during the interviews. The sight of another child in a condition similar to their own child's, a program on television, the sight of the hospital they had so frequently visited, or an offhand remark about birth or newborn care will elicit a flashback to the experiences of their own NICU days. The memories and the emotions are then right there beneath the surface. One mother said (emphasis added)...

> It's funny. The, further away you get from that, the more you forget, *unless you talk to somebody who's been through it recently or something.*

Some parents noted "foggy memories," the need to wipe out unpleasant things, the light years that had passed since they had a baby in the hospital, or the sense that "[sometimes] it seems as if it really didn't happen." One mother claimed that she has had much worse experiences since discharge than at any time during the NICU hospitalization. However easy or difficult the parents' recall, the interview was sufficient to trigger memories for everyone. Interestingly, one mother noted, "...you never know if what you remember is actually what happened."

Generally, families kept discussions about their NICU experiences and the infant's sequelae to themselves as the years went by. As already mentioned above, when responses became complaints, friends and extended family members lost their tolerance for listening to these parents. One parent indicated that their first year after discharge was "an absolute wreck." Certainly not everyone had a medically demanding situation. And although not all families currently have on-going medical issues, the verdict is still out for some.

In our society, normalcy is almost revered. These families were well aware of the need to minimize handicaps, or at least publicly ignore them, and maximize the child's accomplishments. "Concerns about child development, serious sequelae, or handicaps were not issues parents revealed in public places" (Pinch & Spielman 1996, p. 76). As one parent indicated,

> We've got two kids that...that ah...we're going to have the rest of our life and...and ah, I...I have a feeling we're going to die unhappy. That's my feeling, because we're going to be lonely. And what's going to happen to these kids if they do survive after we're not around? These are issues I think about every day. It just gets harder, it doesn't get easier.

Parents also expressed the belief that mature adults should control their emotions and deal objectively with their circumstances when out and about in the community.

Normalcy focused on two areas: the child's development and the family's life. Parents compared their own child and family life to some sort of standard or goal they had set. It was important for the child to be like other children of the same age and for family life to be typical of other similar families. When children or family life did not display this normalcy, parents felt an acute loss. One parent compared her family to another family she met in the NICU:

> They've got normal children now and they've got a family. They've got a happy life. We're still, in that same ICU mode. We're still running to [city] constantly, we're still dealing with medical emergencies...our life is, I don't know, so many. It's, it's affected every inch of our life, from our marriage to our finances, you know, to our family, everything.

In other families, a sense that they had adapted prevailed; according to one father, his four-year-old says that when he dies and goes to heaven, then he will have two kidneys and play football. One parent commented, "I'm where I thought I'd be...married with a family and children."

Although two individuals generally addressed "how time had flown" by since discharge, most people were more specific and related stories about either the child or themselves and their family. Most of the parents focused on the child's growth and development while emphasizing "she's a neat kid," "the miracle of the whole result," "I was impressed with...actually, the way he turned out"; and "There isn't anything I would change about her." Some described the child as a challenge while others emphasized their fear that some crisis could still happen, the possible death of a child, and the handicaps with which the children must continue to live. The families focused on discussions of other children, traveling, moving, divorce, work, stress, and fatigue. A mother said, "This might sound really goody-goody, but I think what stands out is that we actually survived, you know, we, we're, we're not divorced!" The iatrogenic effects of the infant's survival have an impact not only on the infant's future functioning but the outcome for an entire family unit.

Parents were also overwhelmed with their responsibilities since the NICU discharge: "It's just been a real struggle...it's changed our life totally"; "the grind...just the grueling day in, day out, never an end to it"; "I have no vacation time, no sick time left because all my time goes to taking [child]...to the doctors"; "We are not the same people we were back when you first met us"; "acceptance of what we have, handicapped children." Yet at least one parent saw a positive side: "What stands out the most is that we actually survived...we managed to go on and stay basically a whole family."

Parents were asked specifically about the child's growth and development. As in the six-month postdischarge interview, parents initially replied "pretty good" or "doing great" but subsequently qualified that statement. Those more detailed responses were categorized as problematic development given the substantial qualifications offered by these parents (see Table 4.1 for children's status at 4 years postdischarge).

At the time of the four-year interview, only one child could be categorized as having had no problems, and presently is, in fact, in good or very good health. In this case, both parents agreed on the status of the child.

For seven children, parents admitted to serious sequelae or major health issues that were present or ensued since discharge. Three children have cerebral palsy, two had strokes, two have multiple sequelae including profound physical and mental symptoms, and two had serious brain bleeds that account for present developmental problems (multiple issues in some children). In all cases of children with such sequelae, both parents agreed on the child's compromised status.

Of the remaining 21 children whose parents began the discussion by saying that their children were great or doing fine, all showed evidence of problems, delays, or slow development. These problems included both the physical (sitting, walking, motor coordination, size) and the mental (speech, cognitive functioning) aspects of the child's development. Parents most often identified their child (this symptomatology is overlapping) as "underweight," followed closely by poor speech patterns. In addition children had vision and hearing losses. One child has bilateral hearing aids and three are blind in one eye. Seven were identified as mentally "slow" and two were diagnosed as mentally retarded. Parents who have other children (either older or younger than the high-risk neonate), pointed out that they noticed delays or differences from the norm when they compared the NICU child to a sibling, either an older child or a subsequent child who may have caught up with or surpassed the NICU graduate. Parents did not

Table 4.1 ***Characteristics of children in study as newborns and at four years***

No.	Birthweight	Gestational Age	Days in NICU	Current Health Problems
01A	1370 gm	29	72	R
01B	1200	29	71	G&D
03	970	30	68	H, S, G&D
05	680	27	117	G&D
06	1720	32	40	R, S
07A	1220	34	41	S
07B	2480	34	18	G&D, Surgery
08A	1450	31	32	G&D
08B	1680	31	32	H, G&D
09	2600	33	8	**No Problems**
10	3100	36	13	G&D
11	4000	37	29	Mobility, G&D
13	2230	36	12	G&D
14	870	25	110	S, Eye surgery, R
16	1000	28	51	Rehospitalized
18	1060	26	97	Serious
20A	1820	32	27	R, G&D
20B	1920	32	27	R, G&D
20C	1860	32	37	R, G&D
21	3410	35	17	Serious
22	1278	29	37	Serious
23A	700	26	159	Serious
23B	840	26	109	Serious
25A	780	26	96	G&D
26	2020	31	14	R, sinus
28A	950	27	78	R, ↓ mental
28B	970	27	90	Mobility, R, S
29	940	27	79	R, Hearing
30	720	25	96	Serious
32	3011	37	22	G&D, R

Key: G&D = growth & developmental delay; H = hearing; S = speech; R = Respiratory; Serious = multiple complications

necessarily agree on these evaluations, and fathers were more optimistic in their responses than mothers

Some children had been rehospitalized for surgery or respiratory conditions. Respiratory problems were the norm rather than the exception, including frequent colds and related ear infections. Asthma, pneumonia, and placement of tubes in ears were the most frequent etiologies for repeat hospitalizations. Parents generally attributed these problems to the child's premature birth.

Preschool was a theme when parents were asked to discuss concerns that stood out since discharge. Predominant decisions were whether or not to send the child to preschool, when to send the child, whether to choose a regular program or one targeting the handicapped, and what the purpose of the attendance was: learning skills versus socialization. Two families mentioned school concerns about older children. More women addressed the school issue than men. The children attending preschool had often been identified as slow learners, as handicapped, or as having speech problems. Two mothers with handicapped children addressed the issue of deafness and the special school needs of their children. Parents of multiple birth children discussed whether to send all children at the same time or whether they should all be in the same class. One mother addressed her lack of trust in day care.[a]

Approximately 25% of the families addressed discipline as a difficult issue. Knowing "how much is too much" and "how much is not enough," as well as the "how-to" of discipline, was a concern. One parent put the question succinctly: "part of it's because they're twins, part of it's cause they're the first." This issue seemed important to address because parents indicated that the discipline decisions were influenced by the fact that the infant had been in the NICU. These parents wondered whether or not discipline decisions should be different because of this infant's start in life.

Handicap, *disability*, and *impaired* were used as search words in an examination of the interviews, given their presence in discussions of these children and the common use of these terms. We wanted to know if parents actually used these words or some euphemism in describing their children. The paucity of results indicated that these words were not readily used.

Handicaps were discussed by parents whose newborns had been at risk and who were grateful they had been spared or by parents whose children had the most severe impairments.[b] Parents who addressed the fact their children were indeed handicapped or attending school for the handicapped did so with great reluctance. After four years, parents did not appear to have accepted the limitations of their children. For these parents, "hope springs eternal." Parents addressed the stigma attached to the word *handicap*. One parent reflected on the potential dangers of non-acceptance, however:

> I think all of us have certain handicaps, whether they're physical handicaps or mental handicaps, capability handicaps, and many different things. So who's to say why now, if I can't perform to a certain level that everyone else seems to think they want [me] to perform..., [that] I'm not handicapped. Do we start weeding people out?

Two families whose children had serious sequelae did not use the words *handicapped*, *impaired*, or *disability* at all throughout the interview. They either used a general word like *problem* or they specifically named the issue. In Layne's autobiographical account (1996), she labeled her experience as a happy story, partly because "the developmental pediatrician assured us that *disability* would be an optional term for Jasper" (emphasis hers) emphasizing the ultimate importance of appearances. Jasper was only two years old however when Layne wrote this account and she does acknowledge an uncertain future for her child despite his *luck* thus far.

A small number of families continued to discuss the use of monitors. This figure did not match the greater number for whom monitors were ordered at discharge. These were used from four months to one year, a time span that overlapped the interval between the second and third interviews. The apnea monitor represented a form of security for most parents. The most relevant comment expressed by parents was their reliance upon the monitor to decrease their anxiety while they slept at night or whenever the baby slept. Parents readily admitted that the monitor's alarms rang and their child required stimulation to begin breathing again. The emotional response to monitors going off in the middle of the night was the worst aspect as parents gradually learned the problem was not serious in a majority of cases. No parent had to administer CPR. Some parents, especially mothers, found it difficult to give up the monitor. One woman explained that she finally was forced to stop using the monitor because her son learned to unhook the device which made the alarm sound. He loved having everyone run to him. This tactic was amusing for a while but then became a nuisance.

The parental evaluation of the outcome of having a baby born prematurely or spending time in the NICU varied. Most parents commented that if the child seemed to be normal, then everything would be *OK*. One parent stated the outcome and acceptance of their situation might have been a "whole different ball game" if the child could not be considered *normal*. Those who had children with disabilities found life revolved around these children and that their family was totally different because of them. Having a child with special problems was acknowledged as a big burden. Two parents in the same family, expressed dissimilar views of the outcome, with the mother saying, "I've accepted it" while the father said, "There are many, many times that I wish we did not have David." He went on to explain:

> I'm weak at heart you know. I could make that hard decision [to continue to treat], even through David is going to lead a very, very frustrating life. Everything, everyday, he's...that's why he screams. He's frustrated. We, ah, life with David would be infinitely easier, even with all the other things I just mentioned if he was just pleasant, if he was just happy but he's not...when I try to make somebody understand what it's like, it's like, it's like, take a normal child and have them with the flu. Where they're grumpy and...and out of sorts and hard to live with and that's what living with David is like, every day.

This child was born at 25 weeks, weighed 720 grams at birth, and was discharged in 96 days. This father continued:

> We've had a hard time keeping him healthy. Every system he has is weaker and underdeveloped [compared to his younger sister]. He's always had trouble digesting food. We have to put enormous amounts of calories through him at times and he don't seem to use the nutrition that's given to him. He's always been...rattly.
>
> He can roll over with assistance but he doesn't like to be on his stomach. He can move his head a little and he can point. He picks out his clothes in the morning. He seems to hear fine and although he is nearsighted, he can see a smile across the room. His right eye wanders a lot. I feel his mental ability is near normal but he cannot speak. He can't control his behavior and his emotions are right on the surface. He's grumpy all the time, like a normal child with a permanent flu.
>
> We've developed a pattern where Norma [the mother] takes care of him during the day and I take care of him at night and the weekends. So that, when the rest of the world...she's frustrated at the end of the day from constant care. And ah, she says, "I'm glad you're home, here he is. Because I'm going to take care of myself. I'm going to take care of the house and I'm going to do a few of the other things." And on weekends, a lot of the care falls to me, unless there are certain male jobs around the house. And those things are always there. We redid all of our plumbing and stuff like that you know.

The father was asked how this care arrangement came about:

> David was totally dependent upon Norma until Gretchen was born. So Norma more or less decided that she wanted me to feed David. So most meals I'm there feeding David. Part of it's to break him of complete dependence on Norma. That's a whole other thing that we talked about. Part of it was the increasing demands of Gretchen during the day--and, you know, caring for both kids. But he was totally dependent upon Norma. Dad couldn't do anything right, couldn't hold him, couldn't feed him as long as Mom was somewhere in the house. So she couldn't leave. Well, Gretchen came along and that situation was dramatically changed. And since that time I've taken care of most of his meals. And an infinite number of small..., small, hard decisions about his care. All day long, every, every, every day. The grueling day in, day out, never an end to it.

The research assistant wrote the following field notes:

> This man differed significantly from the happy, optimistic mother of David. Norma did break down emotionally during the interview but she finds strength and renewal through her spiritual life.

The research assistant found it very difficult to select the appropriate words to describe the father:

> But, I perceive him to be a beaten man. Very down-trodden. This interview was extremely pessimistic. When I did the first two interviews, these people were both positive in their outlooks, earthy people, living in the country, eating natural food. He was pursuing his dream of independence and work as a carpenter. He was devoted to Pheasants Forever.[c] I heard not one word about Pheasants Forever in this interview. In the earlier interviews I saw a round-faced, pinked-cheeked, happy man. In this third interview, I never saw him smile. I came away with the most depressed feeling about this man and his family, and especially his child. As he walked me to my car he still wanted to talk. He talked, and talked, and talked. His wife had taken the other children and loaded them into the car to go out for pizza. David was still in the house on his bed in the living room. So I finally said to the father, I have some real concerns about you, your health, and how you are nurturing your marriage. So he says:
>
> How can you nurture a marriage when you don't even sleep with your wife? My sole responsibility in this house is baby-sitting. David requires care all night long and it is just easier to sleep with him than to have him fuss and wait for attention until I get awake and go to his room.

The research assistant's comments continue:

> David is such a huge burden for this man, this family. David is by far the smallest child in the family despite the younger age of Gretchen, who is just beginning to toddle around. David has severe cerebral palsy and looks just like an old, anxious, wizened man. And his pained expression never leaves his face. Throughout the interview he was constantly crying or fussing. Nothing his father did pleased him or met his needs. His father got upset and even angry--but I could not blame him as I don't know how I could put up with such a responsibility 24 hours a day.

This was an ambivalent man who felt burdened by what he perceived to be his first and only decision--to resuscitate and treat at birth. As this description demonstrated, not all of the parents' stories have happy endings. In fact, the *endings* have not really been written, given the young age of these children. The integration of a child with special needs into the family, however, can be very challenging. As one father describes the parents' on-going emotional status: "It's a tremendous ball and chain on us, on the family, brothers, and sisters...an emotional drain." Support is a critical ingredient in these situations.

Dimensions of support and the people who provide it were as numerous as the subjects who identified any support. Other parents of high-risk infants that these families met, either while the mother was in labor or during the baby's residence in the NICU, and support groups continued to be the two most frequent sources of strength. Other usual sources of support were mentioned: ministers, nurses, neighbors, and relatives. One parent included the availability of the Ronald McDonald House and another named small-town living. Women found support groups helpful and, if there was no group, they started one. In addition, some parents mentioned their disappointment at the *lack* of assistance from relatives and/or neighbors.

Over half of the parents discussed finances in one way or another. Proportionally more fathers (62%) discussed finances than mothers (57%). Predominately parents were concerned about burdensome hospital bills. At four years after discharge, parents vividly remember their encounters with insurance companies concerning hospital bills. Parents viewed insurance companies as a hassle with repeated submissions and denials, delayed payments, and monumental amounts of paperwork for ongoing medical bills, which continued for months or even years after discharge. In some cases the insurance did not cover entire bills and parents go on perceiving some procedures and tests as unnecessary. They also observed that the bills were not easy to decipher: one mother persists in spending many hours sorting through the bills to determine what expenses were legitimate and then to figure what the insurance would and would not pay. Parents agreed that having an intensive care baby was expensive, requiring them to pay for years on the unpaid balance. Maintaining a job and returning to work remained financial issues for parents. One mother said she just wanted her child to get better and she didn't care what the bill would be. Another indicated the bills were *not* a burden. Other financial concerns centered on family expenses for subsequent infant hospitalization and the relationship between those expenses and the need to keep or get a job. When insurance is tied to employment, your "insurance holds you hostage," one father said. One mother indicated that she was eventually fired because of the number of sick days she took in order to care for her special needs child. She indicated that it was impossible to find another job with this child-care responsibility. Finding day care for children with special needs was hopeless in her situation. Those whose children had special needs face an ongoing financial crisis with possible future hospitalizations, the need for appliances and medications, and the construction of wheelchair accessible housing.

Parents discussed both negative and positive aspects of themselves. Parents generally seemed quite confident and responsible (as opposed to their indecision in previous interviews). It must be remembered that these individuals were now older and had by one means or another survived the crisis of a NICU hospitalization. For some this has meant change, in order to function as an advocate for their children and provide them with the required resources. One father stated, "I can feel...good about myself. I have taken care of and provided for my family no matter what that family turns out to be."

Others note limitations in themselves:

> I mean, here's this professional person and, you know, I mean doctors and god. They're right on the same level, aren't they, in our culture? And, and we're saying, "No, I don't agree with what you're saying and I don't like what you're saying." And...actually we never said that. We just didn't go back.

Some parents were troubled because they were unable to understand their spouse or others at times--their attitudes or behavior--which they connected to the challenges of this child. Others remarked that they still did not feel as well as they anticipated, or they were frightened as they anticipated possible future events. One mother continued to discuss her residual sequelae from the high-risk pregnancy. Another mother struggled with her present symptomatology and its possible relationship to her three weeks in the ICU after the birth.

Parents discussed having other children and the effect of the high-risk infant on this decision. As a result of the NICU experience parents chose doctors and hospital NICUs very carefully with subsequent pregnancies. More often than not, parents stated there would be no more children because of the care entailed by this, their special child. These parents readily admitted that they would like to have had more children, however, they felt that the time, care, and financial limitations of the NICU child were prohibitive. A few others were "surprised" at a subsequent pregnancy while the remainder indicated that they had always planned to have more children and that additional ones were welcome. However, although two women were pregnant at the time of the four-year postdischarge interview, almost all parents were now at the stage where they do *not* plan to have more children. Several women noted their decision to not become pregnant in order to avoid another high-risk pregnancy. One young parent remarked, "Yeah, and in five years I'll be 21 and after I hit 21, I'm going to get my tubes cut, tied, and burnt." Sixteen families have had a pregnancy since the birth of the high-risk infant. In one divorced couple, the father and his present partner had a set of twins but the mother of their high-risk baby has had no subsequent pregnancies; one woman had a miscarriage, and another woman has had two elective abortions.

One of the most profound discoveries I made during this project occurred during the secondary analysis of the data, after all three interviews were conducted and the primary analysis of the data was reported. My experience serves to document a monumental difference in these parents when I was able to compare their discussions at four years postdischarge with their initial predischarge conversation. Drew (1989) discusses the investigator's journal as relevant data in a qualitative study. She particularly targets the phenomenological method but, given my experience, I believe it applies to other qualitative methods as well. Therefore I am including my experience with the data here.

Very briefly the secondary analysis procedures, described in detail in the Appendix, involved rereading each parent's set of three interviews. Chronologically this rereading followed the four-year postdischarge phase of the project. I repeatedly failed to be able to recognize these individuals as I reviewed their description of predischarge events. After several years of research and hundreds of hours spent reading and rereading the transcripts, I was initially puzzled by my inability to mentally identify the parent when rereading the predischarge account. I felt that I had truly learned who these individuals were and had committed many of their experiences to memory. Now I found that these people did not at all seem like the same people we had interviewed at four years postdischarge. My curiosity took over and after a few perplexing experiences, I began to look up the individual's identity in the code book before I read the predischarge transcript.

My bafflement then became shock and surprise as I read these predischarge records. My experience encompassed two levels of response. First, my impressions related to the parents' development, a more scholarly interpretation of my experience. At predischarge parents were in crisis, given the unexpected course of events and the serious condition of the infant. Parents lacked experience with and knowledge of the NICU. Most of them were naive and trusting as they attempted to cope with the hospitalization of their child and their own emotional responses. Over the course of four years these parents became or regained their self-assurance and self-confidence. They were knowledgeable and clearly aware of the effect of this experience and its possible life-long impact. Although some parents still faced challenging circumstances, their embroilment in the crisis of a NICU during the predischarge interview and its immobilizing effect was a past event. Some individuals recognized this change themselves but it seemed to be a most sharp perception for me as I jumped from the "new" self at four years back to the self that started on this journey when the infant was in the NICU. Just how different parents had become was more dramatically apparent when I had the mental picture of the functioning, capable adult in mind as I read the complacent, accepting, passive presentation represented in the predischarge discussions.

On a second level, there was also my emotional reaction to the stark reality of the parents' situation as I read the predischarge transcripts and mentally compared the parents' discussion to what actually happened when they took this baby home and faced the meaning of its birth for their family. Not every family would confront difficulties but basically all families would encounter differences when compared to bringing home a healthy, full-term newborn. Predicting the future is impossible much less knowing exactly what the future will bring. But in a sense, that was my experience as I read the discharge document of a parent, I knew that parent's future. At this emotional level, reading the transcripts was a gut-wrenching struggle. I knew; I was impotent. I could not change their situation and I could not prepare them for the path upon which they had embarked. On several days I felt such a sense of doom that I had difficulty reading more than a few sets of interviews. I wanted to say, "Wake up! Look around. Listen to what you are told. Get ready." But such an opportunity was denied. The future I knew about had already come and gone.

Parents' responses including their passivity during the initial high-risk period can be easily overlooked or rationalized. Parental vulnerability was most acute and obvious when I read about their predischarge perceptions knowing what would ensue for them over the next four years. Their lack of confidence should not be confused with an ability to function. Although parents may temporarily be unable to meet the health professionals' standards of mature, adult performance, such skills and behavior will return. Or, in the case of the very young parent, these skills and behavior can be learned.

Realistically, no health professional knows exactly what will happen to any one individual infant or its family in the future. Yet general predictions are possible. Parental acquiescence to the health professionals' decision-making and care of the infant leaves the parents inadequately prepared for future events. Being marginalized also creates doubts in them later about the initial treatment of their child and its subsequent effect on them. Simply because parents are able to survive, and even grow and develop themselves as a result of these experiences does not absolve health professionals and others from attempting to facilitate parents' involvement while the infant is in NICU.

Memories of the NICU Experience

Present tasks and responsibilities pressed in on these busy parents and crowded out memories and emotions that relate to the NICU experience. In addition, the effect of this experience is something that parents keep private. Parents' remembrances were not far beneath the surface and, once discussion began, parents recalled in substantial detail the events and feelings of the NICU experience. The outstanding events were consistent or similar over time: an irritation, a loving touch, a crisis with the infant, a kindness expressed by another parent, displeasure with staff, a successful outcome, and a "miracle."

At four years postdischarge, the NICU experience was part of a family's history, albeit a compelling one. When asked to relate the story of their infant's hospitalization in the NICU, parents once again put that portion of their lives into context. Stories began with a description of the marriage or family life prior to this pregnancy, the ordeal of infertility, pregnancy issues, or the labor and birth itself. Many comments at this interview were similar to the stories told at the predischarge and six-months postdischarge interviews.

Parents balanced their discussion of the current phase of their lives with a retelling of the NICU experience, as opposed to the six-month interview when they constantly gravitated toward their postdischarge experiences. However challenging the present stage in these individuals' lives, once prodded they were equally able to relate the whole NICU story. The most obvious change from the predischarge interview was the lesser detail in the discussion of the actual NICU experience. Unless these events were recorded in some manner, such details tended to slip away, as indicated by the woman who at the six-month interview discussed the difference between her memories and her previous journal entries. Almost all of the same general themes as addressed by parents in the earlier interviews were included in the later interview. But general impressions were relayed rather than the more specific details in the stories of the predischarge phase.

Among the outstanding pre-NICU admission recollections, a number of women looked back and focused on the pain they experienced during their pregnancy. A greater emphasis was placed on this pain in the four-year interview than in the six-month one, where pain concerns were almost nonexistent. This experience of pain during pregnancy is something that the women believed our society generally negates but that only women know to be *very true*. These women felt that their pain was not noticed nor was it deemed important during obstetrical visits. They were concerned, at four years post-pregnancy, if the pain was related to the high-risk condition of the infant. And of course, in searching for a rationale for their unusual outcomes, it was difficult to determine retrospectively the relationship between their subjective observations and the infant's outcome. However, some women could compare this pregnancy with previous, or more importantly now, subsequent ones and knew that a normal pregnancy does not have the kind of pain they relate to this high-risk experience. One woman who was left with permanent mobility problems attributed her status to ignored pain after delivery. Her family continued to strongly resent the lack of physical therapy during her hospitalization, which may have impeded her recovery.

There were several other outstanding elements in the discussion that will each be examined in more detail below. The emotional response to the NICU experience was among the issues most often addressed at four years postdischarge. In addition, parents continued to emphasize their impressions of the fragility and vulnerability of the infant. Parental perceptions of treatments and procedures were probed and some new observations added. Families spoke more globally about their involvement in infant care in the nursery (or their lack thereof), rather than about details such as diapering, bathing, and the isolette environment, as they had at predischarge. The nasogastric feeding continued to stand out in their memories, however. The infant's pain was important, so too was the relevance of faith and spirituality as the parents traversed the obstacles of their experience with a hospitalized newborn. Parents gave further details about their observations of other infants and parents in the nursery and of the health professionals. A reverse in focus occurred since the issue of the evaluation of parents by health professionals was not addressed in any major way, but more detail was included in their stories about their perception of professional care.

The psychological dimension of the NICU experience was a predominant theme of these parents' stories when they looked back from the four-year postdischarge perspective. They discussed a broad gamut of emotions, documenting the stressfulness of the experience. Most often recounted was the emotional pain parents experienced as they thought about the physical pain of the infant. One father included the importance of their feelings in the ordeal. He recounted a decision-making event in which he was asked to participate during his wife's labor:

> So that's where we tried to base our information off...but we had to put the emotion in there too. 'Cause you can't make a decision like that just strictly on facts.

The compromising effect of emotions was also noted. Another father remarked, "I was pretty upset with them so I was...probably not hearing everything that they were telling me."

The absence of a relationship with the infant during the NICU hospitalization was a common topic as parents reviewed this time in their lives. Only one parent summarized the NICU period as one in which she was busy with infant care, helping the staff in the NICU. A few parents recalled their relative lack of involvement in the infant's life because they had to continue their jobs or schooling. One parent discussed her current insight as she moved further away from the intensity of the experience. She understood now all the "whys and why nots" concerning her infant's care and treatment. During the predischarge phase she was an assertive woman and regularly requested more involvement in the infant's care than she was allowed. She resented her treatment by the staff. She recalled that she was unable to accept explanations or they were not clear to her. Sometimes her requests for additional answers were denied.

> He stayed there a little over 100 days and now that I am away from all the pain and the craziness of the unit, I can see why they did some of the things they did you know. They didn't let us touch our baby. I understand medically now, a lot of the reasons why they don't let you touch your baby and hold him. It's, because it's such a shock to their system. They really need to be constantly watched and kept in a controlled, warm environment. Every time you touch them and take them out of the isolette, their temperature drops. Over-stimulation you know. At the time I couldn't see it, see it their way. One woman even told me that "he's not your baby until he leaves here." And I really resented that. But I...now I realize that she was just doing her job. Just looking out for what was best for my son.

Another mother characterized this period as one without control. Her limited opportunity to interact with her infant only occurred through feeding, "You can be there every three hours to feed them and that was it, you know. That's as much of...their life you could have. It was stressful." Other parents who spent long periods spent in the unit did not discuss any extended involvement with the infant's care. Another mother who wanted to promote a balanced perspective between professional caregiving and the family attachment offered additional insight:

> It's so intense there that you forget that this is a human, this is a child, I mean, this is not you know, a piece of machinery that...we want to make work.[d] It's...it's a child and he...you've got all those dynamics of mom and dad, and grandma, and brothers and sisters. And, and you know, all of those things need to be, are, are just as important, just as important as whether that kid is breathing or not...part of the recovery of this child depends on, and their future depends on dealing with these

> issues too. Because of the attachment that the family has for that child (Pinch & Spielman 1996, p. 77)

Once parents began to discuss the NICU experience in detail, they emphasized the infant's newborn appearance as well as their responses to its conditions and defenselessness. The analogies used by parents and their descriptions of the newborn were quite interesting. Newborns were compared to Barbie dolls, china dolls, birds that had fallen out of the nest, or frogs on the dissection table. Memories of fused eyes, transparent skin, bruises, and no smiles emphasized the fragility of the infants. Hearing the baby cry was a milestone as evidenced by this response:

> Well, when I heard Mary cry for the first time, which was about, she was about six weeks old...I felt that now there was more than just existing. There was a chance to be someone.

When the outcome was satisfactory or acceptable the baby was often viewed as a miracle from the four-year perspective. Mostly mothers described the result as a "miracle baby." One mother who referred to the infant's progress as a miracle very poetically stated "We bonded in a different way [in the NICU] and that was just watching him grow, watching him breathe, *watching the lights blink.*" The regularly blinking indicators on the various machines symbolized stability and survival. She clung to their continuing affirmation of her hopes.

In the case of one family with a severely handicapped child, however, the father's used the word "miracle" to describe the health profession's view of his child's survival, contrasted with his own. "Your miracle, my curse," he says:

> It's a great miracle to read about in the paper but I've got to take the miracle home and...ah, I have to be up with him at two or three o'clock in the morning and then I gotta be up at five-thirty and go to work. Because he was up screaming and uncomfortable and he...we have a lot of, an awful lot of...ah...problems. When all the cameras are gone, the *parents* take home a very sickly child. When the cameras are gone, the burden lies in a very quiet place, you know.

This father also bitterly voiced his criticism of the front-page coverage of the NICU reunion events. He claimed that his family was not welcome at such celebrations because the staff did not want to be reminded of their failures. Paneth (1992) expresses this theme in his censure of aggressive treatment for extremely low birth weight infants. He chastises neonatologists for neglecting to *publicly* acknowledge the limitations of technology and he calls for a "threshold of birth weight and gestational age below which *ordinarily* (there may be exceptions) it is inadvisable to apply the technology of intensive newborn care" (Paneth 1992, p. 155).

Parents basically reiterated their simplistic view of the infant's status in the NICU, the need to gain a little weight, a "little breathing thing." Some parents discussed a few more specific points related to the rationale for admission to the NICU. Most parents had superficial memories of treatments and surgical procedures used during the NICU hospitalization.

Ordinarily, parents continued to be unaware of the rationale for the possible use of common therapies, side effects, or potential outcomes in NICU with some exceptions. For example, several infants had been on ventilators, yet the iatrogenic effects (e.g., cranial bleed) of ventilators were unknown to most parents at this point even when these individuals were facing the untoward outcome of such a treatment in their own child.[e] One mother explained her recollection of a discussion about oxygen use:

> Well, they acted real positive about everything. I mean there was not a lot of...they said they hadn't had a lot of problems with the oxygen usage and all that kind of stuff.

This child was not on oxygen after discharge. One father summed up a common parental perspective on interventions in the NICU: "just everything as needed for whatever they [health care professionals] considered was normal...or safe."

More parents at four years were now better able to discuss oxygen, the rationale for its use, and the possible side effect of blindness. They now discussed treatments, which was an addition to the general knowledge base as compared to earlier interviews. Since this was a therapy continued in the home in a number of cases, it would appear that this knowledge was acquired after discharge. "Well, they explained to us oxygen could quite possibly--the higher the levels the more problems..." Information about this sequela came from a variety of sources, not just nurses and doctors in the NICU. Some parents indicated that their own independent reading was a source of information. One health professional *sent* the parent to her local public library to obtain the information. Another parent was provided with information by the oxygen company that delivered the tanks to her house after the infant was discharged from the unit.

When reassessing NICU care, a small number of parents felt a significant concern about the infants' blood transfusions received in the NICU. The parents' solution for the need for blood had been to offer to donate blood themselves but uniformly were told that it was not an option that the health professionals would even discuss. For a few parents who insisted on a reason, they were told that their donation could not be processed in a timely fashion and therefore could not be considered. One father said that the nurse laughed at them for thinking they could donate blood for their infant. Those who were informed about blood transfusions after the fact were indignant and worried that such a serious measure was done without their being informed. Some parents were quite sure that their infant received blood without their knowledge or permission but understood that they had no documentation for this belief. Parents now asked whether or not it would be advisable to have the children tested for AIDS. This concern stemmed from parental awareness after the infant's discharge, of the risk of HIV transmission due to increasing media attention to HIV and AIDS.

At four years postdischarge, a small group of parents (more than in earlier interviews) were clearly able to name specific drugs such as Lasix, Indocin, theophylline, Diamox, aminophylline, and phenobarbitol and types of drugs, such as antibiotics, steroids, and diuretics. Parents definitely recalled the use of surfactant and decision-making related to it. Some now expressed reluctance to permit the use of this as an experimental drug; others claimed they felt no hesitancy at the time and continued to feel the same. But all agreed, based on the explanation they had received, that the surfactant was necessary for the infant's optimal course. Others simply did not remember details about different medications, only bits and pieces like "something for her heart" or "to help lung development." Few parents recognized the possible side effects of drugs that their children received, such as hearing loss with certain antibiotics.

Parents discussed strong residual feelings related to the gavage feedings for their infants, and the strongest opinions were negative. They believed the gavage was inappropriately used for efficiency in feeding the infants--either nurses wanted to save time or infants were not sufficiently fast in their sucking. Infant discomfort was also associated with the placement of the nasogastric tube. One parent viewed the infant's experience as painful. Watching the nurse put the formula in the tube and seeing it run out the baby's mouth was distasteful. Some parents mentioned their concern for the adequacy of the feedings as well as the debate over breast milk versus formula. One mother now recalled that she was talked into pumping so that her infant could be fed breast milk, while another mother discussed at length her own insistence that she breast-feed her child in the face of staff disapproval. This mother, who was upset with the plan of care, captured her perception of the baby's adjustment and adaptation to feedings and change:

> So they tried putting her on that high calorie formula and every time they'd do that then she'd end up with blood in her stool or vomiting or something like that. And it was...was just...it was stupid to us because being farmers, you don't just change a feed on an animal just cold turkey like that.

Parents again mentioned their concern about possible pain for the infant but their recollections were no different in substance than those they had relayed at the predischarge interview. What parents emphasized at four years was their failure to be reassured when the staff told them either that the infants did not perceive pain or that the infant would not remember the pain. This assurance was diametrically opposed to what the parents observed and as a consequence they had doubts about the truth-telling or competence of the staff. For example, if an infant withdrew a foot during a stick for a laboratory test, would not this be a reaction to pain? It certainly was painful when they themselves experienced such a procedure. The parents were puzzled that they would be asked to believe that the foot withdraw was not an indication of perceived pain. They failed to accept an inability of the infant to remember the pain as a reason for not inflicting suffering.

Parents were more vocal at this third interview compared to the previous two when they were discussing how well aware they were of the other infants in the nursery. They scanned the NICU and compared their child to those infants in neighboring areas, listened to conversations, and tried to read various monitors for other children. For a few, this comparison resulted in feelings of guilt, sadness, relief, or having been cheated. Parents said that a need to "clear the nursery" indicated a crisis for some child. This was a frightening experience. Most often, other babies were viewed as "worse off," smaller, or sicker than the parents' own child. If only someone else was more frail or afflicted, then it was possible that they could manage their own infant. Parents observed that the healthiest babies were those "furthest away from the nurses' station." Parents knew of other families "who have taken home nearly vegetables." One parent asked:

> Are we using that [technology] wisely and do we have the decision-making process that decides when it's time *not* to use our technology...thankfully, the one that we did watch, she did die. But there was nothing there to live. You don't get all the information because you're supposed to respect other people's privacy when you're in a unit.

This need for privacy seemed to result in a code of acceptable behavior that parents imposed upon themselves: "You're not supposed to look over at their *shames*...and you're not supposed to overhear the conversations, and..., but you do [emphasis added]."

In the discussion of the NICU experience, parents evaluated the care that their infants had received. In general, although a perception of good care was initially mentioned, more specific inquiry actually teased out an equal number of positive and negative examples. Some of the examples were contradictory, as might well be expected. One parent recalled receiving support in their tragic situation while another spoke of abandonment during their plight. While parents reiterated the high quality of care their infants received, they included cautionary comments about ways in which their situation could have improved, similar to their discussion in previous interviews. Some evaluated their child's care by comparing their situation with that of other babies in the unit.

Parents discussed the need to trust health professionals either because they themselves did not know enough information to make decisions, or had never had this type of experience before, or because health professionals knew *better* even when parents did have some insight into the situation. Parents specifically compared physicians, nurses, and non-nursing staff. A hierarchy of power and control among the nursery physicians was a perception held most firmly by the parents at this interview. Their additional postdischarge experiences affirmed these impressions. They had to talk to the "right" physician. The most frequent problem for parents was communication and the provision of information, either getting it or not getting it. As one parent indicated, "The doctors never really talked but I did have a real good doctor."

During this interview, few individuals were able to rationalize the physician's reticence. They believed physicians did not want to scare patients or discouraged parents "because they [parents] cannot take losing the child." Challenging a physician's advice was onerous for parents:

> They're the possessors of this incredible technology machine and all of this knowledge and to doubt the medical establishment in American society is a real no-no.

Parents generally had a positive opinion of nurses:. "You know...it's actually the nurses who are with them [infants] and know what they're doing." Some parents believed nurses to be the best source of information, although parents also noted that nurses sometimes knew information they were not free to impart. Nurses were mentioned as instrumental in decreasing stress and helping meet family needs, through personal contact and telephone communication. Among several vivid negative experiences, parents now noted how wary they were of student nurses in the unit and also emphasized their dislike of the nurses' apparent ownership of the child. They particularly remembered the distress these nurses expressed when babies were discharged. Nurses wanted to continue to hold the baby even as parents waited to leave the unit after the infant was discharged. Parents described how some nurses cried as the infants were dressed for home. This observation had not been included in earlier interviews. One woman described her perception of the role of Social Services. She felt that her visits were monitored, and although she disliked the stress and anxiety the NICU produced in her when she went there, she believed if she did not go to see her baby, Social Services would institute measures to prevent her from taking the baby home.

In looking back, a number of people continued to indicate the importance of faith, belief in God, praying for the infant, or the help of the Lord. One mother spoke about her own spirituality in the following manner:

> Well, he's the best thing that ever happened to me and he's also the very worst thing that's ever happened to me. But, I would not be where I am spiritually if he wouldn't have been born. I wouldn't be a Christian at all. And, I would not have had the opportunity to grow spiritually if say, he would have been totally healed you know, from cerebral palsy, early on.

Generally, the infants' stay in the NICU was perceived as a long time ago. When parents drew their final conclusions about the experience, the feeling prevailed that much time had passed and many wounds had healed. Parents felt that, over time, a lot had been resolved; everybody just let go and accepted that life goes on:

> I've always felt like, don't complain about what you get. We were exceedingly poor when I was growing up. I, I developed a philosophy of don't complain about what you get. Just play the cards that are dealt you.

In the previous two phases of this study, parents were usually interviewed together, as described in the Appendix, The Research Enterprise. Data resulting from the strategy of interviewing parents separately revealed only a few differences between parents who both were available for the interview (17 pairs of parents). At this point, four years past the NICU events, the differences most likely represent more firmly entrenched variations.

The fathers' and mothers' stories of the NICU experience were diverse in the starting point or the emphasis, but, overall, the content and the details were the same. Mothers tended to begin the story with the birth experience and women included more discussion of the emotional aspect of the experience. Only mothers discussed the health care professional as a source of solace or comfort for them in their crisis. These women explained that support from nurses helped them decrease feelings of stress. Women reviewed feeding issues such as breast-feeding, gavage, or the central line more than their partners. In describing the newborn's status, women noted the need for weight gain but fathers included a wider variety of factors. When identifying a possible issue of conflict, women focused on children and family, while men targeted job-related incidents or community responsibility as well as finances. Finally, some parents did not agree on the current status of the child. Although both parents were likely to initially indicate that the child was good or OK, fathers were more positive in their appraisal even after probing in detail. Mothers were more specific about the child's status relative to growth and development percentiles and in the exact problems the child had encountered over the intervening four years.

It was our belief that at four years it may be too late to ascertain differences more definitively between the perceptions of mothers and fathers. Since most couples remained together and recounted these events between themselves or with others on numerous occasions over the intervening four years, the stories have probably coalesced. Each version of the experience is likely to be revised to be congruent with new information or coping needs, for example, but the story also takes in and encompasses ideas from the partner as one parent hears the other's story.

Perceptions of Ethical Decision-making in the NICU

At four years postdischarge, once again, most respondents (28 or 70%) clearly indicated that they were not involved in decision-making during the infant's residence in the NICU. The parental role was simply agreeing to whatever offered their child the best chance of survival. One father said, "I guess, you know, I don't know, I don't want to...I don't want to jeopardize his well being because of my ignorance." One father now stated in reference to a delivery room decision:

> But I would be very, very tempted to make a different decision but...you only have five to ten seconds to make that decision, and I am rather certain that I would have still made the same decision to let him live.

Parents were concerned about this secondary role: "And when we start taking authority away from parents, we start seeing a breakdown in every level," one father said. Now he questions, if parental decision-making is impeded when the child is a newborn, at what other point might it also be hindered? Sound families are needed for a sound society. Parents felt a certain level of incompetence because others, in this case health professionals, were in charge. But parental responsibility is not a dimension of family life that should come and go at whim. Parents discussed the responsibility of health professionals to support family cohesiveness during this crisis and help parents feel part of the infant's struggle for life in order for them to love and accept the infant into family life after discharge.

Four years after discharge permission to use surfactant continued to be the decision most readily recalled, although this event was prior to admission to the NICU. Other decisions prior to admission to NICU included having tubes tied, a request for a vaginal birth, and a decision put to one father not addressed in earlier interviews. The woman recounts her husband's experience:

> He was asked...if it came down to it, ah, which one would you rather have us save? He said that he had a two-year-old son at home and he needed help raising him, and he said he wanted both of us to live. He said, but if I have to choose I'd have to choose that I need, you know, I need help raising my...my son.

During his interview, the father of the child acknowledged his wife's dire situation when she was in labor but did not directly state his responsibility to make a choice between the child and the woman. He simply recalled that he was very upset and did not understand the staff's hesitancy in taking action to benefit his wife.

Other examples of decisions parents did discuss four years later were the baptism and naming of the baby, and their own activities: how much time to visit the children in the NICU, whether or not to continue to work or go to school. Several parents mentioned giving permission for surgery on their child (but this was a far lower number than the actual number of surgeries performed). One family continued to recount their decision to remove the ventilator. Several families discussed their *refusal* to agree to suggested treatments: C-section for the mother at birth (this baby was delivered vaginally), immunizations for the child, and circumcision. One parent talked about the request of health professionals for the baby's organs should it die. The baby did not die. Although this respondent indicated that she would *not* have given permission when the baby was in the NICU, since learning about organ donation in the interim she would be willing to give permission for the donation of a child's organs in the future.

One family discussed a subsequent *No Code* decision that they made for their child on a readmission, and another noted the decision to remove their child from a ventilator between the predischarge interview and the six-month postdischarge one. Parents were more likely to identify issues in the postdischarge phase related to decision-making rather than examples from the NICU experience.

One of the families describes the following situation:

> One of our children was readmitted for a fundoplication[f] and the night before the surgery she went into a full code. It was only with great difficulty that the physicians were able to revive her. Her breathing passage had become quite swollen and intubation was onerous. As a result of the code, she was placed on a ventilator. She was not doing very well and a request was made to provide her with a tracheostomy.[g]

The mother explained:

> We said no trach. If she comes off the respirator we don't want her put back on. And I, I wouldn't let them do a trach. I was really, really firm on it. So we went through that for the second time in our lives with her. She had her [fundoplication] surgery and she's doing fine.[h]

The paucity of *ethical* decision-making in this sample, as identified and discussed in the literature, led us to again pursue identification of decisions that people believed were important. Parents were asked how ethics or morality applied to their life and decisions, and what makes an ethical person. Some parents had difficulty understanding or, articulating the meaning of questions related to morality and ethical decision-making--possibly a poverty of moral language. But, in general, morality for these individuals was tied to how one led one's life or how one raised children, as many people would usually understand these concepts.

Religious beliefs or church teaching directed morality for several parents. Moral decisions were those general ones any family might make: reproduction, employment, relocation, birth control, marital status, child custody, child-care, education, and finances. Parents identified such current social issues as drugs and addiction, drinking and driving, and AIDS as examples of moral problems. Within their own lives, parents viewed stealing, lying, lifestyle choices, and alternatives concerning education as moral issues. Most frequently, parents regarded morals, morality, and ethics as somehow sexual in that a majority of responses to questions about ethical issues dealt with infidelity, divorce, promiscuity, vasectomy, tubal ligation, interracial marriage, sterility, contraception, and abortion. The moral responsibility for children was the second most frequent area of response, including disabilities, long-term care, and resources; children's friends; and use of drugs and gang killings. Two individuals could not mention anything that would be a moral issue. One parent summed up: "I'm not used to thinking about my actions as being moral decisions."

Only three parents discussed any relationship between moral or ethical behavior and health care experiences. Those three examples included the decision to *life-flight* the mother to the medical center,[i] the use of fertility drugs, and the increasing number of handicapped children. The latter concerned the individual because of the paucity of resources available for such persons. No parent by her or his own description or discussion correlated ethical or moral concerns with decision-making for their children while they were in the NICU. For the postdischarge situation, specific decisions related to health care which might include a moral dimension were the parents' choice of physicians and health care institutions, and selection of treatment options for the child including medications.

A few parents came to view receiving explanations and signing permits as decision-making on their part. This perhaps reflected their postdischarge experiences in the health care system. Some parents did not view signing permits as playing a role in decision-making but vividly remembered the experience:

> They practically had me signing those papers as they were taking me off the helicopter. They told me about the surfactant on the helicopter and you know, as they were wheeling me down the hall, I was signing papers... I had a nurse tell me...the minute I was put on that helicopter, it was out of my hands, I would have no choices.

Most had little recall about the informed consent process with again the notable exception of surfactant and, to a lesser extent, surgery, circumcision, and blood transfusions. Perhaps such sporadic memory makes this finding significant, given the importance of this process and its relationship to information for decision-making as well as the ethical dimension of consent.

At four years postdischarge, parents held a variety of views about the information they received from adequate, to partial, to totally absent. One parent explained:

> I didn't know about a, a ventilator at that time. I mean, I didn't know, all's I knew is, the magic things that happen in hospitals, you know.

Evidence exists that some parents now possessed more knowledge about the newborn condition and care in the NICU than at six months. These individuals could name medical conditions, tests, procedures, medications, and the roles of various therapists. Although these parents had this knowledge currently, most realized that they had acquired information over time. Parents acquired knowledge after the initial hospitalization of their child, rather than concurrently with care and decision-making in the NICU. Almost half continued to address the perception that they were *not* well informed during the infant's stay in the NICU. Parents clearly differentiated between the kinds of information they received. One category of information related to *curren*t care and *present* tests ordered for the infant, which parents contrasted with another category of information about the neonate's *prognosis*.

Those who felt they were informed received information about the current, ongoing status of the infant in comparison to previous events (weighs more now, recovered from setbacks, feeding better). However, health care professionals did not explain anticipated postdischarge risks according to the parents' perception. Nor did they explain the usual outcomes or expected medical developments for a particular infant weight. Two limitations for parents in processing information were their an inability to evaluate what they were told because of the terminology used, and their inability to articulate cogent questions: "You're just a layperson...I don't know if you would even know what sort of information you need." Parents addressed two areas in which more information would be helpful: skills for family coping while the baby was in the NICU, and guides for behavior in the NICU: when to come, how often, what the *rules* were.

Health care professionals were the most dominant source of information parents did receive, either through direct conversation, or through books and pamphlets these professionals directed parents to read. A few parents sought information on their own from public libraries and friends. Case workers and non-professional contacts were additional sources of information. Only three parents explicitly stated that they did *not* want to be informed. They preferred no warnings of future risks for the child, neither did they want the negative to be emphasized. Parents were emphatic in their need for more information to prepare them for possible future events as the infant developed. They also wanted the doctors to give parents information regularly, in a seated position, away from the NICU.

Advice for Future NICU Care of Parents

Parents have a strong desire to make a difference in the lives of other families with high-risk infants who will use the NICU in the future. They spontaneously suggested various strategies that they would now want implemented should they have another high-risk infant. Some parents had indeed had such an experience and their greater level of knowledge was a comfort to them when a second newborn was admitted to the NICU. It enhanced their understanding and reduced their anxiety about the NICU care.

One family experienced a NICU in another town subsequent to the birth of the child who placed them in this study. At the second NICU, parents were invited to attend daily rounds on the baby. The parents heard the nurse's daily report, listened to the physician's discussions and plans for the care of the infant, and were able to learn from the student nurses' and residents' questions. The parents themselves were encouraged to ask questions. The father found these strategies comforting. He also noted that they were in direct opposition to his perceptions of the first NICU experience. He wanted other parents to have NICU experiences similar to his second one.

Education and provision of information were important elements in coping with this event. These parents wanted future parents to acquire information beginning prenatally (for example, when fertility medications and procedures are implemented), to continue to request material during labor and delivery, and on into the intensive care nursery. Parents wanted information on the prevention of prematurity to be more widely distributed. They advised other parents in the NICU to insist that someone sit down and talk with them about the NICU at the earliest possible point. Parents specifically cited the need for health professionals to provide general information about the birth of a premature baby, treatment modalities, and prognosis. Parents implied that had they known about complications they would have been better prepared. Parents recommended setting up a one-on-one, weekly appointment with the physician once the child was admitted to the NICU. They suggested a "sign-up sheet" or some other mechanism to communicate this need to physicians and obtain an appointment. Parents greatly appreciated the day-to-day reports from the staff who were the infants' primary nurses. One parent was astute in noting that parents particularly need information about possible financial benefits for handicapped children after they are discharged. She did not find out about some of these benefits until almost past her ability to qualify for them. Parents suggested that others request a consultation with the social worker or similar professionals that can apprise them of resources before the infant's discharge.

These parents' advice to parents of other infants in the NICU emphasized being involved. The overall recommendation was to take charge of your infant and his care, to be actively involved by asking questions, and to do so without fear. Parents should seek a second opinion if the situation does not *feel* right and should educate themselves about their baby's condition. Support groups following discharge were also advised for parents, particularly for parents of handicapped children or those who had multiple births. One mother specifically indicated a need to have a professional more closely and frequently monitor the parent's completion of the treatments for her baby, especially in the beginning of the learning process prior to discharge. She also indicated that, as a parent, completely non-versed in any aspect of professional caregiving, she needed more time to learn the procedures she was expected to master and implement at home for the infant. This mother felt pressured into independent responsibility before she was ready. The absolute need for follow-up home care by a professional was stressed in the cases of children with ongoing treatments.

Finally, parents wanted information in various supplementary forms: books, pamphlets, and videos. The videos reflect our current lifestyle and today's visually oriented society, and therefore were more appealing to this group of people.

Most parents had some comment or other to add at the end of the interview. Parents expressed gratitude for their child's survival, the care their child received, the availability of surfactant, and the existence of NICUs. Parents grieved with and for parents whose children had not survived. Two parents mentioned the death of the baby in another family who participated in the project, and their concern for the parents. Negative comments included concerns about the increasing use of the NICU and the questionable results, and the sheer difficulty of living through a NICU experience. One parent was concerned about the ability of medical technology "to interfere in God and Mother Nature's plan."

Interestingly enough, almost half of the comments were related to our research:

- some gained satisfaction from participation in the project
- others were grateful that someone was conducting such a study
- many were pleased someone actually wanted to listen to them, and
- a number had various questions about the results of the project, especially how professionals would use the information or what other parents had said.

Parents gave us the impression that the interviews provided them with a chance to vent feelings. Some parents were concerned about the "flip side." A father noted the increasing number of stories about the NICU in the media, which he said included a lot of congratulations and back-slapping: "Boy isn't this great." However, in his experience, the outcome was not great. Instead, he identified with children who had a "whole host of physical problems, kids not meant to live."

The other major category of advice was spiritual in form: parents should have faith, pray a lot, take one day at a time, appreciate the good things in life, or simply "hang in there." One parent requested pastoral counseling, another was still confused and could not think of any advice, and two advised not to get pregnant under circumstances similar to theirs (at age 13 or while single). Finally, one comment from one of the women, an *inside joke* symbolic of parental assertiveness and control, was "just dump the bottle!" (see Alma's story, *Case of the disappearing formula*, Chapter 2)

Expectations for the Future

Several years have passed since the four-year postdischarge interview with these families. The specific extent of the effect of the high-risk birth may not be known for many years. Should funding be obtained, additional interviews will be conducted with the parents and the high-risk infants who are now of school age. Some speculations can be posed about the future of families with high-risk newborns based on various research projects and the families' own stories as they are publicized in one way or another. Four factors that could influence the future for high-risk infants and the care provided in the NICU will be discussed in Section III. Medical factors certainly include progress in the greater understanding of the functioning of the high-risk neonate, and the devising of new procedures to aid the newborns as they recover from their crises. Technological factors will influence the number of high-risk pregnancies that occur, which in turn has an impact on the census in the high-risk nursery. Scientific advancements also affect possible NICU interventions. Economic factors are another influential area as well as the more sociological and psychological considerations of the role of the fetus and child, and the family's future structure and function. Together these factors will have an impact on the families of this study as well as other families facing the same experiences in the future.

Several additional families were interviewed specifically for this book and the possible interest of the audience in families with high-risk infants at later periods in their lives. The Epilogue, which follows Section III, includes the stories of these representative families with children who are NICU graduates, but beyond 4-years-of-age, as we now leave the families in this project.

Notes

[a] At the time of these interviews, there was an incident in a local major city where a child was left alone in its crib at a day care center when it closed at the end of the business hours. Panic and concern about the child ensued. Although the child was not harmed physically, the parents we were interviewing were obviously affected by the event.

[b] As Layne (1996) concludes her first person account of a NICU experience, she labels her son "lucky." Although he is not completely free of sequelae from his early birth, induced as a result of Layne's toxemia, he is doing well by his mother's account. The interesting comment is her inclusion of the developmental pediatrician's statement that ""disability" would be an optional term for Jasper." This would appear to be further affirmation of the need to avoid any association with handicap, disability, or impaired for these are the final words that Layne leaves with her readers.

[c] Pheasants Forever is a national conservation organization

[d] This was an interesting observation given Butler's discussion of the neonate patient as machine in "Infants, pain and health care" (1989). Although Butler uses machine in her examination of pain and the neonate, the patient as machine is an operational paradigm in the neonatal nursery that this parent certainly observed and considered as a result of her experience there.

[e] Iatrogenic effects (those outcomes caused by the treatment itself) of intermittent mandatory ventilation include: "asynchronous breathing between ventilator and patient, resulting in irregular systemic and cerebral blood flow patterns, airleak syndrome, pulmonary hemorrhage, neurologic complications (e.g. intraventricular hemorrhage and periventricular leukomalacia), and chronic lung disease" (McGettigan et al. 1998).

[f] Fundoplication is a surgical procedure in which the upper portion of the stomach is sutured around the esophagus (the passageway from the mouth and throat into the stomach) to prevent regurgitation.

[g] A tracheostomy is an artificial opening created in the trachea or windpipe into which a tube-like device is placed to permanently maintain access to the lungs. The tube can be connected to the ventilator to facilitate delivery of oxygen to the lungs. It prevents trauma to the upper air passages which can occur from a tube inserted through the nose or mouth for breathing, the alternative approaches.

[h] *Fine* is a relative term in this case. The child at four years of age is unable to eat or drink and maintains nutritional status through a gastrostomy tube (a permanently placed tube directly through the abdominal wall into her stomach). She basically functions at a two-month level and is unable to make even the most voluntary movements, like reaching out and grasping a rattle. However, she has been taught to use *switch toys*. When positioned correctly, she can activate the switch and, for example, start a device that plays music.

[i] *Life-flight* is a term to describe transportation, usually of an emergency nature, by helicopter to the hospital.

CHAPTER 5

Moral Voices of Parents

Complex health care issues like ethical decision-making in the NICU provide the stimulation for professionals to examine many different parameters. One intriguing aspect of ethical decision-making is individual moral development which includes moral reasoning, and moral orientation. An understanding of the possible moral reasoning of patients would seem to be helpful for a holistic perspective of ethical decision-making.[a]

Moral orientation is the psychological dimension of ethical decision-making. The discipline of bioethics places major emphasis on theological or philosophical examination of issues and the debates that surround those issues. However, clinical decision-making involves various individuals and individuals bring particular sets of values, beliefs, and traditions with them. One approach to understanding the foundation for those values and beliefs is to study the moral reasoning and the moral orientation of those individuals.

Theoretical Background

Until the end of the 19th century, psychology was part of the discipline of philosophy. At that time, some scholars wanted to emphasize the scientific aspect so psychology branched off and became its own discipline. Numerous thinkers expressed curiosity about moral development both within and outside of philosophy. Emile Durkheim was interested in moral development in childhood and the internalization of moral values from the individual's culture. Freud, Adler, Jung, and Sears were all students of morality as are more recent theorists such as Havinghurst, Erikson, Levinson, and Loevinger (Kohlberg 1968; Rich & DeVitis 1985). Some theorists focused on adults; others targeted children's moral reasoning and the development of their reasoning skills.

Kohlberg's Groundwork

Kohlberg's theory of moral development and Gilligan's subsequent contributions comprise one possible foundation for an examination of individual moral orientation. John Dewey and Jean Piaget both had a significant impact on Kohlberg's thinking (1975) relative to moral development. Kohlberg proposed that his research, which began in 1955, would validate and redefine a synthesis of Piaget's and Dewey's work. Each scholar had described three levels or stages of moral development which were congruent. While Dewey was a pure theorist, Piaget conducted interviews with children and observed them at play to advance his stages of development.

Kohlberg originally interviewed young boys, ages 10 to 16, to determine their processes of moral reasoning. As a result of his investigation, he proposed a step-wise, hierarchical, invariant, organized, staged process of moral reasoning (1958). In order to validate his conclusions, he followed his original sample for 20 years and added other groups from various foreign countries. Kohlberg's analysis of moral reasoning is grounded in assumptions about cognition or active thinking and logic, and their development (1975). Six stages of development define three levels of moral reasoning as Kohlberg's participants explored a set of verbal moral dilemmas. Although defining the content of the dilemmas is important, for Kohlberg the reasoning process for each dilemma was the focus. An elaborate scoring method was devised to classify each participant's responses to the dilemmas. Before other investigators were permitted to use Kohlberg's method, they were required to participate in training workshops. The scoring manual included the dilemmas, probes, and instructions for scoring.

The most basic response a participant could have belongs in the preconventional level of moral reasoning, which represents the individual, concrete perspective (Kohlberg 1975). Good and bad are determined by the consequences of the action one might choose--avoiding punishment, gaining rewards. The lowest stage in this level is the *punishment-and-obedience orientation* whereby the individual unquestioningly obeys whoever is most powerful. Physical consequences are to be avoided. In the second stage, *instrumental-relativist orientation*, there is an element of reciprocity, but only because of the desire to obtain goods or gain some favor. This is a very pragmatic exchange with an emphasis on receiving, not giving.

The second level, conventional, is based on the individual as that person sees her or himself as a member of a group--family, neighborhood, community, or nation (Kohlberg 1975). People generally want to belong to some formal cluster and want to maintain its order. Reasoning can be categorized as either *interpersonal concordance*, the lower stage, or *law and order*, the higher stage of level two. In the lower stage, Kohlberg describes characteristic behavior as fitting a *good boy-nice girl* model. Individuals do what is expected, what the majority approves. The second stage also incorporates the sense of duty one must take on to maintain orderly societal groups. Laws, rules, and a certain degree of authority are necessary.

The third or postconventional level requires stepping outside of the group or society and more objectively determining the right and wrong for human life. At the fifth stage, *social contract, legalistic orientation*, a rational examination of the law and legal system is incumbent upon society's members. Through free agreement, rights and standards are determined--the official bedrock of American democracy. In the highest stage, *universal-ethical-principle orientation*, one's conscience and universal ethical principles of justice determine moral preferences. Respect for human dignity and equality of human rights are at the heart of moral reasoning.

Making a judgment does not necessarily mean that an individual will act upon that determination. Although Kohlberg invested significant effort in education related to moral development and the construction of a just community to foster moral decision-making, such considerations are beyond the scope of the present discussion. Before leaving Kohlberg's point of view, a few words are in order to emphasize the idea of content versus structure in moral reasoning. Kohlberg was most interested in the latter. One famous dilemma in his project revolved around the situation for Heinz, whose dying wife needed a particularly expensive drug that he could not afford to purchase. Although Heinz discussed his situation with the originator of the drug, there was no compromise and he had to obtain the appropriate amount of money in order to get the drug. In addition, the sale price was 10 times the manufacturing cost but the pharmacist would not budge. Heinz could not raise the money so he either had to steal the drug or let his wife die (Kohlberg 1975).

Whether or not the respondent decides to steal the drug (content) is not as important as the moral reasoning or judgment (structure) for such a choice. Consider two respondents who both determine not to steal the drug, and remember that this is a most simplistic explanation. One individual discusses the laws against stealing as a rationale for the decision. The individual goes on to say that if everyone simply stole what they needed, we would have chaos (Stage 4). The second respondent replies that he fears that the police would come and beat him up if he stole the drug so he would be afraid to take such action (Stage 1). Both respondents come to the same conclusion, yet the reasoning of one would be categorized into a higher level than the other because of the rationale for the possible action.

For Kohlberg, the ideal decision-maker was the logical, abstract, objective, rational, autonomous individual who was able to step outside of personal circumstances and see how society might become better, more just, more fair. These words are also a reminder that Kohlberg was an admirer of the philosopher John Rawls (1958). The third or postconventional level of moral reasoning is reflective of Rawls' *veil of ignorance* device. In theoretically applying this device, decision-makers are disconnected from their usual roles and environment. Rawls determined that individuals make the most objective and fair decisions when they do not know who they are, how they will benefit, or what they will lose, from the moral rules they devise for the ideal society--a stepping outside of one's character, if you will. For Rawls equal liberty and fair distribution of material goods were two key principles for justice.

Considerable research has been conducted related to moral development. Other investigators and educators, including Kohlberg's students, continued to build on his ideas (Blatt & Kohlberg 1975 ; Fenton 1976; Rest 1975, 1976; Rest et al. 1969; Turiel 1974). Kohlberg's original research used hypothetical moral dilemmas, and other scholars followed his justice paradigm in devising additional studies (Chap 1985-86; Holstein 1976; Snarey & Lydens 1990; White 1988). Kohlberg's ideas were expanded into instruments to measure moral development (Rest et al. 1969), and his research was applied to the educational setting (Blatt & Kohlberg 1975; Kohlberg 1987; Scharf 1978). Several investigators continued the use of Rest's Defining Issues Test, which is based conceptually on Kohlberg's research (Fitzgerald & Hyland 1980; Little & Robinson 1989a, 1989b; Rybash, Roodin, et al. 1981; Rybash, Hoyer, et al. 1983/84). Another instrument was the Sociomoral Reflection Measure (SRM) which the originators claim to be a contribution to measurement in moral judgment that is less cumbersome than Kohlberg's method (Gibbs et al. 1984). A shorter version of the SRM was developed later (Basinger et al. 1995).

Obviously Kohlberg has his critics, and limitations to the analysis of moral development exist. A major criticism aims at his use of descriptive data from an exploratory study to formulate a theory and advocate its use to evaluate individuals, develop educational curricula, and promote widespread application. The critics contend that the way things are is not necessarily how they should be. Additionally, as indicated above, the connection between what people think and what they do, based on Kohlberg's work, is not clear. However, the purpose of using Kohlberg's ideas here is simply to describe and explain--a limited application. Overall, it is a fairly reasonable explanation of the basis for decision-making by a large number of people in this society. Kohlberg's theory is more popularly known as a justice paradigm, and his ideas will subsequently simply be called a justice orientation.

Gilligan's Contributions

Carol Gilligan was teaching a section of Erik Erikson's course at Harvard when Kohlberg read her dissertation, which focused on cheating (Robb 1980). In her project, *Responses to temptation: An analysis of motives*, Gilligan examined how stories influenced children to cheat or not cheat (1964). In 1968, Kohlberg invited Gilligan to work on a project in which he was investigating high school students' sexual attitudes and their moral reasoning (Gilligan, Kohlberg et al. 1971). While working with Kohlberg, Gilligan eventually observed a noticeable gap in his original research--an absence of females. Additionally, although girls and women were included in subsequent studies by others as well as Kohlberg, females generally did not score as high as males when Kohlberg's method was used. Another significant element was the factor of context. Fabricated vignettes might enable respondents to examine their possible future action and moral resolve, but an actual ethical dilemma would certainly reveal data possibly closer to the moral values and beliefs to which the respondent ascribes. In the 1970s, a real life drama was the Viet Nam war and Harvard students were facing a moral conflict as a result of the draft (Nair 2000). Although Gilligan herself began an investigation into moral reasoning by studying these students, the war ended and the draft issue was no longer viable. However, another rich area of moral conflict presented itself in 1973 when the U.S. Supreme Court legalized abortion. Gilligan was on leave from Harvard in 1975 when she and a colleague, Mary Belenky, first conducted their interviews with women contemplating abortion (Blackburne-Stover et al. 1982; Robb 1980). Through this work (Gilligan 1977; 1979, 1982a, 1982b, 1988) Gilligan came to realize that the developmental psychology she had studied and was teaching was a psychology of boys and men (Gilligan 1979; Carol Gilligan presents 1997). The women who were making decisions about abortion did not think about the political aspects of abortion, the right to life, or the right to choose. Rather, they were concerned about how their decision would personally affect themselves and others.

Gilligan identified three levels of moral development as a result of her interviews with these women: individual survival, self-sacrifice, and interdependence (1982a). In the first level, individual survival, there is a focus on self-interest and self-preservation--selfishness, if you will. Decision-making is pragmatic--how can I take care of myself, how can I avoid being hurt by others? The individual feels alone, helpless, and powerless. In fact, persons often isolate themselves to prevent the hurt that is possible from the treatment by others. At the second level, self-sacrifice, goodness is defined in terms of caring for others, much like the self-sacrifice often associated with maternal relationships. This is a conventional development, as the expectation of self-sacrifice equated with goodness comes from a shared norm of society. The societal norm is internalized and is most frequently associated with females. Persons at this level want to be accepted and to have their actions valued by others. They are able to maintain their social role by meeting the expectations of giving and selfless behavior. These attributes are also true of minority and other disenfranchised groups--crossing gender boundaries. The highest level, interdependence, embraces the ability to balance care for self and care for others. Decision-making is a reasoned process, but compassion is an essential element. At every level of development, relationships and how the decision affects these relationships are central issues. Morality in general is seen as a responsibility to others rather than a focus on the rights of the individual. The context of the situation is important. Usual roles and environment are pivotal considerations as moral consciousness develops which is diametrically opposed to Rawls' analysis and Kohlberg's theory.

Moving from selfishness to conventional behavior requires the development of self-esteem. Being responsible for others at the second level necessitates a shift in orientation from self-concern to taking care of others, being able to put others' needs ahead of one's own. Feminine goodness is often equated with caring for others, so moving from the second level to the third level again requires sufficient self-esteem to reject the conventions of society. Caring can extend to all, but it is balanced with an honest appraisal of one's own needs. The individual needs to acknowledge that one's own energy and internal resources need to be replenished in order to fulfill the needs of others. One can expect care as well as give care. Gilligan's paradigm is often simply identified as a care orientation.

Gilligan (1977) initially interviewed women who were contemplating a real life ethical dilemma, abortion; both she and others expanded upon this context. Adherents to her caring paradigm enlarged the research base (Brown 1991; Jack & Jack 1988; Rogers & Gilligan 1988). Additionally, researchers developed a specific methodology to examine these paradigms and conducted studies comparing the two moral orientations, justice and care (Becker & Burke 1988; Brown, Argyris et al. 1988; Lyons 1983; Pratt et al. 1991; Walker 1989).

Gilligan is also the object of criticism from a variety of sources (Crigger 1997; Jecker & Reich 1995). Two major sources are from traditional philosophical theorists and feminists. Philosophical criticism is based on the observation that Gilligan's paradigm lacks rigor. While developing arguments for resolving an ethical dilemma, the precepts of the caring paradigm do not readily transfer to a scholarly discussion of the issues in the dilemma, particularly at the social and institutional level. Feminists are concerned because the theory, if used to guide behavior, leads to the promotion of attitudes and actions that place or keep women in a vulnerable position. Feminine traits such as caring and maintaining relationships are not formally valued in our society where authority, power, and prestige are rewarded whether those traits are displayed by men or women. Therefore, the use of the caring paradigm simply keeps women (and others who exhibit caring behaviors) in a subservient, devalued, inferior position (Pinch 1996). However, for purposes of this project, these limitations were judged to be no more of a hindrance than the limitations of Kohlberg's work.

Despite the view of the caring paradigm as less intellectually sound than traditional philosophical theories, the reality is that the *general public's* definition of relationships and caring, and its actual use by individuals facing personal moral dilemmas does exist. More often than not, individuals do make ethical decisions based on relationships and context and do not systematically apply a traditional ethical theory to reach a decision. Caring is context sensitive in that it is a context driven process with context dependent outcomes (Sabat 2001). Therefore when one brings a caring orientation to morality, objective analysis is antithetical to the basic premises of a caring approach. As ordinary groups of people act on these caring values and beliefs, they can make a difference. Numerous successful grass roots efforts to institute change have not always been based on formal, philosophical examinations of the right or wrong of the situation. Therefore the use of both paradigms was judged to be legitimate for purposes of this project.

Gilligan's methodology provides one approach by which moral conflict and choice can be examined (Brown, Argyris et al. 1988). As Gilligan continued her projects and students expanded upon her work, a particular approach to interviewing and identifying moral orientation developed. This method was based on the early interviews of Gilligan and Belenky (Blackburne-Stover et al. 1982) and the later work of Lyons (1983) when she was a student of Gilligan. The process is based on the assumption that for the majority of individuals, moral choice is determined by one's perspective, which can be described by either a justice or a care orientation (Gilligan & Attanucci 1988). Therefore, a justice orientation as defined by concerns for fairness, individual rights, and adherence to standards or principles would be central to moral choice, based on Kohlberg's research. Relationships in a justice orientation are either equal or unequal, and are characterized by reciprocity. In the care orientation, relationships are characterized by attachment or detachment with an overriding desire to maintain relationships, stay connected to others in the situation, and avoid abandonment. Issues in a care orientation are clustered around a focus on context, a *particularistic* concern for knowing and understanding as much as possible about the characters in the dilemma, as identified by Gilligan's research. Through a process of interviewing and interpreting a personal conflict of the participant, those values and beliefs that are relevant to the moral domain of the individual are explored and categorized when applying the methodology developed at the Center for the Study of Gender, Education and Human Development (Brown, Argyris et al. 1988).

Several other premises should be kept in mind in reviewing the above brief description of moral developmental theory and the available methodology to determine moral orientation. Justice and care orientations are not mutually exclusive but are rather shifts in perspective depending upon how the individual interprets the situation and how the relationships among the individuals are defined. Some theorists have likened the two orientations to the classic reversible figure or the ambiguous stimulus that combines two images: the combination of a vase and human profile in one drawing or the old woman and young woman in another. Each is a single picture, but depending upon the gaze or the focus of the viewer, the image in the picture changes. So the single individual faced with a moral conflict (gazing at the drawing) has the potential to see the situation from two perspectives, one justice (the vase is discerned), and the other care (the profile is detected). Individuals generally determine their moral choice based on one view or the other, not usually both for a single dilemma. The different orientations are not integrated when an individual is attempting to resolve a moral dilemma, but rather one orientation is preferred over the other depending on the situation, although both orientations may be represented in the whole discussion. The paradigmatic decision-maker has a different agenda depending upon the moral orientation. Additionally, although the care orientation is generally associated with females, this was not Gilligan's conclusion despite the number of studies her group conducted with girls and women (Hekman 1995). Females are able to interpret moral conflict through a justice lens, while males are able to construe the moral problem as one associated with care. Finally, although it may be more difficult to accept, one orientation is not posed as better or worse than the other. However, voices are aired and heard within a social and political climate which may impose a layer of judgment upon the value and authority of the orientations.

Current Research

The parents of the patient, the newborn, who are involved in ethical decision-making are the focus of the present portrayal. There are many possible sources of moral conflict for parents while their infant is in the NICU. One example of a conflict in the ethical dimension described in earlier chapters is informed consent. Informed consent is a pivotal process for parents in terms of their involvement in infant care. Moral orientation can potentially impact a parent's perspective during that process. How do parents perceive their relationships with the health care providers? Are parents concerned about rights? Do parents depend upon logical and rational thinking when conflict arises? Or, are parents focused on the caring aspects of the situation? Health care professionals are responsible for facilitating the decision-making process in the NICU. If physicians, nurses, and other care givers believe that knowledge about possible parental responses to the NICU experience would enable them as professionals to respond sensitively and cogently to parents, then a description of the moral orientation could contribute to that process. Not only would such a description provide insight for the informed consent procedure but it could enhance the understanding of other moral conflicts as well.

Moral development is of interest to health care professionals (Ketefian 1988), with much of the research focused on examining the moral orientation of the health professional. Some have framed their research within Kohlberg's paradigm (Baldwin et al. 1991; Candee et al. 1982; Crisham 1981; Ketefian 1981; Krawczyk & Kudzma 1978; Munhall 1980; Murphy 1976; Self 1987), while others have included Gilligan's perspective (Chally 1992; Millette 1994). Little if any research has centered on examining the patient's level of moral reasoning, especially as that reasoning is related to a real moral conflict. In my own previous research on moral orientation, healthy elderly persons were asked to consider possible future health care dilemmas and were not patients during the study (Pinch & Parsons 1993). During a literature search, no research was identified that explored the moral orientation of parents of high-risk neonates.

The moral orientation of parents will be reported here within the four dimensions of the reading guide as described in the Appendix, The Research Enterprise.[b] First the stories of the participants will be described, followed by reports of the moral voices which they used, the alignment of the moral voices (either justice or care), and the perceived relationships of individuals in the dilemma as voiced by the participants. All of the examples come directly from the narrative descriptions that were prepared during the secondary analysis of the interviews. In the secondary analysis, these in-depth, narrative descriptions of the entire scope of evidence were based directly on all parental interviews. That material was distilled and interpreted to represent parents' voices in this account of the results.

The Parents' Stories

Many parents' stories have already been discussed, but since the secondary analysis depends upon summarizing these stories as a first step, this aspect will be recapitulated. Stories of the NICU experience were most generally formulated in the context of many other family events. When requested to describe "a time in their NICU experience when they weren't sure what was the right thing to do." parents included difficulty with conception, problem pregnancies, or birth events. Parents also addressed many concerns which arose during the neonate's hospitalization, but very few of their worries matched the prevalent ethical dilemmas that scholars have addressed in the literature. For example, common issues long debated in the literature include the moral status of the newborn (Engelhardt 1978; Fletcher 1979; McCormick 1974), treatment decision-making for infants with compromised physical or mental status (Duff & Campbell 1973; Ramsey 1978), locus of decision-making for newborns (Ellison & Walwork 1986; Shelp 1986; Tyson 1995; Weber 1976), and determining *best interest* standards for neonates (Dunn 1993; Smith 1974). Parents instead vocalized their decision-making in the context of determining whether or not to breast-feed, balancing their on-going family responsibilities to include visits to the neonate, and keeping their lives on hold to accommodate whatever neonatal outcome resulted from the experience. Parents definitely perceived themselves to be in a conflict; it simply did not initially encompass the traditional, neonatal ethical dilemmas.

Across all three phases of this study, parents did not perceive that they were involved in the ethical dimension of decision-making for their infant when it was in the NICU. Prior to discharge they did not object to such a circumstance. In the later two phases (six-months and four-years postdischarge), parents began to voice disagreement about their lack of involvement as they realized the impact of the decision-making on their own lives and family functioning. Only a few would have actually wanted to change the decisions that had been made for them. However, all of the parents wanted to be more suitably informed and better prepared for the events that would face them as they took their baby home and began to integrate it into their family life. Many parents were provided with information, but they lacked the skills to interpret what this information meant for them specifically as individuals and a family.

Presence of Voice

Which voice was present in the interviews? Was only a single voice (care or justice) represented in the comments, or were both voices displayed? An interpretation of the presence of voice was possible in all of the participants' interviews (32 mothers, 20 fathers; neither = 0). Both the justice and the care voices were present in the majority of the participants' interviews (mothers, $n = 27$, 84.4%; fathers, $n = 12$, 60%). That is, there was evidence for both rational, logical, objective reasoning and contextual, interconnected, relationship-based reasoning. The care voice alone (no evidence of the justice voice, or a *pure* care voice) was present in 2 mothers (6.3%) and no fathers. The justice voice alone (no care voice or *pure* justice voice) was present in 3 mothers (9.4%) and 8 fathers (40%). (See Figure 5.1)

Figure 5.1 *Presence of Voice in Participants*

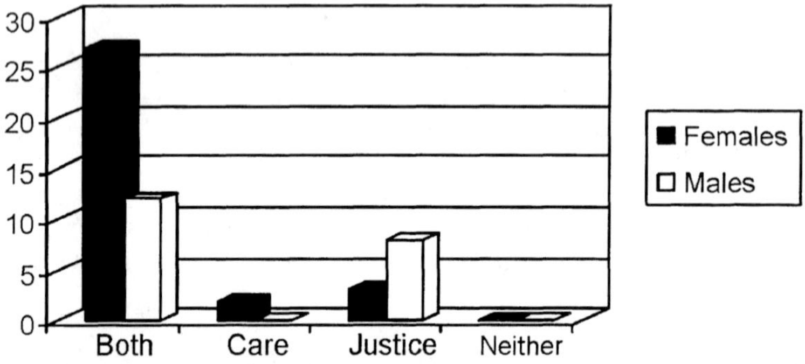

An example of a care voice occurred in a father whose whole life was revolving around an extremely needy child. In the interviews, his relationship to this child and his connectedness to the child's life were abundantly addressed and increased across the interviews as he assumed more and more direct responsibility for the care of his child. Connections to other people were very important to him as well. Family and friends were frequently mentioned as he described his life and its highlights relative to the NICU experience. Although he wished his child had not survived the treatment, he also knew in his heart that he could never have said "**no**" to the aggressive measures that were used. He described his pain and angst at his son's condition as emanating from his perception that if he were in his son's position, he would not want to live. The father frequently referred to the personal price he had to pay for doing the right thing, and the emotional toil his life takes on because of this child.

From the perspective of one woman, who represents a care voice, moral problems depend upon the specific situation. She thinks that there is no moral objective right or wrong but rather describes decision-making as a personal action. She used an example of another baby in the NICU who needed a liver transplant. She decided whether or not the transplant should have been provided in the context of that family and the situation, which may have been different from her family and her situation. She described how she and her husband would try to place themselves in the baby's position if they had to make such a decision. They would ask themselves if it was morally good to make the baby bear such misery and pain, knowing that it might not survive. This was *not* described as a rational process of weighing risks and benefits. Her discussion emphasized the family's circumstances and how that would determine the final decision. Connections among members of the family were of primary significance for her across all interviews, but in the predischarge interview she placed the greatest importance on her connection to the baby. This was her rationale for remaining near the hospital, rather than returning to her home once she herself was discharged from the hospital.

A justice voice came from a father who focused on the image he wanted to present to the staff as they visited the child in the NICU. He wanted to be perceived as a mature person, a good father, and faithful husband. The evaluation of his actions and behavior, as he described it, came from standards for these roles as determined by society. He also mentioned the importance of being a good citizen. The church was an important part of society and was singular in determining right and wrong for him. However, he was adamant that health care decisions were not moral ones. Decision-making in the NICU for him was simply *logical*. Physicians and other staff persons in the NICU were sources of information and, provided this was logical, then the decision was acceptable. In all three interviews he was consistent in his emphasis on the logical, objective nature of decision-making for the treatment of his baby. When medical decisions and explanations were logical, there was no conflict regarding right and wrong.

A justice voice from a mother is represented by the regular inclusion of references to her feelings of intimidation throughout the discussion of her NICU experience. There was a clear portrayal of the staff in a position of power and authority relative to her role as the infant's mother. She was reluctant to make any requests for information and perceived the staff to be unwilling to spontaneously sit down and talk with her. She felt rejected when a blood donation was needed for the baby and the staff rebuffed her when she first volunteered to give it herself. Permission was needed for the transfusion and when she appeared to hesitate in providing it, she indicated that the staff threatened to take her to court if she denied the permission. She said that she understood the need, but she really only wanted to be able to sit down and talk about the baby's condition. This mother wanted to be able to comprehend why a transfusion was necessary. However, she believed that she did not have a right to question the professionals' authority. She voiced her perception that there were *rules* to follow in order to be the *good parent*. She wanted to be that good parent. Being the good parent included her felt need to be "up there [in the NICU] every day" as she discussed the predischarge experience in the first two interviews. She also took a secondary role in the discussion relative to her husband, but even during the solo third interview, she appeared to defer to his authority or to church teachings as the sources for decisions she needed to make.

Predominance of Voice

Which voice was present most frequently during the entire set of interviews? The justice voice predominated in the majority of both mothers' ($n = 16$, 50%) and fathers' interviews ($n = 15$, 75%), although the mothers' results were certainly marginal. Thirty-four percent of the mothers ($n = 11$) and 15% of the fathers ($n = 3$) reflected a care voice predominance. Neither voice predominated in the cases of 5 mothers (15.6%) and 2 fathers (10%) (See Figure 5.2)

Justice can be identified as predominant in a father who discussed morality in terms of what he *thought* was right based on standards he had accepted or developed for himself. In a conflict he discussed, he focused on a need to examine the effects of a decision. One had to take each option and anticipate what each might bring before a decision

Figure 5.2 *Predominance of Voice in Participants*

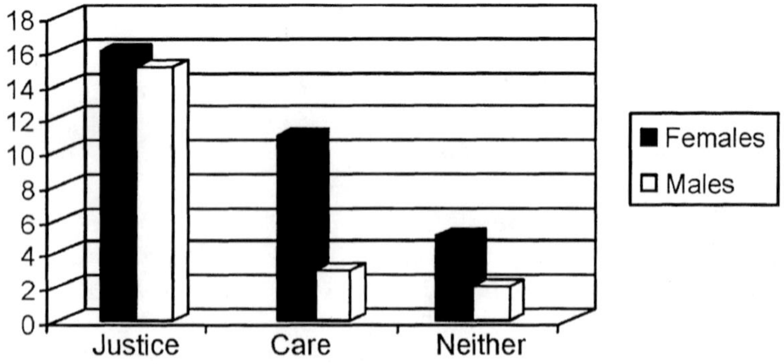

could be made. The older he gets, he said, the more important are the principles that he derives from Biblical teachings. He accepted the decisions of physicians in the NICU because they were the experts and it was their responsibility to take care of the infants. These themes of standards and principles recurred throughout the interview. He focused on thinking, looking at rights and outcomes.

Caring was predominant in a father who related his experiences interacting with the staff as he and his wife visited their newborn. Caring professionals listen to you, he said. In fact, healing can only occur when they do listen. To him the staff was like an extended family. He described long conversations with the staff in which there was a lot of mutual sharing. Because the professionals shared their own lives with him, he knew that they really had heard what he said. He said that the staff went out of their way, went the second mile, doing more than professionals needed to. By his observations, suffering was an experience everyone in the NICU had in common regardless of nationality, finances, or other factors. The unit was a *leveler* of everyone who had a child there. He believed that one needed to love and be charitable to be morally good. The reciprocal nature of relationships this man created for himself in the NICU represented his caring orientation. It dominated his discussion and was his preferred orientation.

One woman whose discussions were dominated by justice had a strong sense of the hierarchical structure of the NICU and her very unequal relationship with the health care professionals. The lack of control in the situation and her recognition of decision-making by others for *her* infant were frequently addressed. This woman consistently referred to herself as *just the mother*. She recalled how the mother of another infant told her that "he's not your baby until he leaves here." Although the justice orientation dominated her descriptions, clearly she did not prefer this orientation. Given the circumstances, she is forced into this perspective. From her affect, tone and emphasis, she definitely aligned with the caring orientation. Distance, inequality, and objectivity were antithetical to her preferred relationships in moral conflict. Nurturing and bonding are of primary importance to her in her relationship with this child and in her adult relationships as well, although she talked of suffering grievously in her choice of marriage partners.

Caring dominated the interview of one of the younger women in her descriptions of conflict and the actions that she took when she recognized a problem. Most of the examples she used represented a priority of relationships, connections, or caring. This was especially true when she recounted her understanding of organ donation. The possibility was brought up when the staff thought her baby might die. At the time, she was very much opposed to the idea of a transplant and would not have been able to give permission for it. Later in the third interview, when she actually raises the issue for the first time, she said that she now more fully understood what organ donation means. She would most assuredly give consent because it would make someone else happy, it would give them life. But it would also help soothe her own loss of a child and connect all of those involved in a very meaningful way.

Alignment with Voice

Which voice was most frequently selected for self? This voice is designated as the alignment for the individual. Most mothers' discussions (n = 17, 53.1%) aligned with the care voice, while 10 mothers aligned with the justice voice (31.3%). The designations were based on evaluation of parents' *I* or *me* statements to determine which, if any, were associated with justice or care. This estimate reflected not only the degree to which self and justice or care were combined but also the participant's preference for one or the other. Most fathers (n = 14, 70%) aligned with the justice voice, and only 3 (15%) with the care voice. Three mothers (9.4%) and 1 father (5%) aligned with both equally; 1 mother (3.1%) and 2 fathers (10%) showed no alignment. In the cases of no alignment, for example, the person's use of *I* statements could not be placed into one or the other framework. In one interview, it was not possible to make an interpretation of alignment (the material was too scanty) (see Figure 5.3).

One woman's interview showed a definite alignment with caring although neither care nor justice dominated the interview. The woman talked about how she had been taught ever since she could remember, to give to others, to sacrifice. She believed that her needs are least important whenever a conflict arises. This woman was genuine in her claim to choose to make sacrifices because they made her feel good. She loved to do things for other people, she said. She had no complaints about others receiving and her going without when necessary. She framed the self-sacrifice in terms of a choice, a freely chosen way of life that the interviewer had difficulty believing. But, in the end after three interviews, it was clear that self-sacrificial caring was a philosophy upon which her life was based. Justice was also evi-

Figure 5.3 *Alignment of Voice Among Participants*

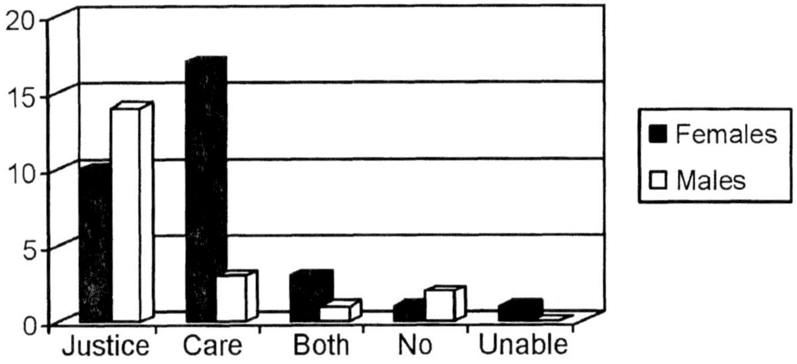

dent. Interjected throughout the discussion of decision-making was her process of "wagering all things." She used this to depict the weighing of the good and bad, determining the risks and the outcomes when faced with a problem and her need to make a decision. In looking at the interviews as a whole, both paradigms were represented equally but the caring statements were more frequently attached to *I* or *me*, making caring the preferred orientation, her alignment.

A father's alignment with caring was apparent from his descriptions of his family life and the relationship with his wife. His alignment was also reflected in terms of the connections he expected to initiate with his twin boys and in the course of 4 years had in fact established. He was able to resist the external pressures to conform to a societal imposed role of the instrumental father. Relatives questioned his involvement with childcare and his preference for an active role. This man thoroughly understood hierarchical structures and associated them with the functioning of the armed services, which he did not like. His discomfort and unhappiness at work were quite strong. He definitely aligned with care and was more than willing to sacrifice his own needs and desires to make time in his life for his children.

One woman's alignment with justice was influenced by the advocate role she carved for herself, representing her handicapped children. When faced with a decision, she liked to put everything down on paper. She made a list and weighed the odds, then came up with a solution. Although this woman may have been a different person before the experience with high-risk twins, she became an assertive, forthright person who made her needs known, sought ways to have her rights honored, and went after her due (or rather what was due her children). She was not hesitant to ask questions and find necessary information. Before the children were discharged, she did not know that she had options. On her emergency life-flight to the hospital before the delivery of the children she was told that everything was out of her control now. The lack of fairness in losing their insurance coverage was also a particular complaint. She felt that her life was full of frustrations from dealing with bureaucratic institutions and people in power.

One father, clearly aligned with justice, framed his discussions within his role as head of the household and financial provider for the family. All conflicts that he could discuss were within his role as employer or husband or father, hierarchical structures by his own account. Who was in authority was an important aspect for him. He saw the NICU as a situation of power relationships, and that was the reason for his failure to perceive any decision-making relative to the infant. The health care professionals knew what they had to do, knew what was best for the baby, not him. There was no need for him to be an active participant while his child was hospitalized. His job was central to most of his discussion. His wife's job was to be mother to his children and keeper of the home. It was the way he had been brought up and it was the way things should be. For him a problem was created when he knew what should be done and other people did not think the same way. There were routines and rules; it was not difficult for him to know what to do.

Relationship Description

The relationship of self to others is the last interpretive decision to be determined from the analysis of the interviews. More mothers' discussions (n = 14, 43.8%) reflected a relationship defined by inequality/equality, as did most fathers' (n = 14, 70%). Such an association was representative of hierarchical structuring. Attachment/ detachment represented the descriptions of 12 mothers (37.5%) and 2 fathers (10%). Connections to other people within this type of relationship could be distant or close. The presence of both types of relationships in decision-making was articulated in an equal manner by

Figure 5.4 *Relationship Descriptions of Participants*

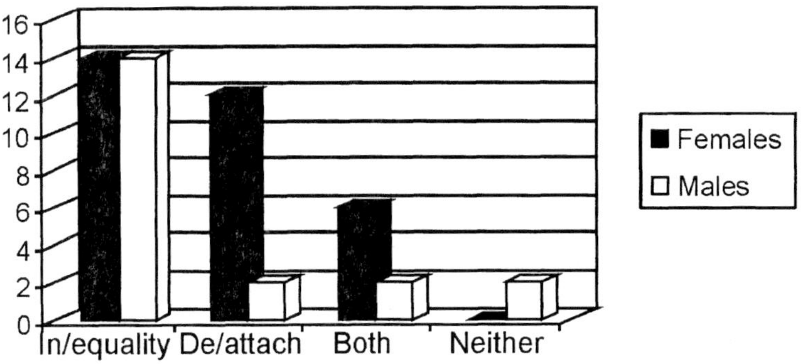

6 mothers (18.8%) and 2 fathers (10%). Neither relationship could be identified in 2 father's interviews (10%) (see Figure 5.4).

For one mother of twins, all examples of decision-making were oriented toward situations in which there were hierarchical relationships. There was always an authority figure present in her descriptions as she moved among examples of herself as a child in relationship to her parents, as a parent toward her own children, or with health professionals who were seen as authority figures. For her there were standards or rules for guiding decisions and behavior (religious teachings, for example). Decision-making was an objective process, according to her. One needed to sit down and talk in order for people to understand each side of the story. But she was careful to disclaim the strategy of putting one's self in the other's role in order to understand that side of the story. Overall she was judged to have a justice orientation for decision-making over the course of all three interviews. There was no evidence for a caring orientation under any circumstances.

One father definitely had problems with questions of control and frequently addressed his points in terms of hierarchical structures. On the one hand he said that all he wanted was the best for his child, yet he discussed his constant resistance to what was done and how it was done. He felt that no one listened to what he thought. All the staff did was evaluate him, and what right did the staff have to judge his behaviors and actions? The staff seemed to have rules for parental behavior in the NICU, but why should he have to conduct himself the way the staff determined a good parent should behave? He felt trapped by the bureaucracy of the health care system. If he took his son home against medical advice, his insurance would not cover any problems that subsequently developed, so he was prevented from acting in the best interest of his child--from his perspective. Additionally, the hospital later sued him for unpaid hospital bills, which he believed was unjust. He pointed out many items that were ordered and not used or used on another child, the unrealistically high price of many products, and unnecessary tests on his child. Finally, he felt he had no choices when it came to his divorce and child custody. The judge controlled his life and did not see his situation in the same way he did.

Relationships were central to the life of one mother as she described her connections to others through friendships, marriage, and the birth of her child. Being a wife and mother was the focus of her life--either in her marriage or with her *miracle* baby. She saw caring for her infant as a moral responsibility, as the child was completely dependent upon her. She noted an especially close relationship with her husband given their 5 years of attempts to become pregnant, their mutual thrill with the pregnancy, and her husband's concern as she developed toxemia. The baby's status was clearly more important when the decision to perform a c-section was made. Her caring for the child included any sacrifice she needed to make for the infant's health.

One father's interviews included equal discussion of relationship frameworks: inequality/equality and attachment/detachment. This man had a clear differentiation between how he perceived relationships within his family for decision-making and relationships for decisions made outside his family. His connection to family members dominated family decisions, while with neighbors and in an impersonal example of "kids trashing K-Mart carts," he made decisions based on a perceived hierarchical structure of relationships. Concern for his infant daughter's suffering was interpreted to be caring oriented in that he discussed it in terms of trying to put himself in her place. Additionally, he held himself to this standard because of his relationship and connection to her. In discussing his financial situation, he lamented being "held hostage" by the insurance coverage, which he attributed to the rules for the policy and eligible participants, an impersonal, unequal relationship with the company.

Commentary

Given the focus on decision-making or circumstances arising in the NICU as a structured health care setting, it was not surprising that a justice orientation dominated discussions by 50% of the women and 75% of the men's. A similar finding in the category of relationships then also seems logical; 43.8% of women cited inequality/equality as a predominant characteristic of relationships, as did 70% of the men. These results can be tied to the parents' perceptions of health professionals as authority figures and of physicians as the leaders among those caring for their child.

One of the most important results from this investigation of moral orientation is the evidence from parents that the NICU is a setting wherein they perceived objective rules guiding actions and driving decision-making. Relationships were arranged in hierarchical fashion and parents believed they were at the bottom of the pyramid. Health care decisions did not particularly have a moral dimension for these parents as information was presented to them. The plan of care for a baby was determined by the physician, who carried out procedures or directed others to follow the orders. Health professionals were definitely authority figures, even more so the physician, and it seemed impossible for most parents to be active participants in decision-making related to their children. The majority of the interviews over the entire course of the study were directed at the NICU experiences, so for most of the discussion, a justice representation of relationships is considered to be prevalent. All but 2 parents were able to articulate experiences that represented this justice framework (39 included both perspectives and 11 were *pure* justice oriented).

This finding is in direct contrast to some research where results indicate a caring orientation in health professionals, especially nurses (Chally 1992; Millette 1994). Evidently many parents do not experience these relationships in the same way professionals claim to interact, or the relative influence of the physician-parent relationship determined the orientation the parent described. Messages sent are not necessarily the same as messages received. Although professionals may have thought they sent *caring* messages, the status of the professional in the NICU may have led to a different decoding by the parent. Parental feelings of distress or vulnerability may have prevented a majority from perceiving caring behaviors in the professionals that surrounded their child.

Some parents did separate relationships with physicians from relationships with nurses. Although nurses were not considered as authoritarian as physicians, the parents understood both the importance of the day-to-day care nurses provided and the control these nurses had over their children. Parents did not want nurses to dislike them or find them inadequate in their role. They believed that such a judgment would lead to a compromise in the care of their infants.

Most women (n=17) were aligned with care and most men (n=14) were aligned with justice, as might be predicted based on previous research on moral orientation. However, as Gilligan emphasizes, orientation is not always gender-specific. The variety of orientations represented in this sample attests to this factor (See Figure 5.3). Ten women were aligned with justice, 3 men with care, 4 parents with both, and 3 showed no preference, for a total of 20 (38.5%) individuals who did not have orientations predictable by gender.

Health professionals need to be cognizant of the possible orientation parents assume based on the situation. Effort is needed to facilitate parental involvement in decision-making, to overcome the hierarchical perception. To accomplish this, a recognition of treatment decision-making as more than medical or nursing decisions is necessary. As long as ethics is *medicalized*, parents will feel inadequate and be reluctant to take a legitimate role in the process (Jennings 1988). Yet professionals are left behind and the baby goes home with the parents to live for many years to come. The professionals in the nursery become less and less important as other events subsequent to the NICU experience dominate the life history of the family. The parents' own roles as they relate to the child and recall previous situations are those that are foremost in their perspective. Their own perception that there was a lack of involvement or preparation for this special child is clearly a critical factor.

Notes

[a] For some additional, basic material related to moral development see the Appendix, The Research Enterprise. Table A.2 summarizes two prominent, contemporary paradigms of moral development.

[b] A review of the description of the method and the sample found in the Appendix, The Research Enterprise, might be helpful at this point as definitions and descriptions will not be repeated here.

CHAPTER 6

Interpretation of the Three Phases

> If [people] define situations as real, they are real in their consequences.
>
> William I. Thomas (n.d.)[a]

A perusal of the various phases of this study will use three lenses. First, the resulting data will be examined relative to existing theoretical work, mostly that of Reich, with which the data seemed to resonate. Second, the men's interviews will become the focus and again, include some observations about their stories. As James May stated, the father tends to be the forgotten parent (1996). However, fathers were included in this project and they offer us some insights that were developed prior to May's assertion. Finally, some feminist commentary will be proposed relative to the women as caregivers of the NICU babies. The latter two sections will include both comparisons and contrasts between the genders.

A Theory of Suffering

At a 1990 meeting for the Society for Health and Human Values, Dr. Warren T. Reich was invited to present a paper and I was one of a panel asked to respond to his paper.[b] The theme of his presentation was compassion with emphasis on his theoretical insights. Although Reich's early descriptions of his theory linked the Biblical story of Job with modern pain management and human suffering (1987b, 1987c, 1989), a number of his other papers examined bioethical dilemmas related to the neonate (1987a, 1991). Given the theoretical constructs of his paradigm of suffering, adult patients were assuredly the models for analysis in his theory, but he was also interested in neonates. Therefore, I was aware of his global interest in the continuum of health care from newborns to aging. On the panel responding to his presentation, I represented nursing. Reich's corollary theory to suffering centered on compassion as a foundation for moral reflection and moral conduct, and this interest in compassion paralleled the interest by nurses in the concept of caring as an ethical framework for professional practice. My responsibility was to reflect on Reich's remarks and compare his concepts to caring as it was espoused in nursing.

We had just completed the analysis of the interviews from Phase II of the project, so data from both the predischarge and six-month postdischarge events had recently been the focus of extended labor. As I listened to Dr. Reich review his Theory of Compassion, I believed I was on track with my prepared remarks. I framed my presentation around one particularly extensive analysis of caring in nursing (Morse et al. 1990). I planned to begin with the tension in nursing between the traditional understanding of caring as nurturing, its association with mothering, and the challenge for the profession to formalize the caring dimension, to legitimize caring interprofessionally. I planned to review the various contributions from the scholars in nursing as they researched caring theoretically and empirically, emphasizing the bioethical investigations (Brody 1988; Fry 1989; Gadow 1990; Reverby 1987; Roach 1987; Swanson 1991; Watson 1985). Carper (1978, 1979) posited an ethic of caring in her work on the epistemology of nursing. For her, the functional dimension of practice requires a particular relationship between the caregiver (nurse) and the object of caring (patient). Other scholars in nursing made caring an integral part of their nursing theories or based successful practice on incorporating caring relationships with patients (Leininger 1981, 1985; Paterson & Zderad 1976; Travelbee 1969; Watson).

I sat in the room at the conference, listening carefully so that I could augment or change my remarks as Reich explicated his theories. The panel had not been given his paper in advance. He addressed his Theory of Compassion first, then he moved on to pain and suffering. After presenting some background with the story of Job, he explained each stage of his Theory of Suffering (See Table 6.1 for a summary). Mute suffering was described as being speechless, struck dumb. Some sudden sort of event was so painful that it completely overwhelmed the individual. Reich quoted Simone Weil, who portrayed such suffering as a *silent* cry in the heart of the sufferer. "The self disappears and suffering takes over," Reich remarked (1990): "All else fades and the person is mute." His words dramatically resonated with my understanding of the parental perspective in the predischarge phase. I

Table 6.1 *Reich's Corollary Theories*[a]

THEORY OF SUFFERING	THEORY OF COMPASSION
Mute Suffering	Silent Empathy, Silent Compassion
Being speechless in the face of one's own suffering	A presence for the sufferer not in a void but quiet as a sign of respect for the *extremis* of the situation
Communication about one's suffering cannot occur	
Expressive Suffering	Expressive Compassion
The sufferer seeks a language to express his or her suffering	Assist sufferers to become conscious of and connected to the wider spectrum of meaning and and value (diagnosis, story, translate, interpret),
Lament or complaint first as it relates to their experiences. past and then look to the future	
A New Identity in Suffering: Having a Voice of One's Own (Regained Autonomy[b])	Having a Compassionate Voice of One's Own
Transformation into the new self identified through the construction of the story of suffering.	Decides at deeper level to be compassionate, conversion to compassion. Develop a *habit* of compassion and stories.

[a]Reich, W.T. 1989. Speaking of suffering: A moral account of compassion. *Soundings*, *72*(1), 83-108. The subgroups are phases in this description.
[b]Reich, W.T. 1987. Models of pain and suffering. *Acta Neurochirurgica, Supplement, 38*, 117-122. The subgroups are originally stages. Earlier, alternative title for Stage Three.

could hardly believe my ears. Was suffering, the way Reich described it, a possible contributing factor to the parents' inability to articulate the ethical dimension of the NICU experience? Was their general lack of understanding of so many aspects of the situation due to the crushing pain they felt, their responsibility for the birth of a distressed, compromised newborn? Parents sensed utter helplessness as they faced an experience with an infant who needed the most sophisticated care and monitoring the health care system had to offer. I waited as Reich continued the report of his theory.

"A dynamic incident is necessary to move on to the second stage," he resumed. A turning point occurs as the individual realizes, for whatever reason, that "this cannot go on." The person understands the contrast between the present experience of pain and suffering, and what it would mean to be without pain. The second stage of suffering--expressive suffering--can then be penetrated. Muteness ends and the sufferer regains some voice. There is a desire to be heard and the story of suffering is generated. The story is constructed to deconstruct the pain. The individual is able to stand somewhat outside the events, gain distance from self, and recount the critical events. It is also necessary to dialogue with others about the suffering, Reich continued (1990).

I felt as if I had been struck by lightening! That's why parents had so much to say in the first postdischarge interview. They had been catapulted from muteness to expressiveness by the jolt of the infant's discharge. They had gained a better understanding of the direct effect on them of their infants' NICU hospitalization, now that the infant was home. They had a desire to be heard. They needed to put their stories together, to be affirmed in their perceptions in order to move on. I was amazed. I hastily revised and expanded my own remarks to include the empirical support from my study for Reich's theory.

The panel was well received. Dr. Reich acknowledged each member's contribution to the session and we all left feeling that we had succeeded. But I left with a gem that has been incorporated into my work ever since that moment. At least one question remained. Reich's theory has a third stage, a new identity in suffering: having a voice of one's own. We had not yet conducted Phase III. Would the congruence hold? Only time would tell. Let us first examine Reich's initial two stages in a little more detail.

Theoretically, it was exciting to note a fit between the inductively derived data from this research project (Sandelowski 1986) and the concepts identified by Reich in his Theory of Suffering (1987a, 1987c, 1989, 1990). In his theological examination of suffering and loss,

Reich originally worked from the Old Testament story of Job. He also incorporated Tolstoy's *The Death of Ivan Ilyich* into his comprehension of pain, suffering, and compassion.

In mute suffering the person in crisis is unable to speak and experiences a loss of autonomy. The sufferer may wonder if anyone could possibly understand the pain and agony of the situation. How frightening it must be to think that no one knows or discerns this suffering! At this point, people lack a voice or words to express the events and the feelings. It does not mean they cannot speak, it means rather that the crisis cannot be articulated. Reich is firm in distinguishing mute suffering from the more commonly understood "suffering in silence" (1989). For him, communication about the suffering at this stage is simply not even possible.

Autonomy is affected in mute suffering because the self is threatened. The loss is not so much in freedom of physical movement but in the ability to make choices, in self-determination. The individual feels that events are out of control, self-control is not possible, and her or his own destiny is endangered. Individuals are preoccupied with suffering and are unable to act on their own values, beliefs, and traditions in the way they had previously done. People feel abandoned and isolated (Reich 1989, 1990).

Reich's model of the sufferer is the adult patient who has experienced a crisis. Although parents are not patients, their response to an imperiled newborn was sufficiently similar to that of a patient enduring her or his own predicament that the theory seemed theoretically appropriate and in fact matched the empirical data. In the predischarge phase of this neonatal study, the parental perception of the NICU experience was called the *medicalization of parenting*. To us this meant an inability to clearly articulate a role as parents for their child. Parents had been catapulted into the maze of neonatal intensive care by a disaster. Few if any were prepared for the ensuing sequence of events as the newborn experienced an emergency, whether it was during pregnancy, birth, or subsequently in the nursery. Babies were whisked away where experts could provide the critical care. Parents were helpless to provide for any of even the most basic needs. The complex care and minute-to-minute adjustments necessary to sustain life were beyond nearly every parent's knowledge and skills. Intimidated by the professionals and overwhelmed by the events, parents' voices were silenced. In some cases, attempts to develop a voice were quelled. At least parents perceived that to be the case. They waited and bided their time, caught in a cycle of ups and downs as they hoped the infant was progressing to possible discharge. Who could possibly comprehend their predicament? Initially when discussing these results and attempting to provide a rationale for the parental perspective, we stated, "The rationale for the distancing that these parents created or were led to develop relative to the ethical decision-making dimension of care for their newborns is unclear" (Pinch & Spielman 1990, p. 717). Until the connection with Reich's work was made, there was insufficient emphasis on the experience of the parents during the NICU hospitalization as being existential pain and suffering. The parents' silence, their lack of voice became significant as we analyzed and discussed Phase II, and the relationship of Reich's theory to the parental perspective was discovered.

Reich posited a transition to Stage Two, Expressive Suffering, based on the person's ability to change, or an event that forces the person to reanalyze the situation (1989). People do not have to change, of course they can simply endure suffering and be stoic, or become apathetic, resigned to life's vagaries. Morally, according to Reich, a person realizes the evil of suffering and accepts the necessary work to free one's self from the confines of suffering. Looking back over the parents' trajectory, bringing the infant home provided a startling moment for parents to begin to come to grips with the impact this infant would have on their lives. Discharge provided them with the impetus to examine the whole series of events and begin to construct their stories. For some parents, relatives, friends, and community members provided the ear for these stories. For others, it was obvious in the postdischarge interview that they were using that event to begin to piece together the meaning of the NICU hospitalization.

According to Reich, in expressive suffering the person starts to communicate the meaning of the crisis experience in the form of lament, complaint, or condemnation. Additionally, the sufferer may create a story or may develop an interpretation of the experience. Composing a story provides sufferers with an opportunity to organize the events they have experienced, gain a more objective perspective on the effect of these circumstances, and then make a place for it in their personal or family history. This process is ever evolving over time and does not separate the past from the present. Portions of the narrative may always remain in close contact with the present. Telling the story serves as an act of acquiring affirmation for the experiences and facilitates the formulation of a new self. A new life is created, and the new voice is necessary for passage to the third stage (Reich 1989).

Although Reich did not use the analogy, expressive suffering can be compared to the process of the Phoenix rising from the ashes. Much has been destroyed, perhaps not always literally, but certainly past expectations for pregnancy, birth, or the newborn were not fulfilled. For many parents there is simply a delay in reconfiguring future plans. Eventually, normal development is a reasonable expectation. For a few parents, the fact that a normal newborn failed to materialize leaves little hope for a normal childhood. Life plans may have been completely shattered.

In Phase II, parents at 6 months postdischarge were just beginning to be able to communicate their experiences and the meaning of the events in the NICU. Parents were more emotional at this point than in the predischarge phase. As they opened themselves to personal reflection, parents responded with both positive and negative feelings about their situation. They were sorting out their experiences and working at putting the NICU events into perspective. Most were in one way or another searching for an explanation for what had happened to them--why them, why at this time. Now that the baby was home and parents were totally responsible for its care, they were faced with the astonishing reality of the effect of this newborn on their lives. At 6 months postdischarge, the stories were not completely constructed (Pinch & Spielman 1993).

Having a voice of one's own marks Reich's third stage of suffering which he calls a new identity in suffering. The individual has faced the pain and suffering of the crisis. Through introspection the sufferer has examined not only the earth-shaking events of the past but also personal qualities and characteristics, values, beliefs, and traditions. The events are tentatively shared at first. The waters are tested, so to speak, as the sufferer begins to engage in dialogue about the experience and its meaning. As voice is gained, the story is revised. The cycle of construction and reflection is completed again and again until gradually a precise new self is formulated. An acceptable interpretation is uncovered. Radical transformation is possible, according to Reich, when one's suffering is accepted by another individual who provides caring and compassion. Reich emphasizes the relative nature of the new self and the fact that pain and suffering may not be eliminated. In regaining autonomy, however, the individual is no longer "submerged in the anguish, the grinding destructiveness, of the suffering" (Reich 1989). "The suffering is translocated and is of minor significance" to the new self (Pinch & Spielman 1996, p. 80).

Was support for Reich's theory sustained by the empirical data collected in Phase III? In the last phase, named *life goes on*, parents did accept or adjust to their crises in some manner or another. They went on to meet their own needs and responsibilities as parents of this *special* newborn. Parents had a comprehensible story at 4 years postdischarge and were able to relate their narrative to others. At four years from the experience, parents incorporated the chronicle of the NICU into their history. Although many initially protested that the hospitalization seemed to be quite a long time past, it was easy to tap the memories and procure substantial recall. Some have positive or no residual effects of the experience; others were permanently and negatively affected. The revisions and additions to the initial stories from the six-month postdischarge phase were quite apparent in the four-year postdischarge interview. The importance of a compassionate recipient for the story was also evident. Parents mentioned their gratitude for being able to participate in this research project. To them it was confirmation of interest in their experience and an attempt to make a difference for future parents' experiences in a NICU. At this last interview, many parents described a new identity of self and had moved on (Pinch & Spielman 1996).

A Theory of Compassion

The importance of a compassionate response to suffering is critical to Reich's understanding of the entire process of recovery. He constructed a Theory of Compassion (see Table 6.1 for a summary) that encompasses three stages of compassion parallel to the stages of suffering:

1. Silent empathy, silent compassion
2. Expressive compassion
3. Having a compassionate voice of one's own.

In silent compassion, no words are necessary. Communication of empathy, respect for the extreme suffering of a fellow human being, can be accomplished by simply being present, *being with.* As Reich indicated, silence indicates receptivity and acceptance of the other (1989).

In the second stage, the compassionate person assists the individual sufferer to construct the story. Reich stressed the importance of information and knowledge for this process. Although a diagnosis such as cancer may be bad news, a diagnosis is a concrete name, a precise term upon which the sufferer can begin to assemble the narrative and make sense of the painful experience. The caregiver can assist by sharing her/his own perception of the experience or the experiences of others from the caregiver's history of contact with similar persons and events. From these examples, the sufferer can compare and contrast personal perceptions and formulate her/his own version (Reich 1989).

With parents at the six-month interview, it was apparent that one of the restrictions imposed upon their attempts to create their stories was the lack of sufficient information about the infant from the NICU experience. An inability to name the infant's problems or articulate the procedures of the NICU hampered them in constructing their own narratives and put the experience into perspective. Such a limitation emphasizes the importance of education in healing--not simply providing the information as documented in the charts of the infants, but also assessing comprehension of the knowledge and its retention.

The compassionate person need not understand the suffering to be effective, however. Recognizing profound suffering and indicating to the bearer of such pain that there is a desire to understand, may be sufficient evidence of empathy and permission for the sufferer to attempt vocally to describe the distress. To indicate a willingness to remain with the suffering person in spite of the misery, and to accept the struggle, not flee from the pain, is a critical role in recovery. Examining the crisis, interpreting its meaning, and defining a new autonomous self are not easy tasks.

Gadow (1980) discussed a similar approach to suffering that she labeled existential advocacy. Individuals are "*assisted* by nursing to *authentically* exercise their freedom of determination" (her emphasis). This means working with individuals to determine what they want to do, not what health professionals or others determine they should do. The nurse, for Gadow, should help protect patients' rights to do what they want to do. It is the nurse's responsibility to assist patients to explore their own values and beliefs in order to determine what they clearly want to do. Self-determination can occur only after self-examination and a reaffirmation or recreation of one's values.

Finally, the compassionate person her/himself is changed (Reich 1989). Intimate engagement in the process of constructing a story of suffering gives the compassionate person new insight into patients' experiences. The caregiver's world view is shifted, somewhat based on this pursuit of understanding. The compassionate person takes the new perspective into every future situation, at best being better able to serve another individual who is suffering at some other point. Mutual involvement with the sufferer augments the ability of the compassionate person to continue to appreciate the subjective dimension of grief, illness, and dying. It helps to enable the health professional as a compassionate person to appreciate the content and context of illness as the patient or the family experiences it.

Loss, Grief, Anger, and Rage

For a few families, the crisis of a NICU experience represented such profound loss that transition to and completion of tasks like those described for Reich's Stage Three may not have yet occurred. Although statistically speaking only occasional families may be affected by extreme morbidity in their children, for those families so touched, it means 100% of their lives are influenced by the residual effects. Some moral distress of parents seen in the interviews of this project relates to the conflict between being the *good parent* for this helpless, needy, afflicted newborn and the outrage they feel for lost dreams and hopes.[c] Part of the expectation of being this good parent is self-imposed. The other portion is how parents interpret society's expectations but more immediately what they believe health professionals in the nursery expect. Parents described their need to be mature, in control, stoic, devoted, caring, loving, accepting, attentive, and other similar attributes, as parents of this child. Parents do not always have the inner strength of resources or external support to meet the expectations of being the good parent when confronted by such significant losses.

The loss for these families may mean the loss of their entire future. The entire set of expectations that parents may have set for themselves has been wiped out. For most couples, the expectation that they will have children and their families will experience the normal developmental milestones is likely present when marriage vows are exchanged or commitment is made to a partner, although such a phenomenon may not necessarily be articulated. More precise expectations may have developed and been voiced if couples encountered infertility. As early as months or years prior to the NICU admission, they may have begun the efforts to become pregnant. The prospects of a normal newborn and postpartum recovery are certainly gone once admission to the NICU is completed. Loss can expand as more crises are encountered and the hospitalization of the infant is protracted.

Loss, as we are aware, can lead to grief, and certainly grief is present in the NICU. Loss, grief, sadness, and more frequently the concept of chronic sorrow have been extensively discussed in relation to parents whose children bear lifelong compromises to their health and well-being (Eakes et al. 1998; Hummel & Eastman 1991; Mallow & Bechtel 1999; Olshansky 1962; Teel 1991). What is also possible in these parents, and what we are less likely to understand, be willing to recognize, and ultimately confront, is the resulting anger and rage that the parents' circumstances create in them. Yet it was anger and rage that a few parents felt and expressed when they were given permission to do so.

Sadness, suffering, and loss have been a part of our description of these parents as we explored their perception of the NICU experience over the entire course of our research endeavors. The resonance with Reich's work on suffering was recognized after the six-month postdischarge interview and was immediately incorporated into discussions of the results. However, the moral significance of the parents' anger and even rage for the process of reconciling the challenge of their circumstances eluded us until more recently.

Kleiver's contributions (1989, 1995) to an understanding of suffering led him to investigate the relationship of anger and rage to pain and suffering. Kleiver did not examine parents of imperiled neonates but instead discussed the situation of Dax, the burn patient who has been celebrated as the icon of a patient's right to die.[d] Kleiver takes exception to such a rights interpretation of the interview with Dax in the film *Please Let Me Die?* and rather focuses on the chronology presented in the film and the veiled emotions in Dax's voice. Dax's case, according to Kleiver involves a chronic condition, not an acute situation, and despite the regular modulation of Dax's voice and his cogent responses to questions of the psychiatrist who converses with him in the film, Dax is suffering acutely. He is angry, but it is carefully masked. Prior to reading this analysis of suffering and resulting rage and anger, I failed to give the anger, and indeed the rage in some parents, the importance it deserved in my research.

It would behoove us as health professionals to remember the experiences that parents expected to encounter as opposed to those that they are actually facing in the NICU. Instead of joy, happiness, pride, and relief, parents feel sadness, fear, anxiety, and trepidation. Rather than viewing experienced health professionals as kind and loving caregivers for their normal newborn, personnel rescued and salvaged a shattered dream. In their suffering and pain, parents can also encounter anger and rage at this toss of the dice. Yes, such a crisis does not happen to all parents, not even a majority of them--but why should they be objects of this twist of fate. Distress and frustration engender anger and rage.

Generally speaking, as health professionals, we are not ready nor willing to confront anger and rage in patients. Anger and rage are generally unacceptable emotions in our society. Yet anger and rage abound, not just in these parents but in many other individuals as well. Our society tends to attempt to sanitize emotions in real people. There is a narrow range of acceptable emotions for even the most devastating experiences, especially when we have to personally confront such emotions. Religion or spiritual experience is one of the few outlets we have to offer. Some of the parents did turn to their religious beliefs, pastors, priests, and rabbis in order to cope with their losses. But we have no other rituals or ceremonies to assuage the havoc created by the loss of the normal newborn when religion and spirituality are an unacceptable refuge for parents.

As a society we have put much emphasis on youth, beauty, physical perfection, and normalcy. The handicapped, imperiled, and disfigured continue to battle for acknowledgment of their rightful place in society. Such a place can be sculpted when sufficient resources are guaranteed to sustain an adequate quality of life for such individuals, and society's attitudes become more accepting related to disabilities and handicaps. In the meantime, we are morally obligated to address the parental experience with children who have severe morbidity, parents who are filled with rage, living in a private hell of profound loss. This is the shadow side of the consequences of a NICU hospitalization.

Another element that has particular impact on the subjective perception of the NICU experience is gender. Content and context are often shaped by the socialization processes that one experiences as either male or female. Mothers and fathers of high-risk newborns bring their own gendered perspectives to the NICU events, just as they do to any ordinary or other extraordinary episode in life. For health professionals, their individual gendered views also shape an often unacknowledged dimension of decision-making. Assumptions and stereotypes can play an unexamined role in the family-infant-professional triad. A closer examination of the high-risk situation with a focus on gender can be enlightening.

Gender as an Ethical Ingredient

Interest in gender as an issue in this study began as we examined material on families or parental responses to the NICU experience. I made two observations. One, both the health care professionals and the women in the study appeared to make the assumption that the mother would be the primary caregiver for the infant, regardless of the volume and complexity of care the child would require when discharged. Second, although parental or family reactions were the focus of the study, it became increasingly apparent that the concept of a *family* response was difficult to develop--not a unique discovery in research. Although we claimed to examine parental perspectives in this project, we discussed issues with either fathers or mothers, together and/or separately. We did not immediately recognize the disservice committed by collapsing data in our own primary analysis into parental perspectives rather than addressing mothers' and fathers' perceptions separately. However, the analysis of moral orientation was specifically completed based on examining data from the women and men separately. Until this secondary analysis and many months of subsequent work on the meaning of that analysis, the need for gender distinctions was not apparent.

In a very early set of articles on parents, Caplan (1960) and associates (1965) described how they set out to conduct research with families. Eventually they decided that they were not doing family research even when they examined both individuals. They regretted that the methodologies available to family researchers were inadequate for measuring the holistic perspective necessary to accurately portray the family and saw the need for development of such methodologies. Therefore they focused exclusively on the mother as she faced the crisis of a premature birth and "other family members only insofar as they affected her and her relationship with the baby" (Caplan 1965, pp. 152-153).[e]

Although the situation has improved since the 1970s (Miles, Funk et al. 1992), some reviewers are still critical of research labeled parental or family (Cardwell 1993; Holditch-Davis & Miles 1997; Moriarty & Cotroneo 1993). Family research is biased in terms of the mother-infant relationship which is vastly over-represented. Cardwell scrutinized 91 studies and concluded that *none* qualified as *family* research. The perinatal studies she examined favored investigation of the mother 2 to 1. *Parenting the prematurely born child* was a review of research published in 1997 (Holditch-Davis & Miles). In every section of their analysis, these reviewers recognized the limitation of neglecting fathers in the investigation of parenting and the need to include them more in the future. Nevertheless, what the authors themselves said was somewhat biased. In one section they stated that fathers were involved in *many* studies conducted during hospitalization, an actual count showed that 11 of 15 studies used only mothers as subjects. Even with such small numbers, four does not seem to be *many* studies involving fathers.

Realistically speaking, in order to investigate a phenomenon in a target population, both the phenomenon and the population have to be present. In many cases where fathers are present in neonatal families, they do not take caregiving roles or implement them extensively. Certainly such circumstances need to be acknowledged. So when we speak of the *burden* of care and the sacrifice women/mothers are expected to make on children's behalf, this contention may reveal more about the failure of men and society to be responsible for children than about problems inherent in the disabilities or special needs of children (Asch & Geller 1996). In other situations, fathers are simply not present in the family. In fact, in one study it was noted that 41% of families with disabled children were headed by a single parent, the mother (Gallagher & Bristol as cited in Gartner et al. 1990, p. 50, note 6). This included separated, never married, and divorced circumstances. Another report included the case of a father who flatly refused to acknowledge his role in the conception of a newborn with physical and mental disabilities. He accused his wife of having relations with the father of another affected child (Palmer & Noble 1986). Of course now we can determine genetic links and such disclaimers can be corrected.

I searched a major index for studies on parenting, families, and caregiving in order to update this situation for myself after the collection of the data for the project was completed.[f] Forty-seven articles were identified that appeared typical of issues related to high-risk neonatal care, and most did in fact target mothers. Of those that used "parenting" or "families" in the title, most were not specific in the abstracts about whether the authors actually considered both parents in the study. One, despite a general title related to neonate care, included only the mother's perspective, and in most pieces, mothers were over-represented.[g] At the extreme, a researcher who claimed to examine parenting actually included 24 mothers and only 1 father (Hall 1996).[h] Marital status for mothers was omitted in a several studies, which limits the information that may be relevant for considerations of support when planning neonatal postdischarge care.

I will provide one exemplar case of the distortion in *parenting* research to show what may be described even if both genders are represented. In the article "A Theory of Transformed Parenting"

(Seideman & Kleine 1995), the abstract indicated the sample was divided into 29 mothers and 13 fathers. In the body of the article, the researchers regularly referred to "parenting" when in fact far, far more of the material related to mothers than to fathers. On 3 of the 6 pages in the article, there were references to only "parent" or "mother," so fathers were not even included in half the material. My own research with parental decision-making also has more mothers represented than fathers, and I too have combined the data in many instances, unaware of the full meaning of this strategy until recently.

In summarizing this literature, it would seem important to appreciate women's roles as caregivers in a majority of families, recognize the absence of fathers in certain situations, and make an effort to include fathers when they are present in the household. Although not all fathers of babies hospitalized in the NICU are present or responsible for parenting the infant, health professionals need to consider the role of fathers if we are to provide holistic care to these families. Conversely, mothers of disabled infants invariably take on disproportionate responsibility for their care and consequently relinquish all other economic and social roles (Asch & Geller 1996). The very survival of these children depends mainly on women, mothers certainly, but also nurses, attendants, and baby-sitters (Pierce & Frank 1992). Generally, women are viewed as responsible for family life. The evidence is overwhelming that mothers are in fact predominately caregivers of these infants; at least, discussants/researchers assume they are, given the target populations of the studies.

Professional caregivers need to be careful not to perpetuate stereotypical thinking. Traditional role-taking by gender should be understood and initially taken into consideration when assessing the parents. Information about motherhood should not be generalized to fathers, any more than results of research targeting males should be applied to females. Professionals can then begin to educate parents about the options available to them relative to their roles. Ideas about more collaborative caregiving can be explored. Some parents may be open to such suggestions because of their family values and beliefs; others may reject alternative recommendations. However, the seed may be planted and traditional parental roles may begin to be viewed differently as the expanding family takes a new place in society. Opening parental eyes to shared caregiving would seem particularly important in cases where newborns are severely compromised and lifelong, special interventions for even activities of daily living are required.

A compelling reason for considering gender differences from a bioethical perspective can also be posited. Despite claims of neutrality or objectivity, or at least claims of justice and fairness, most of us would acknowledge decision-makers and those who would opt to influence parents come to this discussion with values, beliefs, traditions, knowledge bases, goals/objectives, and myriad other factors that render us far from neutral or objective. Some possible biases and prejudices have been addressed. Medical and/or nursing personnel, as well as other health professionals, may have a bias to save and in that process overtreat infants. Parents may be immature, suffering, in grief, or physically incapacitated. Anyone can be prejudiced or ignorant about life with a handicap or disability, or an acceptable minimal quality of life. Withdrawing or withholding treatment for the benefit of family or society rather than in the best interest of the child has also been noted as a serious concern in ethical decision making (Cantor 1995; Kopelman 1995; Weir 1995). But this perspective may prevent reasonable considerations of withholding or withdrawing aggressive therapy. Other biases and prejudices have not been addressed.

It is my premise that we could benefit from further examination of decision-making, particularly from a feminist perspective. Decision-making for children has been a topic of interest and concern for as long as people have discussed or debated the value of children. When disability or some compromised status affects children, the thrust of the debate takes on an especially weighty responsibility. Disability, delayed growth and development, or threats to survival often accompany prematurity, traumatic birth processes, congenital anomalies, and other high-risk newborn conditions.

A child's birth and its subsequent life, whether normal or especially if not normal, have always had specific, significant meaning for women. And the special issues for women related to reproduction--conceiving, child bearing, and birthing a child--have been widely addressed in the feminist literature. It is time to move beyond these basic issues of reproduction, and begin to examine some immediate and longer term implications of ethical decision-making, especially related to high-risk infants and their mothers.[i] Because NICUs appear to have a permanent place in health care systems, what are the possible implications for women in their roles as mothers, especially mothers of infants with long-term sequelae? But first, the father's voice as represented in this project.

The Father's Role: Oft Forgotten

Two concepts are foundational to an understanding of the fathers' perspectives. First is the epistemological aspect, which reflects the idea that examinations of parental issues should address fatherhood as separate from motherhood. What do we presently know about fathers, and how is that different from our knowledge about mothers? Second, is the axiological dimension or the morals and values associated with fathers' beliefs of fathering roles related to the newborn and its subsequent development.

The Fathers' Profile

Few fathers have felt inclined to create and tell their own stories about the NICU experience. One notable exception is Robert Stinson who with his wife, Peggy, coauthored *The long dying of Baby Andrew* (1983). The diary of another father was published as part of a special issue on the NICU in *Second Opinion* (Buchanan 1986). Later, Jerry Adler, a reporter for *Newsweek* magazine, wrote his own story "Every parent's nightmare," promoted on the magazine's cover (1987; 1988). A small first person account on kangaroo care and a story from the father of twins have also been published (Anner 1994; Bartrick 1983). One father, in collaboration with a nurse, discussed his perceptions and recommendations for nursing care in the NICU (Long & Smyth 1998). Max De Pree (1994) wrote about his experience as a grandfather and surrogate father for a 24-weeker delivered by his daughter. A conference on the future of perinatal health care included a presentation on *The Father's Role in Perinatal Care*, a promising development.[j]

Clearly, in the professional literature it is still somewhat difficult to ferret out paternal information. Some material on parents or neonate caregiving does not identify the gender of those involved. For purposes of our study, parental or family research that used only mothers as examples was deemed inadequate. It was especially disappointing to find parental or family research in which marital status was not indicated, gender of participating parents was not cited, or a gender breakdown was not provided. Although this lack may represent a deliberate effort to present data in a gender-neutral manner, conflating the information makes it impossible to discern gender differences.[k]

I am convinced by psychological and sociological principles and my own research results that mothers and fathers are in fact different, and information which simply indicates "parents" is woefully inadequate for understanding fathers or defining nursing interventions for them. Unfortunately, the research foundation of much family and parental data is based only on mothers. I am just as opposed to generalization to fathers based on data from mothers as I am to generalizing to women based on theories and research targeting men. On one hand, gender-neutral language supports the current politically correct approach wherein the parental role is viewed as potentially fulfilled by either gender. On the other hand, there is a disservice to both men and women in ignoring the reality of their present situations by conflated data gathered from individuals and reporting it as parental information. The former, politically correct language, is more or less philosophically ideal while the latter, conflated data, is the empirical base upon which we should be making decisions--the latter is a problem.

What can we tease out about fathers? In about 26 articles on parenting or families of high-risk infants that I was able to access (not including those on decision-making), some gender specific notes were made about fathers. Sixteen articles compared mothers and fathers, and two focused solely on fathers. The findings are summarized below.

Prior to the NICU experience, the developmental tasks of a pregnancy are assigned to the expectant woman for the most part. A wide range of anticipated responses exists among various types of men. Men do pass through several stages however: (a) announcement, which occurs between first suspicion and confirmation; response varies with desirability of pregnancy; (b) moratorium or distancing of self from process; and (c) focusing, with changes in attitudes and redefinition as parent. Some men experience couvade. When preterm labor occurs, the process of becoming a father is shortened, and this can result in anger, distress, grief, and fear for the child (Conner & Denson 1990). Fathers also feel anxiety for the wife related to the complications, hospitalization, and tocolytic medications (McCain & Deatrick 1994). Men feel vulnerable and sense high levels of anxiety during this period as they perceive a need to be a strong support for their wives. One study showed that an opportunity to tour the NICU prior to the newborn's hospitalization results in benefits for the men; the environment became familiar and familiarity is comforting (Griffin et al. 1997).

For most men, the child in the NICU does not belong to them; a child is a reality only after they meet face-to-face and reality is further cemented when the child comes home (Conner & Denson 1990;

Schraeder 1980). Men have concerns for the infant's problems, but these may differ from the mother's focus (Hawkins-Walsh 1980). Although fathers experienced significantly more emotional distress than normative values, they were more well-adjusted and less anxious, hostile, and depressed than mothers (Doering et al. 1999). Fathers are more accepting of health care professionals who indicate the child will be potentially handicapped. Fathers tend to be more concerned about the outcome for child, while mothers were concerned about infant's presenting gestational age (Lee et al. 1991). Affleck and associates (1990) found fathers to have less concern than mothers over possible mental retardation but equal concern for other problems and disabilities. Brown, York, and colleagues (1989) found that fathers were found to actually visit the infant less over time, although Marton and associates found fathers visiting more than mothers prior to the fifth day of the infant's life (1981).

Fathers also expressed a perception of less control over the infant's recovery than mothers and in fact behaved differently toward the infant. Others showed less nurturing behavior (Novak 1990), less touch, and less talk (Harrison & Woods 1991; Thurman & Korteland 1989). They emphasized the small size of the infant (McCain & Deatrick 1994; Novak 1990), lack of clarity about their role, and a competing need to support the mother rather than focus on the baby (Novak). The less intimate behavior by fathers extended through approximately the first year of the infant's life (Harrison & Woods; Thurman & Korteland). However, one study found fathers of newborns with health problems performed significantly more infant care activities at 1 month postdischarge than fathers of healthy newborns study (Brown 1987; Brown, Rustia, et al. 1991). At 3 months postdischarge, activities were not significantly different. Additionally, fathers of infants with health problems had higher adjustment to parenthood scores indicating better adjustment.

In general, fathers feel less prepared for the NICU experience and have a less intense emotional response to it than mothers (Blackburn & Lowen 1986). However, studies of stress and anxiety have shown somewhat mixed results. In most reports, fathers cited less distress (Affleck et al. 1990; Benfield et al. 1976), and less stress (Hughes et al. 1994; Jeffcoate et al. 1979; Miles, Carlson et al. 1996; Philipp 1983; Trause & Kramer 1983). However, mothers and fathers reported the same stress in research by Shields-Poë and Pinelli (1997). Miles and associates (1996) found similar levels of anxiety but Shields-Poë and Pinelli found anxiety higher in fathers, with the anxiety related to perceived morbidity of the infant as well as its ambiguous diagnosis and treatment, and the unclear parental role. Fathers showed less coping difficulties than mothers (Trause & Kramer). The men's use of instrumental activities is associated with their higher emotional well-being (Affleck et al.). Men used less escapist coping strategies.

Spouses are usually the main source of support for each other, but according to Blackburn and Lowen (1986), mothers rather than fathers indicated that their needs were not met. In Miles, Carlson, and Funk's study (1996), nurses were the first line of support for fathers initially and then the spouse became the primary support person. Fathers need less support than mothers and seek it less frequently (Affleck et al. 1990; Miles, Carlson et al. 1996). Spouses agree on the extent of personal harm that ensues from this crisis of a high-risk infant hospitalization.

The lesser degree of stress felt by fathers (Goldberg 1990) and their lesser need for social support (Heaman 1995) continue into the postdischarge phase. Fathers feel less empty (unfulfilled as a result of a premature baby rather than a normal one) and are not depressed by the behavioral problems of their children (Fraley 1986). Fathers have more depression and stress connected with cognitively impaired children than children who have physical handicaps (Clubb 1991). In Lee and associates' study (1991) the majority of parents of both very low birth weight infants and healthy term infants supported saving all infants regardless of the outcome, however, fathers were less likely than mothers to disagree with saving infants predisposed to be severely handicapped or mentally retarded. Generally fathers less frequently than mothers express specific feelings after the preterm birth, although the 10 feelings most frequently cited were the same for both groups (Hummel & Eastman 1991). In that research, the only significant difference found was in frustration, which was higher for mothers. Fathers actually indicated that they try to keep feelings out of problem solving (Heaman). Self-control is an important issue for them. In the study by Hummel and Eastman, 10% of the mothers mentioned that they felt isolated once they were home with the baby, while no father indicated this. Mothers were more frequently the caregiver, while fathers take on an instrumental role (Clubb). Fathers were concerned about finances (Heaman) and being able to hire baby-sitters in order to get out of the house with the spouse alone, without the baby (Fraley; Heaman).

Fathers and Ethical Decision-making in the NICU

I was unable to identify any previous research in ethics that specifically targeted the fathers of high-risk newborns. A few studies about decision-making separately identify mothers and fathers in the description of the samples, with subsequent quotes attributed to fathers when appropriate (Able-Boone et al. 1989; Barber et al. 1992; Benfield et al. 1978; Raines 1996; Rottman 1986; Schlomann & Fister 1995; Walwork & Ellison 1985). Few themes or implications are attributed to fathers rather than mothers even when data were collected separately from each parent (see Benfield et al. 1978 on resulting grief from decision-making/death of infant). Some studies indicated the inclusion of *parents* but either failed to treat parents separately, or simply emphasized or used only mothers' responses (Bodgan et al. 1982; Harrison 1986; Kirschbaum 1994; Mason 1986; Post 1987; Rostain 1986; Rue 1985; Watchko 1983; Zaner & Bilton 1991). Other articles discussed parental perspectives, although this was not indicated in the titles (Duff & Campbell 1973; Evans 1989; Mellien 1992; Swyter 1984). Again these examples of research or discussion may indicate the gender of sources of specific perspectives or quotes, but do not contrast one gender's viewpoint with the other's, or extract fathers' perceptions.

Father's Perceptions of Their Role in the NICU and Beyond

As a reminder, a total of 20 men participated in the project presented here.[1] For about half the experience was their first as a father, and for all of them, it was the first time they had had a seriously ill or critically ill newborn.

Concern for the condition of the woman was the initial crisis most often cited by these fathers as they told their stories of the NICU experience--despite the fact that most of their concerns arose prior to the infant's hospitalization in a NICU and we did not ask parents to recite pre-NICU incidents. Fathers were overwhelmingly concerned about their partner's/wife's status during pregnancy and birth rather than the condition of the fetus/infant. One father described his situation:

> It was terrible...something I wouldn't wish anyone to go through. She laid there for 7 hours hemorrhaging - which is probably the worst part. I mean, I told them I was getting real tired of waiting. If I had to, I was going to call in another doctor to give me another answer because I

> didn't feel that this was right. By this time you know, she's not in very good shape. I thought the decision [to wait] was wrong right there at that particular time. That will be my feeling for the rest of my life even though she is fine now.

Another man remarked how he thought "they knew what they were doing" and "had things under control" despite the early labor and delivery. He understood that his wife's infection was a problem and felt that his stay in the hospital was stressful, but that she was in good hands.

A few men even mentioned that they perceived a possible bias in the health professionals' recommendations toward the fetus's survival rather than the woman's life or health, which actually alarmed them. One man addressed this in terms of a belief that health professionals were "sacrificing the woman." Another noted that he needed his wife at home to continue helping to raise their other children after this experience. By his standards, the birth was relatively unimportant in comparison to the competing needs for the life and health of his spouse. This concern for their partners continued into the NICU experience and was especially strong in cases wherein the woman herself was hospitalized in the postpartum stage for sequelae from either pregnancy or birth. The men worried about the effects of prolonged bedrest and tocolytic drugs on the woman as well as the potential recovery from these events.

A few brought up distress over decisions in the labor/delivery phase, mostly because the woman was not in a position to decide. These men seemed to want to be sure that we knew that their partner's inability to participate in the decision-making was the rationale for their solo role in the process. It was almost as if they felt guilty about not sharing decision-making with the woman, especially in relation to baby issues at delivery.

One father recounted an intense experience when he was asked to make a decision about his baby immediately after birth. The woman's membranes had ruptured early and the professionals were not sure the fetus was of sufficient size to survive. The parents refused a c-section and wanted to let nature take its course. The parents also agreed that no extraordinary means should be used at birth. They did not want aggressive interventions. The father continues to recall to this day how the staff called him into a separate room where they had whisked the baby immediately after the vaginal delivery. The baby was somewhat larger than they had anticipated and the staff was actively resuscitating him. The father speaks:

> They said, do you want to keep him? He's real responsive you know, there is every indication that he is very viable. What could I say? I didn't have the heart to say no. But I never understood why they saved those kids. So I went back into the delivery room and told my wife, but of course by that time the decision was long out of our hands. We told them we didn't want any heroic measures to keep him alive. That's why we didn't have the c-section. Looking back, I couldn't make that hard decision even though [our son] is going to live a very, very frustrating life. I didn't know, all I knew was the magic things that happen in hospitals, you know.[m]

Fathers' descriptions of their newborns focused on the relatively small, fragile appearance of the infant. Although this does not mean mothers were unimpressed by such a small living creature, parents' attitudes about the size were different. Size worried mothers, while fathers expressed their amazement and wonder. One of the more radical differences between spouses provided a striking example which was already described in Chapter 2 (see *Contrasting Perceptions*).

After admission of the infant to the NICU, fathers as a group were no different from mothers in their perception of ethical decision-making about the infant. They were firm about their nonparticipation in decision-making for the infant as described in detail earlier.

While the infant was in the NICU, the fathers were more concerned about getting back to work, continuing their own education, or getting on with their normal/usual role than about interacting with the child or being present in the nursery. Some statements made by fathers were:

- They know what they are doing in there and I can't help.
- I wouldn't know right from wrong, so why worry about what is going on.
- My wife [or other relative] can better do what needs to be done while the baby is in the NICU.

No fathers expressed a desire to be *more* involved than they were in the child's care while the baby was in the hospital.

Fathers also agreed with mothers in their requests for health professionals to sit down and talk with them about their infant and their own expected roles in these circumstances. Most fathers (70%) and many mothers (44%) alike perceived a hierarchical structure in their relationships with professionals, with their own position inferior to that of the professional (see Chapter 5). Men were far less likely than the women to seek comfort, solace, and support from the nurses, however. Also, fathers were more negative about the physician relationship than about their discussions with nurses, and more vocal about these negative perceptions than the mothers.

Looking at their situation from the perspective of living with a high-risk newborn 4 years after discharge, most fathers found the children's outcomes acceptable when initially asked about the child's health status. They were accepting despite the fact that only 1 child out of 30 was without any problems surfacing since discharge; 6 were in serious condition with multiple complications; 15 others had delays in growth and development; and other incidental problems among the whole group included hearing, speech, and/or respiratory issues, or mental impairment. In one-third of the couples, parents disagreed about the child's health status; the men were the more optimistic about the status of the child when parents did not agree.

A strong theme among these men was that, looking back, they wished they had been better prepared for the possible events of a high-risk pregnancy and/or birth. And they certainly wanted to be informed about events prospectively rather than learning after the fact. Several men were able to make this judgment quite clear, based on their later examination of the infants' charts, which they secured after discharge. From their interpretations, they believed that in many cases health professionals had already drawn a particular conclusion or actually made a decision about the child before they as fathers were informed of the circumstances. They perceived that it really did not matter what parents thought or believed at the point when they were brought into the decision-making process, although they had been led to think they were making decisions. It was not that *no* information had been shared but rather that the whole story was not revealed.

It must be added that, although mothers were not much different in their perceptions of being informed by the professional staff about their own particular baby, mothers were more likely to mention that they had sought out and read additional material about a high-risk pregnancy or a multiple birth. They found information in pamphlets, magazines, and books, as well as from other women. Women were more likely to say that they regretted having not asked enough questions. Two men actually said that for certain aspects of their experience, they would *not* want to know. No woman ever said that to us.

Responsibility for child-care was noted by only a minority of fathers. For the majority, work and community involvement were central to their role responsibilities. The men were far more concerned than the women about finances, including keeping their jobs and maintaining insurance coverage. When discussing their moral responsibility, these fathers represented gender stereotypical thinking: Their role was to provide for the family and the family's material needs; mothers were to take care of children (even when a number of these women had employment outside the home and for some women, insurance benefits were tied to the woman's employment status). In one case where the infant died, the father found the experience so intense he was unable to leave the house and go to work for some time. He expressed his guilt over the inability to function in strong terms as he declared his profound grief at his infant's death.

In many cases, the fathers focused on the joy and fun of their child, while the mothers of those same children cited the work connected with the child as a first concern. Enjoyment came second for the women. The fathers generally viewed child problems as less serious than the mothers, and this was probably the area of greatest disagreement between parents. Fathers were more apt to focus on a fortunate aspect of the outcome despite some grim possibilities or on the miracle of their situation, while the mothers worried more about both present and potential problems. In fact, some men noted that people generally worried too much. They based such judgments on two observations: one, the reactions they detected in friends, family, and neighbors, and the other grounded in their experience observing other parents in the NICU. Women more often noted the responsibility to sign various informed consent forms which may have triggered their awareness of interventions. After discharge, children were taken to the physician's office or clinics for additional follow-up by mothers rather than fathers.

The findings that more mothers than fathers were involved in caregiving does not mean that no fathers provided care. One outlier case is a father who had complete responsibility for child-care once he came home from his employment. His situation at 4 years postdischarge is discussed more extensively in Chapter 4. He lamented his situation and continued to feel distressed about the burdens of care. Another father of twins with serious sequelae was headed down the same path when he and his wife turned their mental attitude around. His remarks were included in Chapter 2.

Another area of importance to some fathers but not included by a majority of men was the place of prayer and faith in the experience with a high-risk newborn. This spiritual dimension of life is noted here because of the emphasis that these men placed on this aspect of their lives, especially given the challenge of the NICU experience. One father explained how the NICU experience touched him.

> ...my life has always been touched by God since very young. I would get into things more like meditation and, you know, sit back and write poetry and be in my own little world. Whereas with [wife] and [baby] up there [in the NICU], I became more open. I saw other families up there struggling. I always knew God had some purpose of calling in my life, so it became real easy for me to talk to people about their problems, ask them how they were doing. And it gave me a lot of inner satisfaction just to be a tree or something that somebody could lean on up there. It was doing what I knew in my heart was the right thing to do.

Another man discussed the support he felt from a prayer group while his children were hospitalized:

> ...there's people from church that were always calling and, we have a couple of different prayer chains. And, I suppose just through the prayer that we just always felt so calm even though...we didn't know if they were going to be dead or alive.

Finally a small group of men emphasized how different life was since having this baby. The difference was far more than they had anticipated. The demands of the new baby impinged upon former activities which they valued, and it affected the time they were able to spend with their partner. Sometimes they deeply regretted these developments, but at other times these fathers also had certain expectations for themselves now that family life involved a child.

One father of twins described his situation at 6 months postdischarge. This man had a serious interest in music. In fact, the interviewer first thought he was a professional musician, given the amount and complexity of audio equipment in the family's living room, along with the hundreds and hundreds of tapes, CDs, and records. There was also a piano keyboard and stacks of sheet music, headphones, and other paraphernalia. During the predischarge interview he had mentioned how much he enjoyed music and that he composed music as a hobby. Six months later he said, "no new tapes or equipment." It was one of the things he had to give up.

> ...And they [children] are so demanding. You never find really any time for yourself anymore. I used to have all the time in the world. Now it's an hour here, an hour there...whenever they let me have it. But as for me being a father, it's very important that I spend a lot of time with 'em. For instance, my family thought it was very strange and very funny that I would spend a lot of time with them. I would change their diapers and I would play with them. I just really enjoy being with them. When I come home at night, it's more or less give them a bath, feed them. That's all the time I really get with them. But I think that's very important.

Parenting is obviously an important consideration for fathers as well as mothers. The available data, however, is certainly skewed. Women may have been more available for much of the research that was conducted in the past, or researchers may have been intimidated by the prospect of involving men in their studies resulting in a preponderance of research about mothering. During this project, professionals had more than an incidental response related to the inclusion of men in our interviews. Some commentators were surprised about the incorporation of men; others pointedly asked whether or not we had difficulty getting men to participate. There was an assumption that men would not want to talk about their experiences.

These experiences are significant for holistic family care. All those involved in high-risk perinatal care need to be aware of *both* parents, the potential similarities and the possible differences. These can be fully understood only if the stories of both mothers and fathers are sought. Additionally there are some special considerations for women as mothers that have seldom been addressed. Certainly such discussions do not appear in the bioethical literature on ethical decision-making in the NICU. It is time for such a conversation to begin.

Some Feminist Commentary

Ethical decision-making does not take place on a neutral playing field. I became especially interested in assumptions about women as mothers as this project unfolded. I believe that such assumptions inform and direct our decision-making. Assumptions can be basic to the process of ethical decision-making yet seldom examined until particularly called to our attention. Assumptions can also act as buffers in the decision-making process. That is, they can help rationalize decisions or even protect us from long-term responsibility related to the outcomes of our decisions. Just as Wolf (1996a) noted the largely ignored question of gender in the usual bioethical analysis of euthanasia, so too the dilemma of neonatal care "cries out for analysis."

Although some neonatologists are females, all physicians continue to be authority figures relative to most patients. All physicians were the object of heavy socialization processes leading into roles originally formulated and supervised by men. Although the role of women in medical education and training programs has increased, women continue to cluster at the lower, less influential roles on the faculty (Rosser 1994). All students tend to be socialized by male authority figures throughout medical education, including residencies.

The parent most likely to visit and represent the neonate is the mother. Sometimes this person is the grandmother, who may serve as a primary caregiver when the mother is a young girl. At least such a trend was vocalized by individuals in this study. Therefore the most common interaction during the decision-making dialogue would be between the physician and a female representative of the infant. In general, most communication is verbal, and information is simply imparted (Smith 1996). Such discourse is not necessarily ethical communication just because some instrumental goal is desired and reached, such as obtaining informed consent or informing the parent about the status or prognosis of the infant. Any parent might feel anxious, stressed, or worried, and mothers in particular could be in a compromised state of health because of the pregnancy, birth, or subsequent recovery. All of these affect the mother's receptivity and contribute to her vulnerable status during communication.

An asymmetrical relationship in ethical decision-making leads to other biased qualities in the interaction (Fisher 1988). The power imbalances in society are heightened in the physician-patient relationship: ethnicity, finances, class, employment, education, and gender unless the physician is female, when women as mothers are the infant's representative. The physician is the one who usually initiates the discussion, selects the topic, and determines the sequence and depth of the conversation. The physician controls the information exchanged because of the complexity of medical practice and the specialized training required to understand the high-risk newborn's situation. The woman is parent but as yet not caregiver. The mother is one step removed from intimate knowledge about her own child. In some cases she may not as yet have even held her child. However, critical engagement in the dialogue is essential for ethical communication to ensue. And, prior to the dialogue, how women and mothers are viewed crafts the development of the interaction and its content.

What and how we think about women and mothers might seem rather obvious. Child rearing follows immediately upon childbearing, so it is sometimes arduous to separate the biological from the cultural and sociological imperatives. We often conflate these and simply view the woman's role as *natural* without carefully teasing out a woman's destiny as predetermined by anatomy and physiology from the overlay of social, cultural, and psychological issues over the millennia. The forces of role prescription from the past 180 years most shape our current attitudes (Contrattio 1984). Given, then, the pivotal functional status of women in reproduction, it is quite easy to allow this function to take precedence over any other aspect of the woman's life. Further, as humans in community with one another, we have sought to idealize the function of mothering, even to memorialize it, sentimentalize it, romanticize it.

Consider how we have been taught to think of *mother*. We can fail to view mothers as persons with individual goals, life plans, values, traditions, and beliefs. Instead of seeing a person, we might see mothers only in terms of their responsibilities for an infant or infants because women have been central to caregiving for most infants besides the NICU graduates. We look at mothers of NICU babies and focus on what these women can do or ethically speaking what they *should do,* rather than *who they are.* Rothman (1986) describes mothering as "the ideal of unqualified love and acceptance of children, no matter what they turn out to be" which can provide a rationale for aggressive therapy in high-risk newborn care with little consideration of the outcome. I think that the role women embrace deserves special examination, because the NICU event might be a woman's first experience in her role as mother. The role of mother is compounded by gender biases. We have a particular set of assumptions regarding females' morality, decision-making capacity, and role in society, as opposed to similar expectations for males (Morgan 1987). These assumptions about women, aside from the presumptions about mothers, will *not* be addressed here but I ask you to keep them in mind as well.[n]

I am trying to avoid saying that what women have a *right to* is their *autonomy*, because I do not want to rely on some abstract conception of *rights* or *autonomy*. Neither do I want to decontextualize these women's circumstances as they become caregivers for their infants. But I find questionable how decisions can really be self-determined for a woman, given socialization and cultural imperatives. As Adriene Rich has observed, a woman's "choices - when she has any - are made, or outlawed within the context of laws and professional codes, religious sanctions, and ethnic traditions, from whose creation women have been historically excluded" (1976).

My exploration of mothers will include two dimensions, since the place of mothers as caregivers in discussions and research projects related to neonates was reviewed earlier:

1. The myth of the mother--a multidisciplinary perspective on motherhood.
2. Some insights about ethical decision-making in the NICU related to the woman's role.

The Myth of the Mother

The institution of motherhood cannot be touched or seen (Rich 1976). Nevertheless very strong forces are at work--some rational, some irrational (Bernard 1975). Assumptions about mothers can be found in numerous sources that impact a female's development across the life span and program girls and women to generally believe that only in mothering can they be fully authentic. Within the context of this chapter it is not possible to include all likely examples. There are toys, media, advertisements, comic strips, jokes, *how-to* magazines, news reports and magazines, literature, poetry, fairy tales and myths, art, sculpture, various scholarly disciplines, physiology, health assessments (history taking and physical examinations of women in the context of health care), and so on. But the prevailing social mythology of American culture posits the presence of an exclusive mothering person who will offer unconditional love, meet all of her children's needs and provide full-time compassion (Chesler 1972), an ideal fantasy that in reality is impossible to achieve (Hoffnung 1989). A mother is completely unselfish (Kolbenschlag 1979), noble, and by some standards, holy (Dworkin 1974). Mothering is the universal element of the sexual division of labor (Chadorow 1978); however, there is no payment for this job and independent wages and Social Security benefits are not accrued solely on the basis of years of mothering.

Motherhood is *sacred* so long as the offspring are *legitimate*--that is, as long as the child bears the name of a male who legally controls the mother (Rich 1976). Only *real* women are mothers and society praises women more for having children than for other accomplishments (Chesler 1972). Because, patriarchy could not survive without motherhood and heterosexuality in their institutional forms, they must be treated as axioms, as *nature* itself, not open to question (Kaplan 1992; Rich 1976) --an assumption. So how do females learn to desire this outcome?

From childhood onward girls and women are taught that females bear *and* raise children. "Everything in a girl's socialization and training was designed around the expectation that she would someday be a mother" (Shaevitz 1984). Even female *dolls* have infants and children as epitomized by a recent advertisement in a mail order catalogue. The Mattel Company was promoting a Barbie doll complete with small child in a shopping cart. Needless to say, Ken was not shown with any children. In the same catalogue's Playschool housekeeping set, a female child is shown at the kitchen sink with a toy baby doll in a high chair. There were no males with these *baby* dolls or play-size kitchen furnishings (Service Merchandise 1997).

Fairy tales also influence children and help shape their concept of mother. In fact both fairy tales and myths serve as tutorials for many of our expected behaviors, certainly for females and mothering. The mother and the good woman of fairy tales is passive, beautiful, innocent, and a victim.

> They never think, act, initiate, confront, resist, challenge, feel, care, or question. Sometimes they are forced to do housework...Catatonia is the good woman's most winning quality...the evil mother, is repulsive in her cruelty. She...must be destroyed... [but remember that] she is evil because she acts (Dworkin 1974).

In our culture, views of mothers have shifted over time. The 20th century has been labeled, *The Century of the Child* (Ehrenreich & English 1978). At the end of the 19th century, a combination of sharply falling birth rates (Shields 1984), and the shift from a view of the child as miniature adult, sufferer of early mortality, and victim of child labor, to an exaltation of childhood activated a reappraisal of the responsibilities of motherhood. If a child was to be society's key to the future, educated and comfortable with the growing technological advancements of the century as it unfolded, then the vocation of motherhood required "tremendous effort of will, continuous inspiration" (Ehrenreich & English).

Theodore Roosevelt in 1908 said, "But...the woman who, whether from cowardice, from selfishness, from having a false and vacuous ideal shirks her duty as wife and mother, earns the right to our contempt...." (Ehrenreich & English 1978). However, at the same time a group of child *experts* arose who doubted that women could embrace this responsibility and effectively carry out the necessary tasks and actions. They replaced the advice-giving clergy and physicians of the 18th and 19th centuries (Contrattio 1984). Since motherhood required knowledge and skills, there was hesitancy to allow it to occur willy-nilly. The psychologists moved in to fill the bill and provide the needed directions for mothers to function effectively in their care of children. After all, behaviorist John C. Watson remarked astonishingly, that he "grasp[ed] the basic, vexing problem: How could *women* raise *men*?" (Ehrenreich & English). Without supervision, he asserted, women would only be able to produce a generation of lapdogs.

With all the advice from experts, and grounded in a structured, rule-driven philosophy, motherhood by mid-century consisted of a woman in constant attention creating the nurturing, loving atmosphere that enabled a child to fulfill its potential. But then, motherly instincts became very important. Once again formal education of a woman was viewed as a threat to motherhood, not because of the earlier belief that it would cause *atrophy of the uterus* and compromise childbearing, but rather because it would alienate a woman from her instincts necessary for ideal child-rearing. Quickly emerging out of this child-rearing atmosphere was the experts' drive to blame every child defect, neurosis, or problem on the mother--guilt, guilt, guilt--magnified over and over again (Ehrenreich & English 1978). Mothers were guilty if they were overprotecting and guilty if they were depriving.

In the 1970s, the cult of motherhood went somewhat downhill. Although single life was idolized and the *looking out for #1* mentality was widespread, this was still not basically meant for both sexes or at least could not be applied as readily to women who were mothers. Women continued to be socialized to put others first and feel guilty when they did not. The marketplace psychologists of the day were saying that if women wanted to have children, let them. If they don't want to raise the children themselves, then let *them* lobby for day care centers or other support (Ehrenreich & English 1978).

As we now see, in the 1990s, women's responsibility for children actually expanded as adult children failed to *leave the nest* or came back home because they could not find jobs, or their employment was insufficient to allow them to independently live the lifestyle to which they were accustomed. Added to this was the lengthening life expectancy which includes a woman's own parents on her list of caregiving responsibilities. The sandwich generation was born.

Today women still choose maternity for both traditional and male-imposed reasons: to survive economically and psychologically, and because contraception and abortion are still inadequate, illegal, expensive, dangerous, and morally censured for most women. Romantic love is seen as justifying the inevitable female destiny of marriage and children. Maternity has been glorified and feared, mothers have been eulogized and their labors have been destroyed in battle as their children are killed. Mothers are trained to mount the sacrificial altar willingly. The mother-woman gives up whatever ghost of a unique and human self she has when she marries and rears children. Most children in contemporary American society invade their mothers' privacy, living space, sanity, and selves to such an extent that women must give up these things in order not to commit violence. Modern men say they envy the maternal option but remain in positions which focus on accumulating money--without children underfoot. Despite the *gloriousness* with which men discuss maternity, they fail to be maternal themselves to wives, children, mistresses, secretaries, housekeepers, or even each other (Chesler 1972, p. 22).

Over the years, what has changed? Women can choose to have or not have a child; the age of bearing children has become more flexible. What has not changed? Expectations of mothers. Today's mothers are still responsible for all the same functions as yesterday's mothers, in spite of the fact that many mothers today are employed outside the home and intensely involved in children's activities. Nor have the expectations of businesses and organizations changed for employees--child-free job responsibility of the worker is the norm (Shaevitz 1984). In the extreme, it can be said that "...motherhood as an institution has ghettoized and degraded female potentialities... under patriarchy, female possibility has been literally massacred on the site of motherhood" (Rich 1976).

We continue to sentimentalize mothers--Renoir's blooming women with rosy children at their knees, Raphael's ecstatic Madonnas, a Jewish mother lighting the Sabbath candles in a scrubbed kitchen, the Christ figure on the lap of Mary. Just read Mother's Day cards with a cynical eye sometime. For example:

> It's Mother's Day - a day to relax, a day to be honored, a day to be treated with Love, Affection, and Respect? A day to wonder why this doesn't happen more often...

Gender biases are not always blatant and the negative impact on women as mothers continues. A list prepared by the Children's Defense Fund (1994) summarized *One Day in the Life of American Children.* The list consisted of 29 facts about children related to child abuse, poverty, runaways, arrests, and other problems. All of the information was presented in a gender-neutral manner except for two entries. One, referring to women "who had late or no prenatal care," did not blame or criticize in a gender-discriminatory manner. Certainly only women become pregnant, and, although the father of the baby may have some responsibility for encouraging prenatal care or not deserting the mother after conception occurs, men cannot actually get the prenatal care. On the other hand, the second gender-explicit entry is different: "3325 babies are born to unmarried women." Why specify women? Although the 3325 fathers may in fact be married, they are apparently not married to the pregnant women. The fact that babies are born to unmarried fathers is often forgotten or ignored. A more neutral entry would be a statement such as "3325 babies are born to unmarried couples" (or parents), if marital status needs to be addressed at all.

In an article focusing on the ethics of cloning, the phrase *illegitimate chic* was used to decry the increasing obsolescence of males in reproduction (Post 1997). The author identified the acceptable trend among unmarried celebrity women to bear children as a step on the path toward increasing public acceptance of reproductive technologies and a separation of conception from family functioning. Reproduction could eventually be achieved through cloning which the author cited as the final nail in the coffin of fatherhood.

Although the term *illegitimacy* has been used less frequently in recent years with regard to unwed mothers, any use is particularly offensive because the phrase targets the children of a relationship, not the behavior of the individuals responsible for conceiving them. Moreover, women are likely to be the object of social censure related to a child's status as illegitimate, rather than men. *Illegitimacy* is a patriarchal term, a derogatory label applied to children for the socially unacceptable behavior of the parents (or woman?). Illegitimacy, as commonly used, simply means that some male refused to acknowledge his offspring. The persistent use of such a term supports the functioning of a patriarchal society. The first nail in the coffin of fatherhood was not the current practice of single women raising children as Post claimed, but rather the age-old practice of abandonment and refusal to acknowledge. The term *illegitimacy* was applied to control women and reproduction. Its continued [mis]use emphasizes the power at stake in issues of reproduction. Who is legitimately a mother? The question continues to be asked.

The public interest in abandonment provides the final example related to the mythology surrounding motherhood (Cummins 2000; Jerome et al. 1997). In both a magazine report and a television news broadcast, only mothers were noted as people who abandoned babies. Fathers were never mentioned nor blamed as individuals who might bear some responsibility for the discovery of babies in supermarkets, at schools, or in trash bins. Older individuals who discovered they had been adopted as a result of abandonment targeted mothers with their anger, rage, disappointment, and shock. Some indicated that they wanted to find their biological mothers to thank them for putting them where they would be found. Tom Brokaw expressed incredulity at what he perceived to be an epidemic. No connection was posed between the increasing lack of privacy and confidentiality for women who elect to carry pregnancies to term and then put their children up for adoption. There appeared to be little recognition that the desperation and vulnerability of pregnant girls and women might lead them to first and foremost want to put this event behind them. At the moment of abandonment, they perceive the pregnancy and birth as a mistake, and they may not want to live the balance of their lives open to the sudden appearance of their children, a reminder of their mistake. Open adoption and open adoption records can be seen as another way to control women's reproductive behavior. Children continue to blame mothers rather than fathers for failing to accept parenting as a role. Society persists in instilling guilt in women who do not want to keep their infants, even those who elect adoption rather than abortion.

Women as Caregivers

The above are a few examples of the assumptions with which I believe individuals, to one degree or other, come to the decision-making process. No one single element is sufficiently powerful to completely shape our assumptions about woman as mother, but together they create a strong force which can lead to an ideal image of a female person devoted to child-bearing and raising, selfless and even self-sacrificing (Hoffnung 1989), existing for the pleasure of others. Whatever a woman may do, cheerfully serving the family is what really counts. Just as women are expected to control fertility and adjust it to the needs of the economy, society also expects any woman who bears a child to accept these ethical decisions and *mother* the child - regardless of its outcome and its needs, even when meeting those needs is financially, physically, and psychologically impossible for one person. Not only should the woman accept the child but actually welcome it into her life regardless of the problems it creates. Women are assumed to be willing to sacrifice personal or professional goals they may have and their marriages or any relationships with significant others.

Most non-professional caregivers are women. When making community health visits to families with a high-risk infant, as a follow-up from discharge, fathers were not present. Parents in my project perceived an expectation on the part of the NICU staff for moms to visit but dads were not held to the same high visitation standard. Most parents in my study expected women to be the primary caregiver after discharge. Women's protests about their inadequacy in providing childcare or their lack of readiness can be easily dismissed. Professionals often believe that once the baby is home, women will adapt and learn whatever is necessary. Women's hesitancy can be attributed to the delay these individuals experience in implementing the parental role. Bonding may be also be affected by an infant who is hospitalized four, five, or six months and can be different from bonding with a non-hospitalized newborn.

Emotional responses of women can also be used to stereotype them. Strong emotions can be aroused by a traumatic pregnancy, birth, or newborn experience. Judgments can be made about these emotional states that discredit women as stable individuals capable of making serious choices about the care of their infant. After all, ideal ethical decision-making is viewed as a rational, logical, objective process in which information is provided, alternatives explored, and choices prioritized. An emotional labile woman would not be a candidate for this type of activity when these criteria are applied.

Another dynamic can occur with mothers of infants who do not meet our standard of the *good* mother. A great deal of moral judgment is attached to negative attitudes towards young, teen-age pregnancies or single women who may have even chosen to become pregnant. Such a social situation influences the professional attitude which can seriously compromise the interpersonal relationships and the effectiveness of the professional's interactions with these women. It is quite possible to see these women as actually deserving the hardships that a compromised infant may create in their lives.

And society apparently will not *adjust* to the postdischarge situation by establishing long-term care for compromised infants, special educational settings, financial and emotional support for mothers who provide the 24-hour care, respite care, or myriad other services. For many parents, none of these elements are professionally available. It is acceptable for a mother to provide these services and become totally dependent upon another (spouse, parent, welfare) for financial, physical, and emotional support--since that is not a denial of the *normal* or *natural role* (Magezis 1996). In fact, mothers are expected to *normalize* the integration of a high-risk baby into the family so that little disturbance occurs in other family roles and functioning despite unexpected outcomes for the infant and increased demands for its care. This extended caregiving is in addition to spousal support, marital satisfaction, sibling activities and their acceptance of a new (demanding) infant, relationships with the extended family, and family involvement in the community, among other responsibilities. Has there been a non-verbalized expectation that a *good* woman will soothe everything over and life will go on uninterrupted, even in the face of disability, handicap, or special needs--when ethical decision-making occurs in the NICU?

We should be concerned about women and their role in the decision-making process. Caregiving is not just an ideal function it is reality for mothers of infants with disabilities and chronic disease, mothers of NICU graduates.

Women and Ethical Decision-making in the NICU

What does all of this mean? I see these elements contributing to the disenfranchisement of women qua mothers as decision-makers. The omission of mothers as persons in their own right decreases our tendency to recognize their authority. I see assumptions related to mothering as foundational to ethical discussions and research in the NICU. They serve as reasons for the professional's confidence, assurance, or even arrogance to go unchallenged in an all-out effort to save the lives of these infants. Jonsen (1991) called this prevailing philosophy of care in the NICU *rescuing*. Rescuing means aggressive care with little or no decision-making authority for anyone other than the professional. But after infants are rescued, someone needs to care for the infants after they are discharged. As long as professionals can rationalize their rescue with a corollary belief of mothers as self-sacrificing, willing, and devoted caregivers for the infant, regardless of the outcome--all is well in the nursery. Even a more current, moderate position, such as a best interest standard (Weir 1995) for ethical decision-making in the NICU does not bestow full decision-making authority on the mother, or even partial authority.

The best interest standard has been favored in some court decisions (Cantor 1995), and it has become the emerging mainstream position of choice in ethical decision-making for children. The best interest standard includes a caution against the use of information about the broader impact of decisions on family, society, or some arbitrary standard such as normalcy, acceptability, or quality of life (Weir 1995a). A best interest standard is generally defined as an approach which attempts to balance the overtreatment of infants that resulted from the Baby Doe federal regulations with the desire of some parents to discontinue any treatment of an infant.[o] A major characteristic of this approach is an objective appraisal of factors as they focus solely on the infant: medical condition, potential benefits and burdens of treatments, suffering, and prognosis (Dunn 1993; Weir 1995a). If physicians, in their wisdom and with their experience, determined a particular procedure is necessary for this neonate, how can there possibly be any objection? In addition to the medical expertise that sustains support for a particular piece of physician advice, the best interest standard integrates a psychological potency into the argument. How could anyone object to the *best* medical treatment that is simultaneously in the *best interest* of the child? How could the *good* mother legitimately, morally counter both medical expertise and philosophical wisdom (or is she encountering hubris?).

Neither rescuing nor applying a best interest standard actually advocates eliminating parents from decision-making. However, there is disagreement in the practical, clinical sense about how much parents are really involved. For example, Silverman (1979, 1981, 1982, 1992), my research, and several other sources say parents are not actively decision-makers; Duff and Campbell (1973) and others report a *private* decision with parents. In reality, communication, critical to the decision-making process, is often an event that occurs between the mother and the health care professional. Many fathers are absent; they have abandoned the woman, they are at work, they do not see themselves as caregivers and visiting the baby drops off, or they reject the non-Gerber baby. We must also consider women's usual experiences with decision-making in the health care system. As early as prenatal counseling and genetic work-ups, followed by fertility procedures, monitored pregnancies, and childbirth, women are set up as subject in a medicalized experience. Motherhood may be idealized, but the woman as patient or parent of the patient is not so valued.

Although women receive more health care services than men and have more contact with health care providers either for themselves or as representatives of children, spouse, or their own parents, they are accorded neither status nor favor in the reality of bureaucratic organizations of the health care system. Woman as mother is object.

What I want to emphasize is that an all out *rescue* effort and even a best interest standard frequently moves forward assuming that a primary caregiver--the mother--will accept responsibility for whatever needs are present and will love the child for her entire lifetime. Wouldn't the *good* mother accept her child regardless of the outcome? Functioning, nonfunctioning, mentally alert, totally unaware of surroundings, communicative, non-communicative, lively, helpless, smiling, crying?

I believe we need to work toward a greater emphasis on parents as decision-makers, as the neonate is their child and ultimately, unless our social system changes, mothers will bear a majority of the burden of care. In fact, our current health care system's functioning depends upon unpaid workers, such as mothers, who are caregivers in the home (Pierce & Frank 1992). And given some of the current trends in health care reimbursement, the government's view of its role in service/resource provision, and the public's unwillingness to be taxed further, families will be bearing the burden alone. Once discharge has occurred mothers will be decision-makers. How can they be so incapable one day and not the next?

Neither all-out efforts nor our *best* is morally required. Even with newborns, parents/mothers' needs count, and ethically a balanced fulfillment of needs is a reasonable standard decided through a "nuanced understanding of all the relevant particulars that bear on the decision" (Nelson & Nelson 1995a, p. 805). For some critics, either unlimited aggressive care or an objective best interest standard is unethical without consideration of the caregiver and the context of the infant's life after discharge. In the hospital nursery however, parents seldom seem to be regarded as individuals in their own right but rather are seen only in terms of their relationship to the baby. The woman and man who call or come to visit the newborn are primarily seen as mother and father of Baby John or Baby Jill--not as *Sally Jacobs* or *Sean Cutter*. Parents in our study expressed this observation and were surprised when we specifically asked about them, not just the infant. These parents felt they were seldom seen as people apart from their role as caretakers of the child. However, disrespect for the relationship of the infant to others and lack of recognition of the shift of care to unpaid family members, such as mothers, is beginning to receive attention in the bioethical literature (Nelson & Nelson 1995b).

Summary

As with many research projects, a few answers were obtained but new questions were constantly encountered as the data were scrutinized. One way to understand the parents' experiences was identified through Reich's exposition of a Theory of Suffering (1987b, 1987c, 1989, 1990) and Kleiver's extension of this understanding of crisis to include anger and rage (1989, 1995). The corollary theory of compassion is one suggestion for health professionals as an approach to individuals suffering profound losses. Sensitivity to the similarities and differences by gender in parents' responses to the high-risk infant can also evolve from the analyses in this chapter. Full exploration of assumptions brought to the ethical decision-making process will help balance all needs. Awareness is the first step in opening one's self to new approaches while caring for these parents.

Notes

[a] Thomas is an American Sociologist who lived between 1863 and 1947. According to the entry under author biography in Bowker's *Books in print*, he make this statement in a journal article 10 years after the publication of his two-volume set, *The Polish peasant in Europe and America.* No year is available for these publications. This work, co-authored with Florian Znaniecki, was a decisive contribution which showed the importance of including personal documents while studying social change.

[b] The Society for Health and Human Values annual meeting, November 9-11, 1990. Dr. Reich continued his initial presentation, "The experience of compassion: Toward a theory for health care ministry." with a second theme, "Be care-ful! Pay attention!" for the Ministry in Health Care Education Interest Group.

[c] Rushton (1994), addressing moral decision making in her dissertation, labeled the parents' perception as "being the good parent" for the child. How parents behaved and the kinds of decisions they made were connected to the parents' value system, which unquestionably made being good parents a moral obligation.

[d] There is a rich, lengthy history of commentary on *Dax*. Although his situation is not that of a critically ill newborn, the following resources are cited for their parallel relationship to the suffering and crisis of parents who experience a newborn in the NICU (suffering, lack of control, grief, anger, crisis, long-term

consequences). See:

20/20: A man of endurance 1999. Livonia, MI: ABC News

Burton, K. 1999. A chronicle: Dax's case as it happened. In J. D. Arras & B. Steinbock (Eds.). *Ethical issues in modern medicine* (5th ed.; pp. 187-191). Mountain View, CA: Mayfield Publishing Company.

Dax's Case: Who should decide? 1984. Produced by Unicorn Media, Inc., for Concern for Dying.

Englehardt, H.T. 1975. Commentary. *Hastings Center Report*, **5**(1), 10, 47.

Kleiver, L.D. (Ed.). 1989. *Dax's case: Essays in medical ethics and human meaning.* Dallas, TX: South Texas Methodist University Press.

Platt, M. 1975. Commentary: On asking to die. *Hastings Center Report*, **5**(6), 9-12.

Please Let Me Die? 1976. Galveston, TX: University of Texas Medical Branch, Department of Psychiatry.

Rosenberg, E.A. 1994. An interview with Dax Cowart. *JAMA*, **272**(9), 744-745.

White, R.B. 1975. Commentary. *Hastings Center Report*, **5**(1), 9-10.

[e] At this point it would seem important to raise a question about the use of "mother" which is of sufficient consequence to deserve an essay all of its own. As I became engaged in this project and subsequent work that the project led me to, I wanted to know, When does a woman become a mother? The Random House Dictionary (Flexner 1987) defines a mother as a female parent. Does this then extrapolate to conception? Is a woman a mother if her only pregnancy was aborted? Is a spontaneous abortion different from a therapeutic or elective one? Does motherhood begin sometime during the pregnancy? Not until birth? What if the infant is stillborn? Is a woman a mother after donating eggs that are later fertilized, resulting in the birth of a child she has not gestated? In an article on fetal therapy, the female is variously called a mother, a woman, and a parent. In Fletcher's 1986 article on fetal therapy, mother was seldom used (17% of the total mother/woman use)--the female was usually named--"woman." Given possible feminist commentary in this chapter, the use of mother rather than woman provides a different psychological perspective for the reader. The question might be raised as to whether this is a conscious decision on the part of the writer(s). Even more interesting is the use of parents when it clearly means both parents while discussing the use of therapy (fetal surgery) that obviously has no direct affect on the body of the father. While he may have an interest in the decision relative to the outcome for his child, like infertility treatments that solely target the woman, his body is not the object of any direct action. The weight of his desires and opinions must be weighed carefully relative to the woman who must accept the clear, direct risks inherent in fetal therapy. One might partially excuse Fletcher's writing in 1986 based on

a lack of awareness of the importance of language. However, in 1993 using Evans, Robertson, and Fletcher's piece on legal and ethical issues in fetal therapy, the authors should be well aware of the psychological affect from the use of language that incites various emotions possibly created by the use of "mother" which in turn can sway an argument one way or another depending upon the goal of the writer. Although the percentage for the use of woman increased (approximately 30%), mother was used more frequently in the 1993 piece. See Kauffman (1990) for some interesting commentary on the fetus's mother.

[f] The index was the Cumulative Index to Nursing and Allied Health Literature (CINAHL). The search went back to 1982 and was selected based on the belief that the majority of the caregiving literature would be indexed in this body of publications. It was plausible that nurses would be responsible for the transfer of infant care from the NICU to the parent. Nurses would likely investigate the issue and publish both their experiences with this task and their investigations of the process.

[g] The specific results of the search for articles and their identification of primary caregivers by role and gender were as follows:

Focused on mother	24
Focused on grandmothers	2
Family focused or on parenting 3 included both genders 1 mother exclusively 17 mothers were majority	21
TOTAL	47

[h] This entire paper includes discussion of the results as if both parents were broadly included. Finally, however, at the end of the study as an introduction to one quotation, there is a comment "...from the only father."

[i]Non-reproductive issues are the focus of an anthology edited by Susan Wolf (1996b). Another book whose author does not singly focus on reproductive issues for women is Sherwin (1992).

[j] The conference was co-sponsored by the University of South Florida College of Medicine and the National Perinatal Association. The presentation was offered by Wade E. Horn, PhD President of the National Fatherhood Initiative, Gaithersburg, MD. The session was advertised as including a review of the literature on "the positive influence fathers can have during the perinatal period and present effective ways to get and keep fathers involved in the lives of their children."

[k] While attending a conference and listening to the presentations at a session on diabetes, I was frustrated by the lack of gender break-down in the data for the studies. For many of the elements-- adherence to various regimes, weight,

and others--a gender breakdown would have been helpful,. When I asked about the absence of results by gender, the investigator said that she did not want to unfairly target one gender or the other; she wanted to remain neutral. However, the sample size was small and quite possibly she would have needed a larger sample to detect gender differences. Investigators should set goals to include more subjects in studies where gender might make a difference in interpreting results.

[l] For a more detailed description of these fathers, review Table A.2.

[m] This particular description of the delivery circumstances was not depicted by the father during the predischarge or the six-month postdischarge interviews. In validating this observation, I noted that the mother contributed far more to the joint interviews than the father. The third interview was conducted alone with the father at the four-year postdischarge phase and he discussed the birth in the terms quoted here. This outcome does seem to support the need to conduct interviews separately, although it cannot be known whether he would have made the same statements earlier had he been interviewed alone.

[n] A brief reminder about some of the assumptions as presented by accounts on stereotypical characteristics: Women are emotional, physically weaker, irrational, dependent, intuitive, passive, peace-loving, submissive, nurturing, caring, self-sacrificing...(Tavris 1992).

[o] Some historical commentary regarding the Baby Doe regulations and its impact on ethical decision-making in the NICU are included in Chapter 1. Briefly, in 1983, Health and Human Services released "an interim final rule" prohibiting the failure to feed and care for handicapped infants in any facility that received federal funds. See Lyon (1985), *Playing God in the Nursery* for an extensive discussion of this issue.

CHAPTER 7

Reckoning With the Future

Ethical decision-making, even in such a circumscribed area of health care as the NICU, is not an isolated activity. Decision-making occurs in a broader context that has many aspects: sociological, psychological, cultural, theological or spiritual, economic, and philosophical. Parents of high-risk newborns are profoundly affected by these decisions. The future NICU experience can be viewed as a mirror which reflects several elements challenging us in the 21st century. For me, these elements are technological ventures, family life, the child's destiny, and economic trends. The technological developments set the stage for what we are able to do, and they raise the ethical question of whether or not we *should* use the devices or procedures that are available. Speculation about future families and the anticipated prospects for children relates to the *who* question in ethics--what role *should* be the family have in decision-making? Finally, economic trends influence our ethical concerns for justice. Even though a high standard of living is possible in our country, not all individuals are able to attain even minimum standards of living. Resources are not limitless. What decisions *ought* to be made at both the microallocation and macroallocation levels to ensure fair distribution of these resources?

Technological Ventures

One cannot think about future health care without considering technology. In many ways it is the driving force in the regimes that professionals implement for a broad range of patients including compromised newborns in the NICU. Our society in general is dazzled and addicted to technology, as shown in the term "technological imperative" coined by Fuchs in 1968 (Haney 1987). Therefore, it is not just technology in the NICU that provokes ethical debate but also the impetus to apply it. Whitney observed that "Half the work of bioethics is cleaning up after technology" (1998).

As the parents in this project pointed out, infertility issues and the technology applied to resolve them can compound problems during pregnancy, birth, or after delivery. Dr. Samuel Wood, specializing as an infertility physician, has said, "My belief is that in 20 years, no couple will be unable to have a baby...genetically, except for the few on the extremes of reproductive life" (Frontline 1999a). Unless the procedures and the resulting newborns are without problems, there are serious implications for NICU care.

For such a prediction to become reality, the success rate of infertility treatment will need to change dramatically. However, the desperation of many families will undoubtedly remain strong. Several families in this project were extraordinarily motivated to have a child with genetic connections to themselves. For myriad reasons including societal pressure and role expectations in addition to personal desires, women want to experience pregnancy and birth. Women are willing to undergo many unpleasant and painful procedures to become pregnant, even when the etiology of infertility resides in their partner. An in-depth discussion of the ethical aspects of reproductive technologies is beyond the scope of this book, but a few comments are salient.[a]

Mahowald and associates' research (1998; Ravin et al. 1997) supports the premise that, when given the choice, women prefer the gestational experience (51%) rather than only a genetic connection (48%) to a child. The difference is small; nevertheless, gestation is preferred. For men, 74% rate the genetic tie more highly than their spouse or partner gestating their child. Technological interventions will continue to be sought by women and their families to treat infertility despite the personal and financial cost. About 7%-10% of couples of reproductive age have infertility problems (American Society for Reproductive Medicine [ASRM] 2000; Assisted reproductive 1999). Etiologies of infertility are equally divided, with half of the problems in the male and half in the female (See Figure 7.1). Some of the problems are due solely to the male, some exclusively to the female, and the remainder a combination of both. Reproductive technologies are sought for reasons other than infertility as well--nonheterosexual couples and single individuals may also avail themselves of the therapy. Costs of many infertility treatments are not reimbursed by third-party payers, although there are various grass roots efforts to change such policies.

Figure 7.1 *Primary Diagnosis in Cases of Infertility*

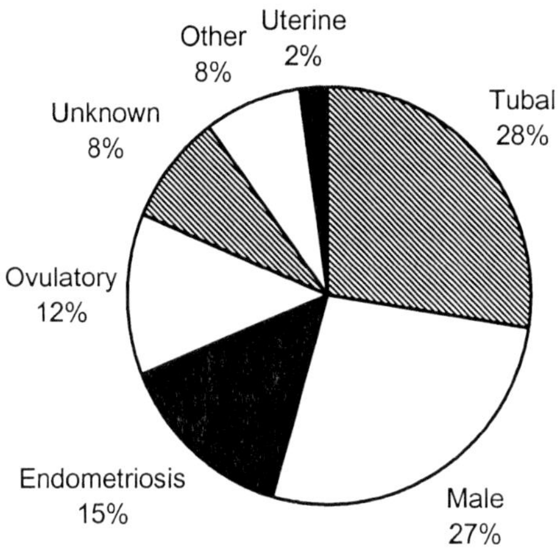

Note: These statistics are based on couples who had fresh, nondonor ART cycles.
Male alone etiologies: low sperm count or other problems with sperm function
Endometriosis: the abnormal presence of tissue, like the lining of the uterus, in other organs such as the ovaries
Ovulatory dysfunction: the ovaries do not produce eggs normally, or the function has diminished
Uterine factor: disorder of the uterus
Other causes: examples include immunological problems, chromosomal abnormalities, cancer chemotherapy, and serious illnesses
Tubal problems: blocked or damaged fallopian tubes
Unknown: no cause determined

From: Assisted reproductive, 1999

Few large-scale, rigorous studies have been conducted to determine the impact of infertility treatments on the pregnancy, birth, and neonate outcomes. As yet there is no official board certification for infertility treatments, so systematic collection of data relating to patient experiences and fetal outcomes are limited (Raymond 1993). Since infertility treatments often lead to high-risk pregnancies, such interventions can increase the demand for NICU beds. A primary contribution comes from ovulation-inducing drugs which over-stimulate the ovaries, resulting in the release of multiple ova and multigestation.[b] Additionally, assisted reproductive technology (ART) includes an increasing armamentarium of interventions such as artificial insemination, *in vitro* fertilization (IVF), gamete intrafallopian transfer (GIFT), zygote intrafallopian transfer (ZIFT), intracytoplas-mic sperm injection, cyropreservation, and *in vitro* ovum nuclear trans-plantation (See Figure 7.2 for data about these procedures).[c] In some of the techniques, standard practice involves insertion of more than one embryo which leads to multiple gestation. Multiple gestation in itself is a high-risk pregnancy, with the likelihood of need for NICU care of the resulting infants.

Treating infertility is a big business with more than 300 clinics in the United States today despite the relatively small number of individuals who are affected with reproductive difficulties (Assisted reproductive 1999). However, the number of clinics does not include those physicians who independently offer reproductive services and therefore are not part of the usual surveys, or who fail to report their data. The government report cited above lists only two clinics for Nebraska. However, none of the women who were given Clomid for infertility in my project attended those clinics, providing evidence for the ability to secure such services outside the sources included in formal reports.[d] However, the widespread availability of interventions is not the only reason for raising ethical concerns relative to reproductive therapies. The particular concern relative to these interventions in the context of this project is the potential outcome--not the services themselves, which contain their own ethical dilemmas beyond simply their availability.

The disturbing aspect of infertility treatment is the failure in many situations to include the whole story, the dark side of the range of possibilities. Many advertisements in magazines, newspapers, and on the World-Wide Web are negligent when it comes to full disclosure. Few mention the details necessary to make an informed decision, details about exactly how the advertiser defines success and what risks for infants are associated with outcomes of the treatments. Also, the media often fails to present a balanced perspective on these issues.[e] The *miracle* baby or the success story is often emphasized, rather than a negative outcome. A program on the Public Broadcasting System's

Figure 7.2 *Types of Artificial Reproductive Procedures*

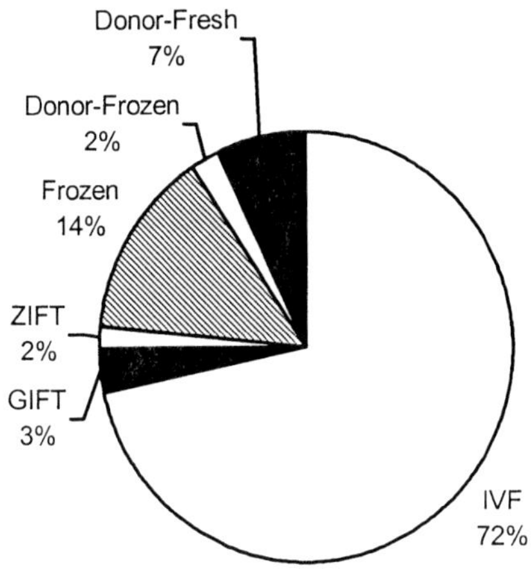

Note:
IVF, GIFT, and *ZIFT* includes fresh, nondonor cycles
IVF: woman's eggs are extracted, fertilized in the laboratory, and the resulting embryo(s) transferred back into the woman, not frozen
GIFT: after retrieval of eggs and procuring sperm, the unfertilized elements are transferred to the woman's fallopian tubes with a laproscope
IVF, *GIFT*, and *ZIFT* using donor eggs or frozen embryos (thawed and transferred in 1997) are included in *donor* or *frozen* categories

From: Assisted reproductive, 1999

Frontline, "Making Babies," included an interview with parents whose twin newborns were admitted to the neonatal unit immediately after birth (1999a, 1999b). They were born 3 months early and weighed approximately 1.5 pounds each. The parents were devastated by this turn of events and frightened by the outcome of their infertility endeavors. As the woman discussed her shock, she mentioned getting a big packet of information at the fertility clinic, but did not recall anything about multiples and prematurity. Yet this woman had had pregnancy reduction from triplets to twins in an attempt to avoid a premature birth. The father clarified their perception: "Well, you get the stuff about the risk of multiple pregnancy but I don't think you really get the full gravity of what that means." As the physician in the program countered, people hear only what they want to hear, and pregnancy is the goal--statistics will apply to someone else. In families who are able to maintain a pregnancy to viability after ART, 50% of the infants need intensive care. A baby's sequelae and admission to such a unit should not be a surprise.

Most cases of infertility can be treated pharmacologically or with surgery (ASRM 2000). As indicated earlier, statistics are difficult to obtain. Although the Centers for Disease Control (CDC) was charged to publish pregnancy success rates for ART procedures, their statistics include only IVF, GIFT, and ZIFT (Assisted reproductive 1999). Artificial insemination and ovary over-stimulation are not included. Additionally, success is defined differently by various programs. The most liberal definition counts as successful every woman whose hormone levels increase as a result of implantation. Some count pregnancies of a particular duration, for example, reaching the second trimester, while for the most conservative an actual live birth is considered a success. Even these figures can be misleading, as a pregnancy is often attained only after three, four, or more cycles of treatment (Some information about treatment outcomes is provided in Figures 7.3 and 7.4). According to the ASRM, the average live delivery rate is 22.5%, the same as the chance for a healthy couple becoming pregnant without using ART. What requires additional factoring, however, is the cost--the total cost. Treatment often requires more than one cycle and each cycle carries an additional fee, while for healthy couples of course, there is no fee for intercourse.

The average cost for one cycle of IVF is about $7,800 according to the ASRM (2000), and between $3,000 and $8,000 as cited by Petrinovich (1998). Artificial insemination costs about $953 for each assist. The total cost of the average course of treatment with IVF has been quoted at $22,000 (Petrinovich). Treatment for infertility is a $1 billion a year industry--and the number of couples using various technologies is growing each year. Since 1981, approximately 70,000 babies have resulted from ART while 45,000 have resulted from IVF alone (ASRM).[f] Risks are associated with pregnancies resulting from reproductive interventions. The very fact that an intervention was necessary to achieve pregnancy frequently places the

Figure 7.3 *Pregnancy Results of Fresh, Nondonor ART* cycles

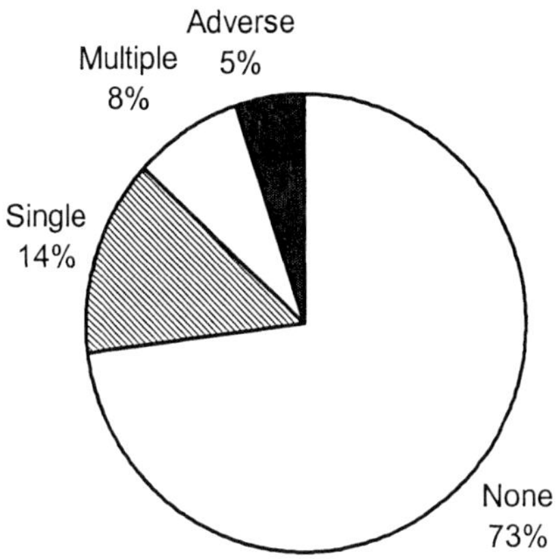

Note:
None - no pregnancy resulted
Single - one infant delivered
Multiple - each multiple is counted as one. The infants are not counted separately in this chart.
Adverse outcome means ectopic pregnancy, spontaneous abortion, induced abortion, or stillbirth. Multiple births with adverse outcomes (requiring NICU admission for instance) are not included in *Adverse outcomes*. Multifetal pregnancy reductions information is incomplete so it is not included here, neither are newborn deaths or birth defects.
The total live birth rate is equal to the total of single and multiple births, 22%
The pregnancy rate is therefore 27%, the total of single, multiple, and adverse outcomes.

From: Assisted reproductive, 1999

woman in a high-risk category for the entire pregnancy. When more than one embryo is implanted, or ovulatory over-stimulation results in the release of more than one egg, the odds are raised that something untoward will occur. Frequently, more than one embryo is inserted so

Figure 7.4 *Outcomes of Pregnancies Resulting from Fresh, Nondonor ART Cycles*

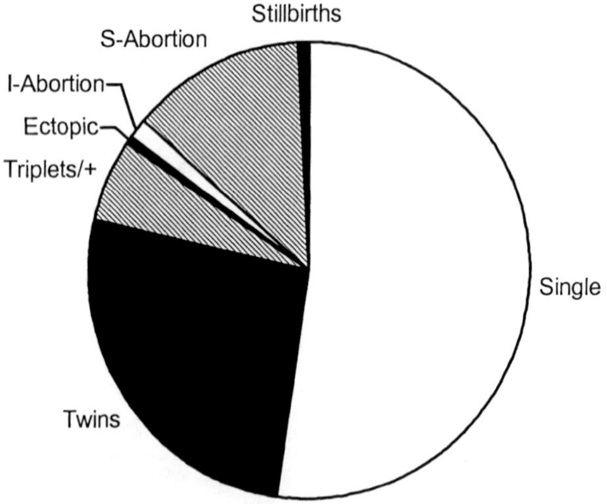

Note:
Outcomes from the 27% of ART cycles from Figure 7.3 that produced a pregnancy:
Single = 52.3%
Twins = 26.3%
Triplets = 5.8%
Ectopic pregnancy = 0.5%
I-abortion represents induced abortion = 1.5%
S-abortion stands for spontaneous abortion = 12.9%
Stillbirths = 0.7%
A multiple birth is counted as one live birth. The total live birth rate represented here was 22%. Thus, 38% of all ART births were multiples compared to 2.7% of births in the general population.

From: Assisted reproductive, 1999

that the physician can be assured that at least one embryo successfully implants. When all embryos survive or all simultaneously released eggs are fertilized, then multiple fetuses develop: twins, triplets, quadruplets, quintuplets, or more. Multiple gestations incur higher risks--medical complications during pregnancy, higher cesarean-section rates, premature birth, low birth weight, and developmental disabilities (Assistive reproductive 1999).

The rate at which multiple gestations are currently produced is staggering. Before 1989 the CDC did not even subcategorize multiple births above triplets because there were so few (Martin & Park 1999). Births were recorded as twins or triplets-plus. Figure 7.5 shows the dramatic difference between naturally occurring multiple births and multiple births in 1996, the most recent year for these rates. The actual figures that follow are based on the total U.S. birth rate for 1996:

- Twins naturally occur once in 90 births (based on the 1996 birth rate, 43,298 would theoretically result) but actually there were over twice as many (101,178).
- Triplets naturally occur once in 8,100 births, which extrapolates to 480 sets expected for 1996 actually there were 5,380 sets, 11 times the normal.
- Quadruplets naturally occur once in 729,000 births, so we could expect 5 sets in 1996, but there were actually 561 sets or 112 times the naturally occurring rate.
- Quintuplets, based on a steady birth rate identical to 1996, would occur once every 17 years or so (1 in 65,610,000 births); however, 81 sets were born in that year alone (Vohr 2000a, 2000b).

I did not calculate the predictable rate for sextuplets, septuplets, or octuplets. One can simply think about the natural quintuplet rate and then consider the number actually born in these higher categories in the last few years. The results are incomprehensible. Almost all of these newborns spend some time in a neonatal intensive care unit. Newborns in multiple births are more likely to die within the first month of life. For twins, the death rate is 4 times as great as for singletons, for triplets the rate increases to 10 times, for quadruplets 13 times, and quintuplets 30 times (Martin & Park). No statistics are available for higher multiples.

Shortly after this project began, an article appeared in the local newspaper celebrating the birth of a set of triplets (Triplets 1988). This was the first triplet birth in that particular hospital in nineteen years. The report also touted the fact that the triplets received surfactant as part of a national trial, to prevent problems from lung immaturity. A 1998 article in the same newspaper summarized advice from four parents of *quadruplets* for the parents of Nebraska's first *quintuplets*

Figure 7.5 *Multiple Births in 1996 - 3,891,494 Total U.S. Births*[g]

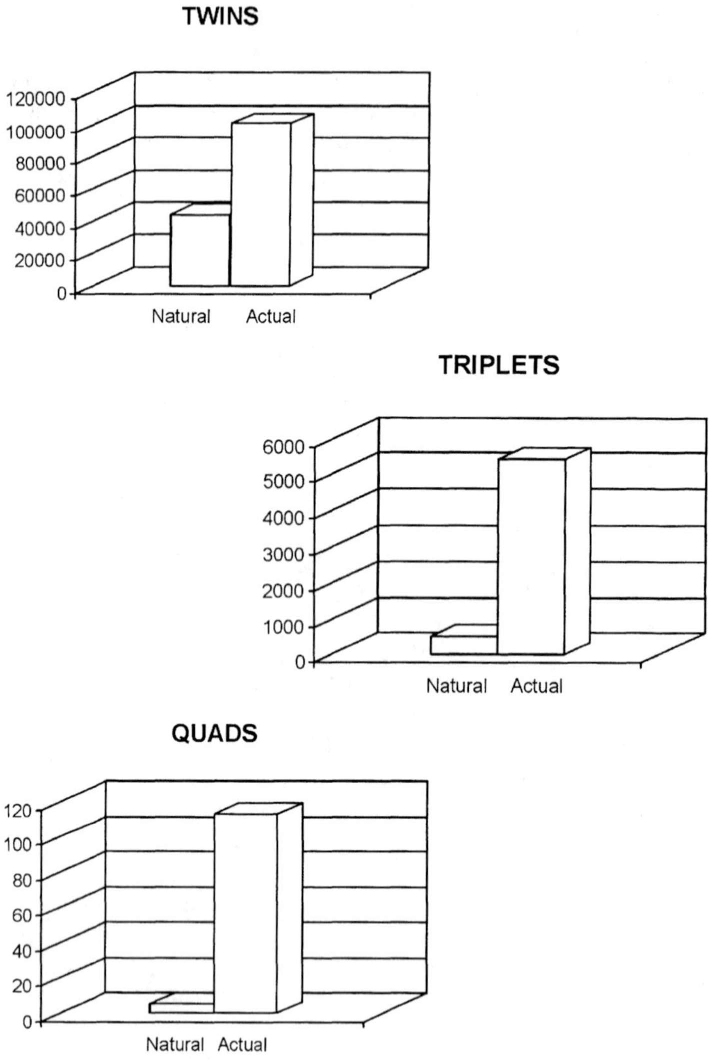

Figure 7.5 *Multiple Births* (Continued)

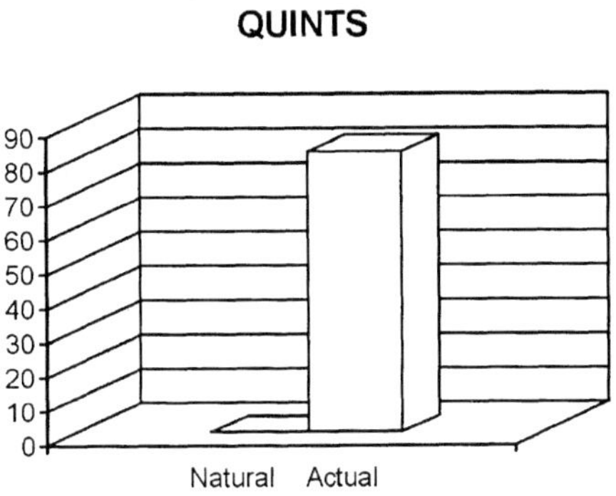

From: Vohr (2000a, 2000b).

(Knief 1998). The presence of several sets of various combinations of multiple births in a NICU on a continuous basis is no longer an unusual occurrence. Given the reproductive technologies, the future potential for multiple births does not appear to be declining.

One set of triplets, as we can see, no longer makes headlines. Instead the McCaughey septuplets (Klotzko 1998), Thompson sextuplets (Gaines 1997), Humair septuplets (Claiborne 2001), Chukwu octuplets (one was stillborn) (Zewe 1998), and most recently the Qahtani septuplets (Kovaleski & Goldstein 2001) capture the public's attention, although interestingly, most of the births were less publicized than the McCaughey developments. In fact, the Thompsons were all but forgotten until the McCaughey set was born (Gaines). Some media writers have speculated about when we will see the first *living* set of octuplets and what sort of public response that will engender.

Efforts to prevent multiple order gestations have occurred as some physicians and the ASRM publicize the failure of such births rather than successes (Trafford 2001). More such publicity is required before the public is no longer thrilled with a new winner of the "Super Birth Sweepstakes." Also in the meantime, surfactant as used experimentally in the triplets born in 1988, became a routine treatment and newborns regularly benefit from its use. That pharmacological advancement significantly reduced the risk of respiratory distress in prematures.

Callahan wrote an interesting report in 1986 about how technology was reframing the abortion debate. Basically, he stated that as abortions become technically safer, especially later in the pregnancy, then these services for pregnant women moved onto a direct collision course with increasingly successful interventions for younger and younger fetuses. Technology and the abortion issue could reframe major ethical debate in the NICU, he predicted. His thesis continues to be germane as interventions for younger and smaller newborns become available. Now even the potential life for stored embryos is debated as stem cell research is a headline issue.

In addressing the possible interventions for the infants themselves, the potential to treat the fetus before birth will ultimately have a significant impact on both the abortion issue and NICU demographics. Currently only infants with life-threatening conditions are candidates for treatment, and, for example, the majority of patients who come to the University of California San Francisco Fetal Treatment Center for possible treatment are not candidates for surgery (FAQs 1997). Conditions considered for surgery include diaphragmatic hernia, cystic adnatone malformation of the lung, sacrococcyxyeal trauma, and urinary obstruction. In another procedure, a surgeon uses a laser to block the flow of blood between fetuses in twin-to-twin transfusion; however, this is technically placental surgery rather than fetal surgery (Between twin 2000). The possible number of surgeries will only increase in the future. At a pediatric conference, Joseph Bruner, M.D., of Vanderbilt University, described 50 cases of fetal surgical repair for spina bifida (Jones 2001). Recently, Bruner completed his 130th case. Physician concern over these surgeries is based on the high-risk, less than optimal outcomes, and the lack of research data from randomized, controlled clinical trials. Vanderbilt's website on fetal surgery is captivating. and parents may decide to take the surgical risk prior to any evaluation of the procedure. However, one post-surgical risk is preterm labor, and as more surgery is conducted with fetuses, more women will be at risk for preterm labor. Of course, surgery presents a risk of death and even further disability for the fetus (Kahn 1999). Such circumstances will potentially increase admissions to the NICU.[h]

After birth, lung viability is one of the sizable hurdles to be overcome. If some sort of technology is developed to *completely* break the barrier of lung viability, then a further test of our ethical responsibilities will require us to face the dilemma of, on the one hand the request for abortion, even very early abortions, and on the other hand, the possible obligation to all fetal life on the other hand.[i] If a process and the necessary devices are developed to totally sustain fetal life outside the uterus throughout a whole pregnancy, ethical debates about the viability factor, frozen embryos (potential fetuses), and NICU care will overlap considerably, even totally.

Jeffrey Fisher (1992), a pathologist, predicted in his book *℞ 2000* that by 2015 or 2020 we will have *in vitro* gestation, extracorporeal gestation.[j] He cited Dr. Stephen Corson, clinical professor of obstetrics/gynecology at the University of Pennsylvania School of Medicine, in pointing out that: the main function of the placenta is to bring in nutrients and remove waste materials, and we already have heart-lung machines and renal dialysis that accomplish similar functions. We can also provide nutrients through the cardiovascular system when the gastrointestinal track is immature or diseased. An artificial placenta cannot be far off. Writers variously refer to this process as ectogenesis, extra corporal gestation, or *in vitro* gestation. We may face the day when *nurseries* are divided into age ranges: artificial placenta-dependent fetuses and physiologically less dependent newborns. Physiologically dependent infants could be further divided into those almost fully functioning and those with problems, possibly the more complex problems separated from the simple ones.[k]

Until ectogenesis is perfected, micropreemie newborns (22 to 25 weeks old) are becoming more common consumers of NICU technologies and a challenge to the knowledge and ingenuity of their care providers (Blakemore 2000).[l] The price of survival is often severe disabilities. One family called the treatment of their 22-week-old infant "medical torture" and sued because they believed the therapies were medical experimentation. But some outcomes are favorable, and another mother of a 26-week-infant is pleased that the treatment for her child was aggressive.

Technological dependence no longer prevents discharge from the hospital to the home (Cohen 1999). As equipment became minaturized, it could easily be accommodated in an ordinary household bedroom and transported as necessary when the infant is moved about. Although the use of highly sophisticated devices in the home presents its own problems, those problems do not curtail the challenge to continue such technological developments for more and more serious conditions.

The ethical questions related to technology will be numerous. As the possible issues are examined, the ethical questions continue to fall into two major categories:

1. the treatment question, and
2. the locus of decision question.

Certainly there will be the question of how the available technology will be used, and whether it should be used, and the questions are likely to arise first with regard to technologies associated with infertility issues. For example, although infertility rates are higher for blacks in the United States, treatment programs are more likely to be available for whites (Berg 1995; Sherwin 1992). What prevents black community members from benefiting from these technologies? Additionally, should every embryo and fetus receive aggressive care? What about decisions to abort based on complex congenital problems? What choices will be available for women when fetal surgery is no longer an experimental option? Not every condition will be amenable to correction by fetal surgery. Avery's review (1998) of the history of medical decision-making in the NICU, concluded that the treatment question remains paramount including issues of efficacy, futility, and harm.

As with many new technologies for prematurity and other high-risk conditions, the effectiveness of treatments must often be extrapolated from the use of the same or similar treatments in other age groups. Although not strictly a technology, the use of "off-label" drugs in the NICU occurs simply because their effects on this specific group of newborns is unknown but possibly beneficial, given the presenting condition or problems in the neonate.[m] New treatments in the NICU are initiated, sometimes without formal clinical trials, based on the neonatologist's estimation of need. As NICU infants become younger or unique conditions or inexplicable complications develop, creative solutions are often posed based on the experience of the neonatologists and their collective ingenuity. And early on, as with all new technology, mistakes will occur. It is very unlikely, no matter how much testing is completed, that every nuance will be understood. What ethical responsibility is incurred for these mistakes?

Futile has been used as a classification for treatments in an attempt to distinguish those interventions that are not benefiting the infant and can therefore be discontinued, or, if suggested as possible options, do not need to be initiated. Tyson (1995) indicated that it is almost impossible to demonstrate futility--so determining what is mandatory in the treatment of the high-risk newborn has not been satisfactory. He took issue with prolonging each and every life, but rather opted for medical reasonableness. Reasonableness encompasses a consideration of more than a modest chance of survival, and for Tyson, survival with serious sequelae is also not justifiable.

Diverse approaches to the questions about technological interventions are possible. The range of possible problems for newborns in the NICU is extensive and challenging. For the newborn, even recovery from untoward conditions during pregnancy and birth trauma may require an extended period. The parallel range of available technologies and other interventions will only grow with the passage of time. One major criticism of technologies can be corrected in the future by rigorous scientific testing of these inventions and how they are used as physicians vary in their application (Horbar & Lucey 1995). Large, multicenter trials are necessary, such as were conducted with surfactant therapy, high-frequency ventilation, and cryotherapy for retinopathy of prematurity. Researchers need to create large data-bases to provide benchmarks for practice. Meta-analyses of smaller studies are also suggested. Research utilization is another barrier, in that not all physicians avail themselves of a practice protocol even when there is strong evidence for its effectiveness. One example is antenatal steroid therapy.

Then there is the question of who decides. Treatment philosophies of the diverse members of the health care team are likely to vary. Not only can health professionals disagree about treatment alternatives in a particular case, but, based on the numerous variables affecting each newborn's condition, approaches to care differ from case to case. Some prefer more aggressive, technological interventions uniformly applied to most infants while others favor a response based on interactive signs from the infant itself (Brinchmann & Nortvedt 2001). Commitment to aggressive interventions in the NICU is less strong in some countries, notably England and Sweden (Harrison 1997). Yet, after discharge, these countries show a far greater societal commitment than in the United States.

Physicians, including neonatologists, can be characterized as generally adhering to a mechanistic view of illness which can be positively influenced by the availability of technological intervention. The patient becomes a means to an end as the professional sets out to win the battle against the disease or trauma. Good intentions motivate decisions to treat the infant until the outcome is certain, yet the aggregate benefits versus the aggregate harms are not always considered as seriously as they should be (Haney 1987; Muraskas et al. 1999). Self-interest of neonatologists can compromise the objective aspect of decision-making. Success in and of itself is an important goal, but there are financial rewards for these physicians as well. NICUs have made some physicians very wealthy (Simpson 1999).

The role of parents in decision-making will continue to be debated. Few parents in the project reported in this book indicated that they had a role in technology and treatment decisions while the infant was in the NICU. Taking an active role is simply not the situation for all parents and acceptance of a passive role is not sufficient ethical rationale for excluding them from the decision-making process. Although one discussant has claimed that unilateral decisions by physicians are "rare" and parents have significant input, that claim is not supported by many parents' stories of their experience (see Chapter 1) and various health professionals' reports (Miya et al. 1991; Silverman 1992). Some effects of the Baby Doe regulations have been to reduce parental authority, reduce considerations of quality of life for the infant, and justify the use of interventions (Tyson 1995). One recommendation acknowledges the physician's need to often make quick judgments about life-and-death, for example, whether to resuscitate the newborn at birth. Otherwise, treatments ought to be discussed with parents and when the physician is in doubt, then it is best to defer to the parents (Stevenson & Goldworth 1999). Tyson suggested that it is critical to allow parental autonomy in decision-making when the treatment is experimental. Communication with parents seems to be as important as the actual decision-making authority. This is not to suggest creating a false inclusiveness that simply makes parents "feel" involved, but rather continuously informing parents and apprising them in advance of interventions for their child prior to their use as much as possible. This aspect of professional-parent interaction would seem to need more emphasis in the future.

The use of technology is not *just* a medical issue, a decision privately determined between doctor and patient. At present, the government is involved in technology, both in funding its development and in regulating its use to some extent. For example, government restrictions exist related to research and embryo use. A Supreme Court decision was handed down on abortion. Numerous private interests in technology and medication development are related to patents and profits. Insurance companies, health care plans, and other third-party payers also have a stake in technological developments in terms of member coverage. Various advocacy groups have their own special interests promoting selected issues that often encompass technological developments: reproductive rights advocacy, protection of the unborn, and others.

Several suggestions and guidelines have been published to assist NICU personnel in making decisions related to technology and treatments. One approach to treatment has been the development of various sets of interventions targeting specific infant conditions, weights, or gestational ages. For example, one investigative team presented an algorithm for infants at 23 to 25 weeks gestational age based on 10 years experience with more than 1,400 extremely low birth weight infants (ELBW) (Muraskas et al. 1999). Another interesting strategy for the use of technology was taken by the Neonatal Comfort Care Study (Catlin & Carter 1999-2001). Through the use of a consensus panel, a protocol for "a dignified, loving, and comfortable death for the dying neonate" was created (Catlin & Carter In press). Determining which neonates are appropriate for this protocol rather than aggressive technological care was part of the study.

Faced with available technology and futuristic trends, bioethical decision-making will be continually pushed to intellectual limits in developing responses to the demands of NICU care and those situations which subsequently require the services available there.

Family Life

A cartoon on the editorial page of a local paper portrayed a modern family (see Figure 7.6). The new baby is featured in a carriage at center stage. The middle row consists of various individuals related in some way to this infant but a key group of individuals occupies the third row--the lawyers. Such was the perception of families in the aftermath of legal hassles involving reproductive technologies and surrogate gestation.[n] Families will undoubtedly be highly varied in structure as we move through the 21st century. Such developments could be threatening or challenging. However, we first need to realistically appraise the past.

Lest we be captured by a romantic image of a long-gone, golden age of family life, we should heed the words of Stephanie Coontz (1992), who carefully examined many nostalgic notions about family structure and function, and refuted them. First, time tends to erase difficulties and hardships so our memories about some past, glorious family life may not be accurate. One myth discussed by Coontz is our conviction that families really functioned or should function as the 1950s' *Leave it to Beaver*-type television programs would lead us to believe. Although the two-parent family was often the icon of the television family, in reality such families were in the minority even in the decades of those popular television programs. In 1960, only 45% of households consisted of married couples with children under 18, while

Figure 7.6 *The Modern Family*

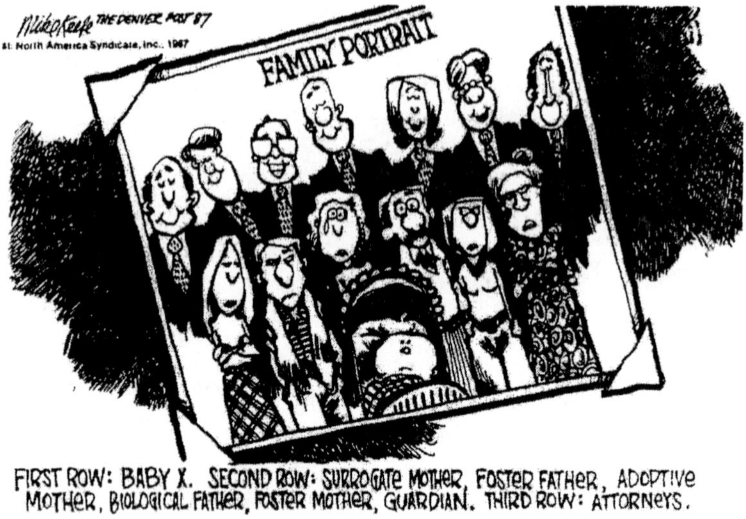
FAMILY PORTRAIT
FIRST ROW: BABY X. SECOND ROW: SURROGATE MOTHER, FOSTER FATHER, ADOPTIVE MOTHER, BIOLOGICAL FATHER, FOSTER MOTHER, GUARDIAN. THIRD ROW: ATTORNEYS.

Reprinted with permission from Mike Keefe, The Denver Post .°

more recent figures set that percentage at 23.5 (Not so many are 2001). The number of women who head households with children grew 5 time faster in the 1990s than the number of married couples with children.

Second, whatever negative aspects of family life are really present in our society, they did not just occur overnight (Coontz 1992). The predicament is the product of the complex interaction of many factors including economic, social, and political phenomena. Changes in family life are not simply changes in gender roles, or women entering the work force, or state intervention in family life, or our materialistic mentality. West (2001) affirmed the above analysis and blamed the disintegration of the family on the seduction of society by sexual exploitation, society's fascination with violence, and the focusing of people's energies on consumption. Fulfilling one's own desires and pleasuring the self supersedes or replaces loving care and concern for others. So in examining the implications of family life for children who graduate from the NICU, especially those who leave with life-long sequelae, we need to confront the reality faced by their families in day-to-day life.

As noted in the discussion of technology, families are impacted by the technologies of reproduction. Multiple roles emerge for all of those who participate. We no longer simply have *parents*. There are many social and ethical implications for various roles: genetic roles (those whose sperm and eggs are used), gestational role (the woman who carries the fetus), and social roles (parents who participate in the raising of the child or children). There is an especially poignant dimension when the NICU is the required level of care and the outcome is less than ideal. There can be a contentious denial of responsibility by all adults for the results of the process. Lawyers and judges may be called upon to intervene. Wright (1998) said that numerous options in reproductive technology have transformed the previous linear path of family roles from biological ones to gestational ones, as couples became parents. A child might now have five parents and still be an orphan (donor sperm and egg, gestational pregnancy, and then the infertile couple who might abandon the newborn when the outcome does not meet their expectations).

With or without reproductive technologies, some families are legally questioning the aggressive approach utilized for their child in the NICU. One couple in Milwaukee filed a lawsuit on the basis of wrongful life against the physicians and hospital where their son was born--a micropreemie who at 1 year of age requires around the clock care (Babies and technology 2000; Micro-preemies 2000).[p]

The major concern, whatever the impetus for admission to the NICU, is that all families will need to adjust to the outcome of the crisis. Many whose children have marginal problems or problems that were amenable to the available treatment may face no long-term challenges. As an ethically responsible community and nation, our focus should target those families who have children with ongoing, special needs. Adjustment of family life to a child with special needs begins in the nursery and continues in the community after discharge. Therefore there are two areas to examine: the initial, acute phase of family adjustment while the infant is hospitalized, and the subsequent integration of the infant into family life and long-term care.

Evaluations of families are made every day in the NICU and will continue, based on who visits the baby, how often they visit, the time spent with the newborn, the availability of parents when consent must be obtained, how bonding develops, and many more aspects of the relationship between the parents and the neonate. Families who do not meet the image of the ideal family can suffer as professionals interact with the representatives of those families and judge them as lacking, not good enough to receive this newborn the staff has worked so hard to heal. Health professionals need to be open to a range of possible family structures and functioning. Family life can be successful within a variety of permutations.

The greatest need related to families, however, appears to depend not on either function or structure but rather on values and commitment. Although Cornel West wrote about black America (1993, reissued in 2001), his observations are also applicable as one examines the families of high-risk infants, albeit on a smaller scale. The psychological depression, personal worthlessness, and social despair he describes for black Americans, are also the problems that can plague families of these high-risk infants. These problems are the result of stigmatism, prejudice, and shunning which are not limited to black Americans are also experienced by families whose members have disabilities or less than optimal health. Of course, a number of families with high-risk infants are themselves black Americans.

The family as a basic unit of society--stable, protective, committed to one another, and cooperative--appears to be needed as much as economic support and political power for this unit of society (West 2001). Such a description of the family is not to be interpreted as an easily dismissed, maudlin, supersaturated saccharine perspective of family life. There are problems in any relationship or group interaction but as long as they have a basic minimum of these intangibles, individuals can grow and develop from infants to adults without serious scars. The intangible elements of family life are required first in the most intimate experiences of our lives in order for those values to be significantly woven into the fabric of community life, thus preventing despair and dread, and the ultimate disintegration of a unified nation. A wide range of family structures and functions are capable of transmitting these values, given the opportunity and support to do so. Rather than setting a uni-dimensional ideal and forcing families into this preconceived mold, efforts should be extended to not simply tolerate or passively accept diversity in structure and function, but to embrace variety within the mainstream of public life. Differences need not be tempered or disguised in order to "fit in," to be conventional. A wide range of possibilities should be accommodated. Then, whatever the structure or function, the goal is to provide the resources to develop and promote stability, commitment, and cooperation in an environment that promotes the full potential of each member, especially the high-risk infant.

These families, then, are the ones who should participate in the decision-making process for their infants--from conception, through birth, and in subsequent situations. Various strategies have been proposed relative to the level of parental involvement in decision-making and the weight that should be accorded their preferences (Weir 1992). Shiono and Behrman (1995) emphasized the need to inform parents and ideally discuss any potential untoward events prior to the birth. If specialized care of the infant is predicted and services are centralized, parents need to be prepared for transport of the infant. This will also entail the need for the family to travel and perhaps temporarily locate elsewhere for a portion of the pregnancy as well as after the birth.

Although few would publicly propose totally ignoring the parental choices, rather elaborate arguments have been developed to rationalize the legitimacy of either minimizing parental wishes or by-passing them. I continue to be deeply troubled by such proposals, whether they be sophisticated theorizing or simple clinical practices related to ethical decision-making. Many health professionals tends to view parents as unable to make decisions based on their lack of education, fear, regression, inability to understand information, capacity for decision-making, emotional instability, pain, and others (Howe 1998; Savage et al. 1993; Waltman & Schenk 1999). A colleague regularly counters my plea for parental involvement with the philosophy as espoused by neonatologists in his acquaintance. These physicians take the position that decision-making belongs in the hands of the professional so that parents can later blame them for any untoward or negative outcomes related to the decisions in the NICU. For professionals to possess such hubris as to think that 2 or 3, or even 10 years later parents will recall the NICU experience and remember the professionals sufficiently to blame them for the decision that led to their present distress, frustration, or unhappiness is preposterous.

Anna Freud's observations about the attitude of physicians toward adult patients put in realistic perspective the long-term memory of these individuals relative to health care. As Freud told the students of Western Reserve Medical School:

> ...you must not be tempted to treat [the patient] as a child. You must be tolerant toward him as you would be toward a child and as respectful as you would be towards a fellow adult because he has only gone back to childhood as far as he's ill. He also has another part of his personality which has remained intact and that part of him will resent it

> deeply, if you make too much use of your authority (Katz 1995, p. 1261).

The project reported here confirms Freud's statements: parents of neonates in the NICU do remember how they were treated, and they do remember when professionals viewed them as incompetent, unable to make decisions for their infants.

Others are more subtle in arguing against parental involvement in ethical decision-making. Howe (1998) would prevent parents from making decisions only when it would cause "substantial, unnecessary, permanent physical harm, or substantial, unnecessary even short-term emotional suffering" in the infant (p. 216). Who determines the potential negative outcome is unclear. Howe, however, is unusual acknowledging that the emotional responses of health professionals, especially caregivers who are women, may influence decision-making! He does not include suggestions for the locus of control in decision-making should the professionals' decisions be emotionally based. In Brinchmann's study (2000a), health personnel were almost unanimous about taking the responsibility for the final decision in ethical dilemmas, which Brinchmann accepted as legitimate, providing a best interest standard is used. Parents varied in their perception of responsibility for decision-making and were ambivalent about being involved, in Brinchmann's study, but they were adamant about remembering their need to live with the consequences. They appreciated the knowledge level that professionals brought to the decision-making process as well as their professional understanding of the uniqueness of each situation. Nonetheless, parents concluded that they need to feel involved. Avery (1998) also reminded those making decisions that it is a complex process and although only professionals and parents may be present in the nursery, the influence of payers (managed care, Medicaid) and regulations including court decisions (and others such as advocates for the handicapped) is strong. Bauman's advice is profoundly appropriate in making ethical decisions, " Issues have no predetermined solutions...there are no hard-and-fast principles which one can learn, memorize and deploy in order to escape situations without a good outcome.......Human reality is messy and ambiguous - and so moral decisions, unlike abstract ethical principles, are ambivalent" (1993, p. 142).

Regardless of the capacity of the parents when the infant is in the NICU, family values need to be clarified and articulated (Savage et al. 1993). Nurses can use their therapeutic communication skills to ascertain the family's perspective. One author suggests that parents need allies not adversaries in the NICU, and nurses can fill this role (Erlen 1994). Problems of "ownership" of the infant need to be addressed, as that issue jeopardizes the nurse's appearance as an ally. When nurses view the baby as theirs and parents also view the infant as theirs, conflicts will arise. Two examples from individuals not in the sample, were shared with us during our research project. Parents described one situation as they observed the discharge of another infant in the NICU. The other set of parents were ready to take the discharged infant out to their car, but several nurses were crying and wanted to hold the baby "one last time." The parents who observed this scene described the other parents as looking quite awkward and at a loss as to what to do as they waited to claim their child. The woman said that as she looked on this drama, she wanted to get up and go over, snatch the baby from the nurses, and give it to the parents saying, "Here, he belongs to you. Just get out of here."

On another occasion, a nurse described a colleague who worked in the NICU. She was particularly attached to an infant who experienced a very bumpy course during his hospitalization. The nurse was planning to be married, and the closer she got to the wedding day, the more anxious the nurse became about the infant and what would happen if she was not there to care for it. She even briefly contemplated postponing her wedding until the infant was stable. Although she did not act on this idea, she did call the NICU regularly during her honeymoon to get information about the infant and its progress. She simply could not let go.

During the NICU hospitalization, families are prepared for discharge. Information is essential as parents move toward discharge, information in addition to that required for any role in decision-making. NICU personnel are certainly responsible for that dimension of care. In addition, parents can benefit from support groups or simply contact with another family who has had a similar experience. Many families now go to the internet for information. It behooves health professionals to familiarize themselves with these sources. Websites should be evaluated and professionals should monitor them and be prepared to recommend those with up-to-date and accurate information.[q]

As found in one study (Hamelin et al. 1997), mothers who were interviewed prior to discharge indicated that they felt supported during the infant's hospitalization, prepared and confident to take the infant home. Not until after discharge, at a 6-week postdischarge interview, did these mothers realize how ill prepared they were. Caplan and associates found similar results more than 30 years ago (1965). Despite such reports, special needs of parents whose child is hospitalized in the NICU continue. Hamelin's group recommended the development of structured and comprehensive teaching plans that are implemented with all parents even through their study included only women, with written materials for parents to take home and review before discharge. Rooming-in for more than one night was also a suggestion. When the mother chooses breast-feeding, extended efforts are needed to ensure her success while the infant is still hospitalized. Lactation specialists should be utilized.

Families face considerable challenge after discharge beyond the initial weeks of adjustment, especially when they have children with disabilities. Families experience various mixtures of success and failure--but common to all is unexpected change. For some, these changes in expectations for their families will be lifelong. The newborn with serious defects dramatically changes the rest of the lives of both parents and siblings. It can potentially alter the quality of their lives to a serious degree (Hardwig 1990). This is not to say that every family's experiences match their plans or that negative outcomes are never encountered by others without disabled children. Problems and disabilities in children are particularly troublesome for families, and in general, this dark side of the NICU episode is ignored. Yet these outcomes should be central to the ethical decision-making that occurs every day in the NICU. Tyson (1995), a physician himself, says it is easy "to demand prolongation of each and every life that requires none of one's own...resources to maintain that life later" (p. 201). Therefore, we will examine some of the reports related to the discharge situation for families, especially those who experience difficulties. Not that success stories are not important. Successful adjustment and coping are very important, as those stories provide valuable strategies for families who are not succeeding. Especially touching are films about these families and their children.[r] More of our focus ought to be on those who did not succeed in order to better serve those families in the future.

Deinstitutionalization, which began in the 1950s, forced families whose children have disabilities to care for them in their homes and become their advocates (Gartner et al. 1990). This phenomenon applied to both those with physical disabilities and those who were mentally retarded. No huge changes are forecast for this situation. Once the child is sent home for care, the question arises: Who cares for that child? In the majority of cases, that caregiver is the mother (Abel & Nelson

1990; Fewell & Vadsy 1986; Fisher & Tronto 1990; Mahowald n.d.; Pierce & Frank 1992; Turnbull 1985; Turnbull & Turnbull 1990). Currently professionals in the health care system assume that women as unpaid workers will care for the chronically ill in the home (Pierce & Frank). Many mothers are already in the work force and after the birth had planned to return to work. The number of women not employed outside the home is declining and more women have different expectations of themselves than in the past. Professionals who direct discharge planning must move beyond the assumption that every mother is "an enthusiastic therapist with time on her hands" (Gartner et al. 1990). For example, in an extensive discussion of withdrawing nutrition and hydration in a premature (36 weeks) born with severe perinatal asphyxia, only an afterthought addressed the mother's position (Johnson & Mitchell 2000). The authors stated "Perhaps it should be added that the family could not obtain affordable child-care and the mother has, therefore, not been able to return to work, which was the source of the family's health insurance" (p. 134). Not only was the mother's employment a non-issue but the relevance of the family's resources for health care was ignored. Lewit and associates (1995) investigated the effects of low birth weight (LBW)[s] and found that this status did not affect whether or not a mother worked. This is contrary to earlier studies, but they remind the reader that services and programs have increased from earlier decades. However, a report in 2001 from Benko indicated that states are limiting children's health care coverage, which is part of the funds available for disabled children. Idaho was specifically cited, but some 42 states have set their eligibility levels for Medicaid at 170% of the federal poverty income level, or higher. More detail about the financial implications will be addressed in the section on economic trends. According to Hamelin and associates (1997), women who attempt to continue employment outside the home find it more difficult to adjust to the care of the child with special needs. Lewit and associates also acknowledged that undercounted expenses in their report stem from the modification of everyday activities in family life to accommodate the needs of LBW children.

Caring for a severely disabled child in the home can extract a grievous toll on everyone, but especially the mother, who is usually the primary caregiver. In some situations her own physical and emotional health can be compromised (Turnbull 1985). Women who devote their hours, days, and weeks to caregiving can experience stress, chronic fatigue, ill health, guilt, depression, and anger (Abandonment case 2000; Mahowald n.d.; Singer et al. 1999).[t] Curry (1995) described her journey with a disabled child as one with two conflicting forces: hope and sorrow. In working toward a resolution of their situation, she posits a choice between despair and redefinition. Mothers' responses to responsibilities for a disabled child are influenced by the degree of chronic illness and the relationship with the child's father (Mahowald). Parents have indicated that the experience of having a child with serious difficulties affects them for many years ahead. Kratochvil and associates' study (1991) of the parent-child relationship 8 years after NICU discharge found 40% of the parents believed they experienced a negative effect, but 12% suggested that they felt closer to the child. Fathers and mothers see the disability in the child differently (Turnbull & Turnbull 1990). Fathers were more impacted when the child is a male and are more concerned about the stigma the family will face, especially when the child is male. Mothers are more affected when the child is female.

Mothers, rather than fathers, are also subjected to criticism about their caregiving (Mahowald n.d.). Sometimes mothers are criticized for not providing sufficient care, and at other times for being overprotective. Certainly a lose-lose situation. Ordinarily homecare for the child is not remunerated and does not garner much prestige. In addition, women who gave up employment outside the home or were unable to avail themselves of career opportunities after the child was discharged, lose that income and prestige as well as the social interactions that occur in the work setting. In general, Cohen (1999) found middle class families experienced a downward trend in income and social status when caring for a technologically dependent child in the home. In contrast, she found that marginalized families had an increase in self-esteem as a result of the skills they had to learn while caring for the child. They also found visits to health professionals a positive experience as it reduced their isolation. Nevertheless, family members can feel like prisoners in their own homes (Abel & Nelson 1990; Brinchmann 1999). Marginalized families perceived less social distance between the professionals and themselves than did middle class families, which Cohen theorized might account for the decreased stress in the marginalized families. Lewit and associates (1995) found that LBW infants were neither more nor less likely than full-term infants to be placed in some kind of childcare, but this circumstance can be interpreted as either positive or negative. On the positive side, it may represent acceptance of the infant and lack of difficulties with its care. On the other hand it may simply mean that the family does not have the resources, either financial or availability of respite care or other substitute caregiving, to take advantage of outside child care.

As a society, we enshrine the characteristic of independence and place far more value on instrumental roles rather than expressive roles (Abel & Nelson 1990). We distance ourselves from basic life events and devalue the activities that women usually accomplish in the home. Caregiving cannot be done without skills--and not just the technological or manual skills required for the disabled child, although the level of these skills should not be minimized (Pierce & Frank 1992). Often the mother is required to be the central coordinator of professionals, services, and supplies when these are available. Self-integrity and connectedness to the recipient of caregiving are essential traits for attentiveness, responsiveness, and personal strength in the caregiver (Abel & Nelson). Good caregiving fosters autonomy and independence, to the extent possible, in those who are cared for. People have some obligation to care for others to some extent--we were all dependent at one point on the caregiving of others as we began life. Reciprocating that care would seem to be a responsibility for everyone. Hardwig (1990) raised a moral question about how far family and friends can be asked to support and sustain the patient rather than simply trying to ascertain *whether* family members' interests are relevant or *whether* their interests should be included. "It is one thing to claim that the ill deserve special consideration; it is quite another to maintain that they deserve exclusive or even overriding consideration" (p. 6). Finding a balance is the challenge.

The marital relationship can also be strained, and siblings of the disabled child frequently have less time with their parents (Pierce & Frank 1992; Turnbull 1985). Fewell and Vadsy (1986) found that 26% of handicapped children were cared for by single women. Eighty percent of women who had handicapped children and had divorced, did not expect to remarry. Extended family members and friends generally lag behind in their adjustment to the disabled child (Curry 1995). In fact, Cohen (1999) found that friends withdraw in situations when professional caregivers are coming and going. Abel and Nelson (1990) also noted that friendships dissolve during family caregiving. Families face financial hardship and part of the permanent damage they experience is a result of monetary difficulties, including bankruptcy for some (Weir 1992). The extent of this financial burden is detailed in the section on economic trends.

Parents have an ongoing responsibility to be advocates for the child (Curry 1995). As time passes, parents race against a developmental clock that is already late for their child. The health care setting can be frustrating. Often parents are patronized and their capabilities underestimated. Whatever lessons the parents have to learn in meeting the needs of this child, whatever hurdles they face in the health care system, the child must live with the consequences of any decisions. However seriously ill the child, Curry recommends that parents learn to treat the child as an individual rather than a health problem. Turnbull and Turnbull (1990) emphasized that services and programs for families of disabled children should be based on assessments of the parents as individuals rather than the assumption that parents will implement traditional roles (fathers taking the instrumental role while mothers take the expressive, caregiving role). In extreme cases, women may be so overburdened that hospitalization is required (Turnbull 1985). Psychological screening, family therapy, and support services should be available for families with chronically ill children (Gottlieb 1998; Singer et al. 1999). One of the discouraging features of family therapy is the problem of reimbursement, since many third-party payers work on the medical model of individual clients rather than groups. Policies in general have been enacted to shift the burden of care to the home and family rather than to shelter and protect the family from the impact of serious and prolonged illness (Hardwig 1990). Services and education must encompass all family members and not simply parents and siblings but even grandparents (Gartner et al. 1990). An interesting suggestion was offered by Horbar and Lucey (1995) who petitioned for meaningful follow-up care for families of high-risk survivors. These authors believe that parents need to have a role in determining the future research agenda. Currently, only a small percentage of NICU graduates are enrolled in formal follow-up studies. Horbar and Lucey would promote a broad evaluation of societal and familial costs and benefits, not simply a narrow examination of the newborn's growth and development. Parents could contribute vital information and a unique, practical perspective as a research agenda is created to make neonatal care and subsequent follow-up effective and efficient. Focus groups would seem to be a viable research approach to obtain such data, as parents might feel less intimidated and more willing to share their ideas as they interact with others who had similar life events.

In summary, Eakes and colleagues' (1998) description of chronic sorrow seems to fit the experiences of a number of families with seriously disabled children. Chronic sorrow is cyclical and continues as long as the disparity created by a loss remains, which is the situation for families who must face lifelong sequelae in the child. These theorists described chronic sorrow as a normal response to abnormal situations and characterized it as pervasive, permanent, periodic, and potentially progressive in nature. The disparity between the idealized and the actual circumstances, when parents are confronted with children who have physical or mental infirmities and developmental milestones are not completed, create the condition that qualifies as chronic sorrow. Another instance for family caregivers that triggers chronic sorrow is associated with illness and events that reinforce the unending nature of the caregiving responsibilities. Chronic sorrow also occurs when there are disparities between self (the parents in this case) and others, especially in regard to developmental expectations, relationship, and abilities commonly cited in this regard. All of these etiologies are potentially present when families are faced with newborns who have extensive needs--in some cases as Brinchmann noted, "a baby that never grows up" (1999, p. 141).

The Child's Destiny

What will children mean to us in the future? I pose this as a combination cultural/psychological question. Over the centuries, children have meant different things at different times. Children have also meant different things in various cultures. The idea of *the child* and childhood is a continually evolving concept. In Western societies, a child is expected to provide little for the family: "love, smiles, and emotional satisfaction" may be all that is given to today's parents (Zelizer 1985). It is not unusual today for children to expect an income from parents. Sometimes chores are arranged so that the child's character is built, so the child does not grow up thinking that money is freely available, but often these chores are not as critical to family functioning as they were in the past. In addition when children do earn money, as in the case of child movie stars or child models, we are very concerned that these children's parents do not benefit from the income.

Is this a healthy approach to child rearing in the 21st century? Or should we return to a concept of the economically useful child? Is the child psychologically more healthy, does it have increased self-esteem when it engages in serious, productive activities while growing up? Is this even a reasonable goal, given the problems that a high-risk infant may face as it grows, possibly with serious limitations in development for its entire lifetime? How much is reasonable to expect in a child that faces burdens the normal, healthy newborn never encounters? Relative to the status of the neonate and its future welfare, particularly the newborn with sequelae that will pose challenges in becoming fully functioning, what effect would a shift to an ideology of a *useful* child have?

We then need to ask, what will the 21st century bring? Will there be changes in how we view children? There is currently profound concern about the welfare of children, but an interesting paradox has occurred. While we value individual children, this special regard for children is often a private concern. Parental altruism seems to stop in some instances at the family doorstep as for one example, child abuse seems to have become more common (Zelizer 1985). Even more important, provisions for children with special needs are not easily forthcoming.

Additionally, many children live in poverty, and a number of those in poverty situations are infants that began life in the NICU. But much rhetoric proposes cuts in welfare and benefits to families for needy children. School systems strive to provide services for children with special needs, voters often reject increases in school budgets, salary increases for teachers, and programs/facilities for these children. Since 1976 there has been a 27% increase in the number of students with disabilities in the public school system (Special Education 1992-1993). Handicapped children often grow up to become adults with special needs. There is much evidence that we as a society are often not ready to integrate such adults into common societal/community interaction.

A prevailing theme continues to propose the institution of strategies that would limit the number of children in the high-risk category. Beginning with prenatal care, Paneth (1995) emphasizes the need to continue epidemiological studies that would "decode the biological expression of social stratification" (p. 31). Low birth weight has been found to be related to social class (occupation, education, income, marital status), but the exact mechanism is still unknown. Paneth quoted research that supports the lack of a relationship between caloric intake or smoking and LBW. For interventions to be successful, the relationship between social and economic roots to the problem must be specific. Paneth asks, "Poverty must alter health through biological mechanisms" but precisely what can we do?" (p. 31).

Tanner discussed the practice of inducing early labor, sometimes as early as 35 to 36 weeks, and contended it should be curtailed except for emergencies (2000). Although surfactant is currently available for lung functioning, kidneys, heart, skin, and other systems are not mature either. Outside the uterus, the infant's status is dependent upon these systems functioning well and being able to integrate with each other.

Physicians should not depend upon surfactant just to schedule a convenient delivery time while ignoring the possible immaturity of other systems. On the other hand, Grossman (2000) recommends education for pediatricians and obstetricians, as they tend to underestimate the survival rate for premature infants. Education would enable the physicians to intervene appropriately in the care of women who go into early labor and to treat the premature infant correctly when no neonatologist is present.

Avoiding death is not the only goal in the care of the high-risk newborn although death is a significant risk for LBW and premature infants. Paneth (1995) reported that in New York City, these LBW infants accounted for 73.7% of deaths of Caucasian infants in the first month of life and 83.4% of black newborn deaths. Tyson (1995) reminded us that suffering, quality of life, and even cost should be considered in addition to the risk of death. This was affirmed by Shiono and Behrman (1995). Pain in the neonate is also a salient issue. Studies now show that premature babies tend to report more pain in their childhood years and their pain response is greater than that of their normal siblings (Recer 2000a).

Two forces are in tension relative to saving these infants' lives in the NICU. On the one hand, there appears to be a mandate for or at least acceptance of providing care for these newborns, even in marginal circumstances. Physicians seem to be more willing to simply treat aggressively rather than grapple with the issues surrounding withholding or withdrawing treatment. Society is generally reluctant to call a halt to interventions for newborns, even fairly marginal ones. However, this does not come without a certain price. Various studies have documented the adverse consequences of the initiation into life, particularly for infnats of lower weights in whom problems can continue into adolescence (Hack et al. 1995; Paneth 1995; Recer 2000b; Saigal 2000; Steward et al. 1999). One of the most contentious issues confronting NICU personnel is whether we should limit the use of life-saving treatment and life-sustaining treatments to any of these infants based on their marginal weights (Weir 1992). One work in progress is attempting to define when hospice care is the most appropriate approach to the marginal neonates (Catlin & Carter 1999-2001).

On the other hand, as a society, we also seem to be reluctant to acknowledge that we basically abandon our interest in these infants at discharge. When they survive, and especially when they survive with serious sequelae, we need to both embrace their presence in society and provide the necessary services for their well-being. We are morally responsible for grappling with our tendency to allow the "tyranny of the normal" to overly influence our attitudes and actions (Wright 1979). These children can neither be ignored nor simply left supported only by the limited resources of their families. Children do not need to be perfect to be valued.

First we need to consider the barriers that face the high-risk infants when problems occur. Although many function within a normal range as they develop, lower weight infants are more likely to have higher rates of various problems, and some of their activities are limited as a result of adverse health. Cerebral palsy is the most common neurological abnormality for infants, with the incidence increasing as weight decreases (Hack et al. 1995). Various possible outcomes for these infants are summarized in Table 7.7. Although their birth status was not reported, interesting results from a small, circumscribed study of children conceived through artificial insemination with donor sperm found them to be well adjusted and emotionally stable (Reaney 2001). The children agreed with the findings. However, most children did not know the conditions of their conception.

As more infants need NICU care, more survivals are likely, which means that morbidity can be higher than it is presently (Wright 1979). Multiple births account for a significant portion of this increase and the number of such births has quadrupled since 1971 (Wright 1998). Health professionals need to accept the responsibility for counteracting the bias which frequently accompanies individuals who we perceive as different and strange--including those with disabilities (Wright 1979). As a society, we have a tendency to weigh negative aspects more heavily than positive ones. Overcoming this bias is particularly difficult, because the basis for our negativity is partly an irrational cognitive process. Rehabilitation psychology is an important adjunct to the ongoing care of the disabled infant and the parents. Caregivers need to be aware as well that acceptance of a child as a family member is rarely based on rationality; rather, parents act on faith and feeling (van Eys 2001). Professionals can interact with parents on this basis so that parents can be informed and participate in decision-making in a mature and responsible manner.

Commitment to these infants should not stop at discharge (Carter 1998; Shiono & Behrman 1995; What is early intervention 1996). Developmental follow-up is important. The earlier the intervention, the better. Services should to be provided through centers, in the home, at hospitals, or in combinations of these settings. An intervention study by

Table 7.7 *Summary of outcomes for high-risk newborns by birth weight category*

Weight Category	Mental Capacity	Developmental Prediction	Behavioral effects	Health Problems
Low birth weight (LBW) <2500 grams[a]	Score lower on intelligence tests and academic ability. Learning difficulties. Mainstreamed but more likely to need special help in school. Reading age impaired. 4 times more likely not to graduate from high school.	Function within the normal range but can have difficulties. Some limitation in activities. Growth is less.	Risk for conduct disorders, hyperactivity, attentional weaknesses--an excess of behavioral problems. Difficulty with social skills. More shyness, unassertiveness and withdrawn behavior. Problems as measured by Rutter behavioral test. More peer conflict. and less social success.	Cerebral palsy (CP). Asthma, respiratory infections, ear infections. Rehospitalized more than normal weight children. Unequivocally abnormal MRI for 50% and equivocal scans for 25%.[b]
Very low birth weight (VLBW) <1500 grams[c]		Developmental disabilities in 25%-59% from intraventricular hemorrhage or periventricular leukomalacia		Cerebral palsy in 5%-15% of infants. Anemia, respiratory difficulties (bronchopulmonary dysplasia and apnea), visual problems (retinopathy of prematurity), gastroesophageal reflux, hernias, cryptorchidism.[d]

(Continued on next page)

Weight Category	Mental Capacity	Developmental Prediction	Behavioral Effects	Health Problems
Extremely low birth weight (ELBW) <1000 grams[e]	Mental retardation. More school difficulties. Fared worse on cognitive and achievement measures especially math. IQs were lower. Need special educational assistance and/or grade repetition.		More behavioral problems than normal birthweight peers.	20% risk of developing a severe handicap. cerebral palsy, epilepsy, blindness, or deafness.
Micropreemies 500-600 grams[f]	Major learning problems.	Severe developmental delays.		50%-70% will have cerebral palsy, impaired hearing and vision and other difficulties. Digestive difficulties.

[a] Sources: Hack et al., 1995; Recer, 2000b; Saigel, 2000; Steward et al., 1999.

[b] Magnetic resonance imaging (MRI) is a complex, diagnostic procedure based on radiological techniques, that requires large, expensive, and complicated equipment. However, it yields precise images of the body based on the varying proportions of magnetic elements in different tissues. Very minor differences can be detected and, as one might guess, a highly trained operator and a specially trained physician are required to complete the procedure (Sternlof 1999).

[c] Sources: Any problem or difficulty listed in the higher category (or categories) of infant weights also applies to all of the lower categories; Babies and technology, 2000; Blakemore, 2000; Paneth, 1995; Saigal, 2000; Trachtenbarg & Golemon, 1998.

[d] Cryptorchidism is the failure of the testes to descend into the scrotal sac. They remain inside the abdomen which can be detrimental to their healthy status. The higher temperature of the abdomen can damage the testes, which later will negatively affect sperm production and result in sterility.

[e] Source: Paneth, 1995; Saigal, 2000.

[f] Source: Babies and technology, 2000; Blakemore, 2000.

Broyles and colleagues (2000) showed that comprehensive care in a follow-up clinic was cost-effective in reducing life-threatening illness among high-risk inner-city infants. Although this study has limited application in terms of the targeted infants (VLBW) and length of the support, the results are promising. The intervention reduced life-threatening illness and total days of pediatric intensive care by more than 42% at no additional cost. The investigators attributed their success to the 24-hour-a-day access to primary caregivers who were highly experienced in the care of VLBW infants. In contrast, a nurse in Davis' study (1994) reported the situation in a large children's hospital where a follow-up clinic was not developed because the director of the NICU was troubled by the problems which the children had after discharge.

One area that is almost unknown is the perspective of the infants themselves as they grow, develop, and reach adolescence and young adulthood. Saigal and co-investigators (1999) surveyed the outcome preferences of adolescents (ages 12 to 16) including 50% who had been ELBW, parents of the adolescents, neonatologists, and neonatal nurses through direct interviews. Neonatologists and nurses had similar preferences and rated the health states of the hypothetical cases as lower than the parents of the ELBW infants. The adolescents also rated the health states lower than parents but their ratings were closer to the parents, than to the health professionals. Based on these results, the investigators recommended the parents as the most appropriate agents when making decisions for their infants in the NICU. The health professionals' preferences indicate they would seem to offer fewer options to parents when infants are severely disabled when in fact, parents would support saving the infant's life despite higher morbidity. Although these data are interesting and may be useful in some cases, there is no better source of information than the children themselves, telling their own stories, with understanding, of course that the most severely disabled may not be able to articulate their perspectives. Future endeavors should be made in this area.

Some additional comment about the best interest standard would appear to be appropriate to close this section, since this strategy is promoted as holding the infant or child central to the examination of the situation as decisions are made for its health care before he or she is able to contribute her or his own preferences (Dunn 1993; Weir 1995). In Rose's concept analysis (1995) of "best interest," the major themes identified in the review of the literature were:

- expert involvement (the health professional who served, advised, and decided for the client)
- incompetence in the client (including children)
- conflict (a choice is required but it need not be a hostile situation)
- intention to do long-term good (even if short-term harm is inflicted)
- wishes of the client (primarily when the client's wishes are not congruent with the experts--as what we wish may not be what is good for us)

When the client is a child, the "wishes" may be those of the parents. Based on the use of the concept "best interest" in the literature, Rose concluded that paternalism serves as a basis for this concept, which is in conflict with autonomy. She questioned the professional's ability to act as a patient advocate and determine what is in the best interest of the patient if health professionals are unable to accept the client's (or parents') values.

Brinchmann's finding (2000b) that professionals use an assessment of infant vitality raises serious concerns about their objectivity if they profess to use a best interest standard. Vitality was found especially important for the professional when outcomes from the continuation of active treatment was ambiguous and uncertain (Brinchmann & Nortvedt 2001). Vitality was assessed through seeing, hearing, and touching the infant. Infants with vitality were described as ones with spunk, sparkle, energy, and extra strength--a judgment of the probable fitness or willingness of the child to survive. This concept has moral significance as the professional's assessment of the level of the infant's vitality has the potential to influence that person's determination of what would be in the best interest of the infant. A judgment of vitality by health professionals at this point does not appear to be an objective assessment. Whether this is a better moral situation in ethical decision-making than the possibility of parents including family interests in their decision-making is debatable.

Economic Trends

What monetary limits are set for NICU care? Should limits be set? If so, what should those limits be? As I understand the situation, few financial limits have been imposed upon the NICU. I predict that this liberal use of finite resources will not continue far into the 21st century. We are concerned not only about the economic situation for the NICU, but also about the long-term financial implications of these high-risk infants and their families.

The Baby Doe regulations resulted in a great deal of confusion about mandated care for disabled neonates. Over the long-term, the effect was the institution of extensive, aggressive care sometimes in situations where it was not warranted nor even required by the regulations. The federal government may have responded to the public outcry of discrimination in newborn care, but it has done little to provide financial support for these endeavors when families are uninsured or underinsured, or have limited eligibility for state aid programs for these children (Weir 1992). The lingering effect of the pressure created by the Baby Doe regulations makes neonatologists feel falsely obligated to provide extensive and aggressive care--and, it might be added, without regard to cost (Kopelman et al. 1988).

Costs and charges for NICU were discussed in Chapter 1, and numerous statistics were summarized. There are more than 4 million births each year and $11 million is spent on health care for infants. Very briefly, costs for NICU care vary geographically, but are definitely going up with no evidence that costs will decline (Weir 1992). Examples include an increase from the 1981 national average of $8000 for each infant receiving NICU care to costs ranging between $14,000 and $40,700 in a Boston hospital for survivors of NICU care. Costs for ELBW infants range from $72,100 to $525,110. Another source indicated that ELBW infants can raise average costs enormously--charges can reach $1 million per infant (Paneth 1995). The lowest weight infants generally require longer stays and the rising number of these infants is partially related to the increased use of infertility treatments. Nationally, nine percent of the infants admitted to the NICU are between 500 and 2500 grams yet they consume 57% of the costs (Harvey 1994). In general, LBW accounts for 10% of all health care costs to children but only 7% of the number of newborns (Lewit et al. 1995). In 1988, costs for children between 0 and 15 years, born LBW infants, were $5.5 billion to $6 billion higher than children of the same ages who had normal needs.[u] These estimates are thought to be low by as much as 10%, as costs of long-term care and institutionalization were not included.

A few highly publicized cases have cited extraordinary financial burdens as a result of NICU care. One is the case of Baby L., who had an unpaid hospital bill of $1 million and also has an estimated lifetime medical cost of $10 million (Avery 1998). In *Hospital Corp. of America v. Miller*, health professionals revived the Millers' child at birth, in direct contradiction of the decision the parents had made prior to the delivery (Willing 2000). The extraordinary measures taken to save the child's life have left her blind, brain-damaged, incontinent, and paralyzed in three limbs. The Millers were awarded $43 million in their 1998 lawsuit, now worth $64 million with interest, and the corporation's appeal is being heard in a Texas court. The Millers claim battery and treatment without consent for their child. Advocates for the disabled are troubled over the idea, that the probability of future handicap would be sufficient reason to not treat and that the case might lead to new legislation supporting such reasoning.

In considering the subsequent care for the most seriously affected babies, Menzel (1990) cited costs of care ranging from modest sums of $40,000 up to $200,000 per year for complex cases.[v] Subsequent care above and beyond that needed for a normal newborn includes rehospitalization and other medical treatments, special child care, early intervention programs, preschool programs, support services, special education, and extra demands on the family (Lewit et al. 1995). At school age, all high-risk infants have the potential for requiring special services. Low birth weight infants use more special educational services, are more likely to repeat a grade--which in turn makes them more likely to drop out of school, have lower job earnings, commit crime, and generally require more social services as adults. Tyson (1995) pointed out that, as the use of neonatal intensive care increases, funding for follow-up and rehabilitation has been restricted or reduced.

Insurance restrictions for NICU care have been present for some time. Some policies held by the parents in my study included options related to newborns: either they were not covered initially, or there was a limit to the coverage including a yearly or even a lifetime cap on reimbursement after the initial ineligibility period. One parent mentioned a special rider or extra policy, available from their insurance company, to cover high-risk newborn care. Fortunately, this family had taken out the supplementary policy. Generally private insurance is incomplete and much of NICU care is uncompensated (McCormick & Richardson 1995). Public financial support includes Medicaid, which is available even for insured parties. Social Security benefits are also available for the medically needy.

Health care reform and the move to managed care will have an impact--probably imposing limitations--but these may be among the last effects because of the values we hold relative to children, especially dependent newborns. These values combined with the ghost of the Baby Doe regulations, mean that more treatments rather than fewer are carried over from handicapped newborns to all infants. Few people want to open Pandora's box again and be responsible for curtailing treatment in cases involving disabled or handicapped newborns, or those with chronic illnesses. One strategy of managed care organizations driven by the need to reduce costs, translates into directing obstetric care into lower level hospitals even when the evidence shows that higher level facilities have better outcomes (McCormick & Richardson 1995). This area needs more research before extensive conclusions can be drawn, however. In any case, one reason for the proliferation of NICUs is financial in that insurance plans and providers are competing for obstetric patients because women make most of a family's medical care decisions. A positive birth experience is highly influential in subsequent care decisions for the entire family, not just for the woman and her future care. Therefore many hospitals want to offer the services of a NICU and have instituted these units to serve their obstetric patients when necessary.

After discharge, health costs continue for high-risk infants. Although development may proceed as expected, more expenses can be incurred during the process. These expenses for LBW infants exceeded the health costs of AIDS and unintentional injuries in children after infancy (Lewit et al. 1995; Shiono & Behrman 1995). For LBW infants, initial birth expenses were greater, utilization of health care after birth was double that for healthy infants and when hospitalized, the LBW infant stayed longer. At school age, these same LBW infants will spend more nights in the hospital and use more health services than children who were normal weight at birth.

Some changes have been suggested for the future. One strongly favored approach would make a greater effort long before the high-risk birth becomes a reality. For every dollar spent on high-risk prenatal care, from $2 to $20 could be saved on neonatal intensive care (Harvey 1994). Horbar & Lucey (1995) claimed that $30 to $40 invested in prenatal care in the first trimester saves one additional life as opposed to the $2,000 to $3,000 required to save an additional life for LBW infants receiving NICU care. They acknowledged that prenatal care will not provide the complete answer to avoiding intensive care for newborns. But from a cost-benefit perspective, neonatal care is the least efficient approach to perinatal care. Given the impetus to seek and use infertility treatments, one must remember that these statistics do not take into account the high-risk pregnancy with multiples as a result of reproductive interventions--these women *do* receive extensive prenatal care.

Other writers affirm the need for earlier intervention and add their own emphasis on the necessity of examining cost-effectiveness, including quality of life which is technically measured as quality adjusted life years (QALYs) (Horbar & Lucey 1995; Tyson 1995).[w] As utility arguments contend, although cost cannot alone determine who should receive care, several interventions are currently offered other age groups that all have *higher* estimated costs per QALY gained than NICU care for even infants in the 500 to 999 gram range. These other interventions include coronary bypass surgery for single-vessel disease, school tuberculin testing, continuous ambulatory peritoneal dialysis, hospital hemodialysis, and liver transplant ($250,000 for each QALY in liver transplant versus <$10,000 for each LBW infant). If we invoke a justice argument, then it seems reasonable on a utilitarian basis to provide intensive care for high-risk infants.

Whether or not changes are made in hospital benefits, we are already making changes in welfare. There will be future demands for resources in school systems and other public institutions to accommodate the needs of children who will live their whole lives with the sequelae of their high-risk birth. Some school systems are struggling to find resources to meet the special needs required. When these children become adults, all community-based institutions will need to be prepared for them. As a society, we do not seem ready to sacrifice to meet these needs and sacrifice may well be required. It will be interesting to see how priorities are set and what will actually be implemented. Just as our views on welfare for single-parent families have changed, so might our views on mainstreaming children and providing accessibility in public buildings. At one point in our country, influential policy makers wanted women to stay home and focus on raising children in accordance with society's idealized view of motherhood. When a single woman did not have adequate resources she was supported as a full-time caregiver for the child. The welfare system was partially founded on this philosophical belief, but in recent years has come around to now promote job training and assistance for single women to obtain employment and support themselves and their children. This change was influenced by a need to restrict government spending. What we spend to provide educational services and various programs to facilitate the maximum development of the child with special needs is as yet indeterminate. We could decide to extend and expand what we currently do. But these decisions will be made in the context of a tax-conscious public.

Conclusion

In conclusion, I hope that I have given you some food for thought. I may have touched on some areas that you did not expect me to address in a discussion of ethics and parental decision-making in the NICU. It is, however, the way I see bioethics--in a broad context, in real life, with a moral responsibility for what actually happens to people. A philosopher friend of mine said that every question and every situation can have an ethical element. Sometimes the ethical element does not pose a problem because everyone agrees or the right course of action is apparent for those involved. At other times quite a dilemma can result. But in either case, ethics is present.

So too for bioethics and neonatal care, ethical issues will always be there. A colleague once asked at a conference on ethical dilemmas and high-risk care,

> Why do you continue to examine NICU problems? There are a number of credible studies and well-developed arguments about the issues. Why not simply depend on the work that is already done? (paraphrased)

The work in this area continues because, despite good work and fine arguments, some aspects have not changed. In addition, each new endeavor adds to the existing body of knowledge and can bring a new perspective to that collection of ideas. However, the major reason for the continuing effort is that ethical problems are still there. Solutions are required. All those involved need to be prepared for them and deal with them. Sometimes it will be easy, sometimes it will be difficult, but in any case, if we are thoughtful, considerate, and give ethical obligation its due, we will have fulfilled our moral responsibility in our professional roles. In that way, the parents of these high-risk neonates will have the best experience possible within the constraints of their circumstances.

Notes

[a] The following are suggestions for the reader: Callahan (1995); Raymond (1993); Scully (1994) and Sandelowski (1999). One of the most interesting reproductive issues for women is that most treatments for male infertility actually

target the woman as the patient even when she has no fertility problems. For such conditions as low sperm count, mobility problems with sperm, or the sperm's inability to penetrate the ovum, *in vitro* fertilization is frequently the technique of choice for treatment. This approach requires harvesting of ova from the woman after over-stimulation of the ovaries, then implanting the selected embryos back into the woman, when **she** has a normal reproductive system and is without malfunction.

[b] Although ova *stimulation* is the more commonly used term, I prefer *over-stimulation* for several reasons. First, the action of these drugs is over-stimulation because far more ova reach maturity than would normally reach such a stage. Women of course, do naturally release more than one mature ovum on occasion, but the drugs are more potent than a woman's naturally cycling hormones. Second, over-stimulation is important to consider, for the long-term effects of such treatments are virtually unknown. Some suspect that there may be a connection between the use of ovary-stimulating drugs and ovarian cancer. (See Rothman 1992; Goldberg & Runowicz 1992).

[c] Definitions for these technologies are listed below:

- Artificial insemination - Sperm from either the male partner (AIH - artificial insemination by husband) or donor (AID - artificial insemination from a donor) is collected and then introduced at the appropriate time during a woman's menstrual cycle to enhance conception.
- *In vitro* fertilization (IVF) - Sperm and ova are combined in a test tube or petri dish containing material that will provide nutrients for the embryos as they form and grow prior to implantation. This technique can use sperm from a donor or the male partner.
- Gamete intrafallopian transfer (GIFT) - Both ova and sperm are inserted into the fallopian tubes through a small abdominal incision so that fertilization occurs in the woman's body, believed to be a more *natural* process.
- Zygote intrafallopian transfer (ZIFT) - Eggs and sperm are cultured outside the body, and the resulting product, called a zygote, is placed into the woman's fallopian tubes.
- Cyropreservation - Material, in this case sperm or ova, is frozen for some future use either by the donor or by another individual through gift or purchase.
- Cytoplasmic transfer - Material surrounding the nucleus is extracted from a egg of a young donor and injected into an older woman's egg. This enhances the chances of successful fertilization and may reduce the potential genetic errors in the older egg (Richardson 1998).
- *In vitro* ovum nuclear transplantation (IVONT) - DNA (cell nuclei) from an older egg is transferred to the enucleated (DNA removed) egg from a younger donor in order to enable the recipient to keep the maternal genetic

material but retain the physiological advantages of a younger, donated egg. In Jamie Grifo's research at New York University Medical Center, chromosomal abnormalities more frequently found in vintage eggs are reduced by using this method (Wright 1998). In theory, this technique could possibly be used to create an embryo genetically related to two men. A donor egg would be enucleated (genetic material removed) and the nucleus from the body cell of one male partner is slipped into the egg. Then sperm from the second male partner would be used to fertilize the egg. A female volunteer is used for gestation (Richardson 1998). This procedure has not been reported as actually occurring at this time.

• Intracytoplasmic sperm injection - After the collection of a sample, the sperm are microscopically examined and the healthiest single sperm is selected for individual injection into the retrieved egg. Some reports note changes in fetal development after such aggressive fertilization and worry about possible sex chromosome abnormalities that may appear at puberty in the resulting child (Newman 2000). One study of 420 children found them twice as likely to have major birth defects of the heart, genitals, and digestive tract (Wright 1998).

• Assisted hatching (AH) - The shell or outer membrane of the embryo is pierced to aid in the implantation process in the uterus (Richardson 1998).

[d] About one-third of the women in my project had infertility problems, and most of those women received Clomid as a treatment for their infertility.

[e] Obviously, reporters might engage in editorial license, although biased and selective reporting is ultimately a disservice to the public. A *New York Times* item reprinted in a local paper had the headline, "Researchers find preemies successful." The report was true as far as the items selected for the report. However, none of the chronic problems for these preemies were noted in the newspaper summary. This gives the public the impression that there are no risks to a preemie birth. The *New England Journal of Medicine* article was a research report from Hack, Flannery, Schluchter, Cartar, Borawski, and Klein (2002).

[f] The first IVF baby, Louise Joy Brown was born in 1978 (Pence 2000).

[g] After Dr. Vohr's presentation at Children's Hospital in Omaha, my husband told me that I would be interested in her research. I immediately contacted her as I was scheduled to make a presentation where I thought the information might be useful. I would like to again extend appreciation to Dr. Betty R. Vohr, Brown University School of Medicine for her willingness to share her data with me which forms the basis for this set of graphs I constructed.

[h] Genetic interventions are another consideration for the future. The potential for genetic manipulation exists on many levels, several of which could impact new life from conception through pregnancy and birth. As with the other interventions specifically noted here, successful cases will undoubtedly by-pass

the NICU but unsuccessful practices could increase the demand for high-risk care.

[i]Liquid ventilation, another strategy which has been under investigation for about 30 years, has been used experimentally to enhance mechanical ventilation. In 1989 the first neonates were treated with perflurochemical liquid. This is one of the most extensively studied revolutionary medical therapies under investigation today (Weis & Fox 1999).

[j] Fisher mentions two different dates, 2020 (pages 37-38) and 2015 (page 129).

[k] Additional evidence for progress in developing artificial wombs (*in vitro* gestation) comes from Liu of Cornell University and Kuwabara in Tokyo. Both are working on prototypes for a womb and the pace of their effort is startling as reported in *The Observer* by Robin McKie, Sunday February 10, 2002. See http://www. observer.co.uk/international/story/0,6903,648024,00.html

[l] A video of this *Nightline* program which aired August 21, 2000 is also available. #N000821-01, "Micropreemies"

[m] "Off-label" means that the drug is approved by the Federal Drug Administration but not for the intended use as in the case of neonatal intensive care. For example, pharmacological studies using larger newborns or older children may have been conducted, but not neonates with low-birth-weight.

[n] Some scholars object to the use of the word "surrogate" and instead prefer gestational mother. As Tong argues, one of the major legal issues at stake is the identity of the baby's *real* mother. Since women can be related to the child genetically, gestationally, or socially, it is preferable to use one of those terms since they all make a claim as the child's real mother. Using surrogate for the gestational mother can imply that she among all the claimants is not the real mother (only a substitute), when *real* mother is precisely her claim (1995, p. 57).

[o] Some would suggest that we need to coin a new term to replace "family," given the assumptions that accompany its use (Calhoun 1997). The application of "traditional nuclear" to define a certain type of family consisting of two heterosexual parents and their biological offspring in coresidency has little representation in the reality of society as the statistics in this chapter show. However, this conception of the ideal family is reflected in several dimensions of our society. Thus the tension created by the differences between the reality and the ideal is problematic. The status of alternative configurations of "family" are often viewed as pathological when the family is evaluated, much as health professionals evaluate the family in the NICU (Bradford & Sartwell 1997). Considerable self-help literature would guide their clients to acquire such an "ideal" family life within their suggestions for improvement. And finally, courts, in custody decisions, reflect an effort to create a traditional family in some way for children in the aftermath of divorce (Robinson et al. 1997).

[p] Micropreemies are defined as newborns between 22 and 25 weeks gestational age rather than the 40 weeks of full gestation or development. About 450,000 premature babies are born each year and 25,000 are considered micropreemies. One must keep in mind that the weeks of gestation are not precise figures and the weight of these newborns can vary considerably which also has an effect on the outcome. Furthermore, lung maturity plays a significant role and the ability of the lungs to function, their viability, reaches an important milestone at about 23 weeks relative to independent operation. Some benefit can be gained by the use of steroids before birth to accelerate lung maturity and by the use of surfactant immediately prior to the infant's first breath.

[q] Using "prematurity" as a search word provides an overwhelming number of possible internet websites. Rather than evaluating every possible site, it would be more expeditious to prepare a list of recommended sites for parents. Some sites include "chat rooms" where more personal information is shared and lay recommendations are included. A number of diagnoses and procedures used as search words also lead the user to websites. Whether professionals prepare their own informational packets and brochures or refer parents to websites, of course, is a decision for the unit.

[r] One such film was directed by Garcia, *A day at a time*, relating a family's coping with twins who are severely disabled with cerebral palsy . This is advertised as "a triumphant film rather than a sad one." Another film is *For love of Julian*, directed by Blaustein (Blaustein & Kassell 1999).

[s] Low birth weight (LBW) is <2500 grams or 5 pounds, 8 ounces (Lewit et al. 1995), very low birth weight (VLBW) is <1500 grams or 3 pounds, 5 ounces (Singer et al. 1999), extremely low birth weight infants (ELBW) are <1000 grams or 2 pounds, 3 ounces (Muraskas et al. 1999), and micropreemies are about 500-600 grams or 1 pound, 1.5 ounce to 1 pound, 5 ounces (Paneth 1995; Blakemore 2000).

[t] The 10-year-old boy with cerebral palsy who was abandoned by his parents in the hospital lobby was a case that should have alerted many to the needs of families who have life-long caregiving responsibilities for a child. This family did not institutionalize the child but did everything for the child who would never speak, walk, or control his bowels. The media did report some sympathetic responses. For some families problems seems endless and there are no holidays from these chores. Although this story presents only the media's version, it is not far removed from others in many towns across America. One only needs to follow community health nurses on their rounds, when their caseloads include families eligible for such a service.

[u] Raising a child who did not have a high-risk birth and who has no major medical problems, from birth to age 18, has been estimated to cost $160,140 for a middle income family (Wynia, 2002).

[v] Converted to 2001 dollars these figures are $54,109 and $270,543 respectively.

[w] A formula was devised to mathematically measure the lifetime benefits accrued by saving a life in order to compare the cost of the treatments or interventions across various programs. When the formula is applied to the NICU, the number of life-years gained from intensive care is reduced by the number of handicapped survivors and the severity of the handicaps in those survivors. When two or more NICUs have the same expenses and the same number of life-years gained, then the number of survivors with handicaps and the degree of disability will be used to determine which unit is better--a lower number of those with handicaps and fewer disabling features improve the unit's rating. This approach is not without criticism (Tyson 1995).

EPILOGUE

A Road Less Traveled

> It's like planning a fabulous vacation trip - to Italy. After months of eager anticipation...the plane lands. The stewardess...says, "Welcome to Holland." What do you mean Holland?? I'm supposed to be in Italy. [Now] you must go out and buy new guidebooks. It's just a different place...but everyone you know is busy coming and going from Italy. And for the rest of your life, you will say, "Yes, that's where I was supposed to go." And the pain of that will never, ever, ever, ever go away. But if you spend your life mourning...Italy, you may never be free to enjoy...Holland.
>
> Emily Perl Kingsley (1987),
> on describing the experience of
> having a disabled child.[a]

Most of the babies born in the United States never see the inside of a NICU. We generally take a baby's survival for granted. Almost everyone is distressed when a birth is not normal and shocked when a newborn death is announced. But out of more than 4 million births each year, approximately 100,000 or 2% to 3% of those infants are admitted to a NICU for various reasons (Doering et al. 1999; Shinono & Behrman 1995).[b] So, families whose perinatal experience includes NICU care are in the minority. Additionally, every year some 40,000 babies die (Shiono & Behrman 1995). Obviously this is not a common experience among families.

Over the years with NICU care, survival rates have dramatically increased. Many infants eventually recover from the experience with little or no evidence of their high-risk entry into life. However, much interest in these fragile newborns has been generated over the years. Not only is neonatology the largest subspeciality in pediatrics, but neonatal nurse practitioners now number 7,800, a large increase from only 171 in 1983, the first year certification was offered (Waltman &

Schenk 1999). People in the disciplines of psychology, sociology, anthropology, theology, and bioethics all contribute to the discussion and debate on high-risk care. And interest is not declining, including mine.

As researchers, both my assistant and I were very curious about the later outcomes for the families of high-risk newborns. In fact, every time we made a presentation, regardless of the phase of our project, people in the audience wanted to know what happened next, or how the family's story ended. As with most family stories, there is no "ending." These are not fairy tales where one can write, "And they lived happily ever after," or novels where the detective solves the murder mystery or the young boy finds his lost dog. Family histories are continually being written so that there are always additional phases to explore and examine--there is really never a final conclusion to be reached.

As yet we do not have funding to formally continue this study.[c] There are few, if any, longitudinal studies of the ethical dimension of family responses to the NICU experience that extend 5, 10, or more years beyond discharge. However, we completed a small number of interviews with families whose children are at various ages beyond the four-year postdischarge stage, the point at which our initial project stopped.[d] The epilogue stories will provide some insight into situations for families at even later stages of development. What is missing here, which we regret, is the children's own stories. As noted in Chapter 6, the children's perspectives are a very important part of the whole area of health care, and discussion of ethical decision-making in the NICU will never be complete until the children's stories are systematically recorded. However, as discussed later, not every child knows her or his own birth story, which in itself is an interesting phenomenon.

The Parents and Their Children

The families represented in the epilogue interviews differed somewhat from the parents who participated in the original study (see Table A.3 for a summary of the demographic data for the original sample).[e] This group was more homogeneous particularly in relation to socio-economic status, education, and ethnic identification. The self-selected group of parents for the epilogue interviews (12 total) all identified themselves as Caucasian and all were currently married, although not necessarily married to the biological parent of the high-risk child. Protestant, Roman Catholic, and Jewish religions were represented. Parents ranged in age between 28 and 53 years, and, given the ages of the children, few women had been teenagers when they gave birth to their child. Nine of the 12 interviewees were women. All of the parents had educational experiences beyond high school, and seven had completed master's degrees. The financial status of most families was currently adequate on all dimensions that we explored, including daily needs, clothing, housing needs, food, health care needs, recreational needs, and others (as they defined or added). A few indicated more than adequate financial resources. One couple had previously declared bankruptcy and two others indicated that they had been "close to it" or had had an uphill financial battle after their infant was discharged. Since the birth of this child, financial status definitely changed.

Gestational ages of the newborns varied from a low of 23 weeks to a high of 38 weeks (see Table A.4 for a summary of the data about the infants in the original study). The smallest infant weighed one pound 6 ounces at birth; the largest weighed 8 pounds 4 ounces. Two sets of twins and 10 singleton births were in this group of families. Prematurity was the major reason for admission to the NICU, but parents also noted low birth weight (mostly correlated with prematurity), twin-to-twin transfusion, respiratory problems, infection, chromosomal abnormality, and a respiratory crisis in the normal newborn nursery as the rationale. NICU residence varied between 8 and 56 days. At the time of the interview, the children were between 9 and 18 years of age. None of the health status data related to the infants was corroborated with a hospital or patient record, nor were any health care professionals sought to verify parental impressions.

A serious limitation of these written accounts of the parents' stories is the difficulty of conveying the emotional tenor of the interviews. Most individuals were interviewed over the telephone but voices disclosed a gamut of sentiment that parents experienced as they recalled their situations. They expressed joy, pleasure, and satisfaction as well as anger, frustration, sadness, and helplessness. Some simply stopped talking at times, unable to speak, and others cried openly. Sometimes parents raised their voices and almost shouted into the telephone. At other times voices were barely audible and I had to ask them to repeat their statements. All of the following accounts should be brushed over with the colors of such feelings as the descriptions are read.

Retelling the Story of the NICU

Stories of the NICU experience readily came forth, reaffirming the various postdischarge perspectives of parents in the original project, as the new group looked back at their experiences from the six-month and four-year standpoints. Actually listening to the stories from these parents' early experiences was somewhat eerie. Although more than 10 years separated the epilogue interviews from the original ones in the project, we were quickly transported back to relive that earlier experience as we heard familiar expressions and interpretations of the NICU events from the new group of parents. Asking the parents to tell us those stories met our goal of confirming or refuting the data that we had originally obtained. Before exploring the long-term postdischarge stories, we wanted some indication that these new families had experiences during the infant's hospitalization in the NICU that were similar to those of our original families.

Only selected observations will be summarized here since the new group's perception of events was so affirming of the previous analysis. This is not meant to minimize the importance of these fresh stories, as they served the critical function of providing evidence for our conclusion that a new group of parents did not interpret their recollections differently. Given the purpose of the project--to examine ethical decision-making by parents whose infant was in the NICU--it does bear repeating that most of these parents reinforced the perception that they had little opportunity for decision-making related to the infant when it was hospitalized. Generally speaking, for most parents there was no moral dimension to the care of the child in the NICU. One parent thought that the staff's persistent questioning of her about possible illegal drug use had moral implications, another parent noted her guilt when she failed to want to bond with her infant, and for some the classic abortion issue was mentioned as a moral issue--but not treatment for premature infants, except in one case. One parent indicated that perhaps physicians did not offer parents choices because later, if the outcome is not good, then parents can blame physicians for their children's problems.

One mother did believe there were moral elements to NICU care and particularly addressed the issue of resuscitation. Part of the apparent rationale for addressing this stemmed from her desire to explain that her position on resuscitation had changed in light of her experience after the NICU experience. Before she gave birth to her children, she believed that physicians ought to attempt to resuscitate every newborn regardless of gestational age. Although she is extremely happy that her very small children were resuscitated, she now believes that such a decision ought to be made in a more discretionary fashion rather than attempting to resuscitate all infants. Some newborns, she stated, are at greater risk for either having unexpected hurdles to overcome or for developing more serious sequelae based on the pregnancy or birth experience.[f] This requires decision-making that is more individualistic rather than policy driven.

Despite the longer interval since the NICU admission and the lesser diversification represented in this group, parents continued to remember their initial experiences in the NICU as scary, overwhelming, frightening, exhausting, traumatic, or extremely emotional. One father called it "a hell of a place," so traumatic and terrible that he has never gone back to the unit as many other parents have done. The ease with which the nurses handled the fragile infant was intimidating for one mother. She recalled, "They were so confident...we felt really alone."

Parents additionally recalled feelings of stress, guilt, inadequacy, failure, insecurity, and anger. Based on professionals' observations of parents in such a condition, they did not solicit the parents' active participation in decision-making. In general, however, parents perceived that they were not sufficiently informed to take that active role. Although a number of parents mentioned being provided with explanations, this was not for any purpose other than to have them know what the staff had done or were going to do. A mother reflected, "They didn't say you don't have a choice. But they were very persuasive about what really should be done." She went on later to say, "We were so overwhelmed with our ignorance. We questioned things to gain information but not to challenge." Questioning, as noted in the original group of parents, was also not always acceptable behavior. One mother viewed herself as an educated consumer and wanted to be informed. Instead she felt she was patted on the head and patronized while being told that "we'll take care of it."

The need for support was emphasized again along with the fact that, often, it was not offered. When support existed, empathetic staff persons and at other times family, friends, and/or clergy were the most likely candidates. The women mentioned being adversely affected by their association with friends who were pregnant or new mothers who had normal postpartum experiences. Pregnant strangers or advertisements that included normal newborns could arouse jealousy or envy as well, which in some women continues to the present. Fathers particularly noted their minor role during the NICU hospitalization, understood the need to focus on the child and mother, but abhorred their own neglect. One father was appalled by the success stories other individuals imposed on him. He believed that there was little appreciation for the variety of circumstances that initiated a NICU admission. In general he believed that people did not understand what "little" and "early" meant in terms of the profound, life-long effect these conditions can have.

Eventually all of these babies were discharged, so we can examine the more extended postdischarge experiences. Few parents were prepared for the experiences they were likely to encounter at home, especially for the possible long-term effects of this high-risk experience on their lives. As one mother said,

> They told me, she'll be fine. And, based on my history as a NICU nurse, I thought too, she'll be just fine. I really felt I had a good comprehension of what it was like for parents emotionally to go through being in the NICU. It was very arrogant of me and I was completely humbled when I had my own child in the NICU. I know now that it's an extremely traumatic situation. Previously, I told many, many parents, well, it'll be hard for the first year but you'll be OK. Do your best to treat them like a normal baby. Here's how to take their temperature, and feed them, and yada, yada. And--see you later.

However, even under such grave circumstances as an intensive care hospitalization at birth, expectations are often not based on reality. It has been said that we make the most consequential decisions based 5% on fact, 15% on hearsay, and 80% on fantasy.[g] In some cases, perhaps if we knew the unvarnished reality of parenting and other monumental choices we make in life, we would never choose to try.

The Great Divide

The one major difference among families after discharge is between those whose children do not have residual effects from the NICU experience and those who do. For parents whose children face on-going sequelae, the families can usually be categorized as belonging to one of two subgroups. First there are those who adapt, manage the challenges of their special children, and adjust to the required changes in their lifestyles. Obstacles are encountered, but the strengths of the family and the available resources appear to sustain them so that they avoid major disasters. Life is certainly not ideal, but given the situation, it is more often as good as it could be rather than a complete failure. Certainly, not every moment is glorious. But on balance, life events are mostly manageable. Second, there are those who do not adapt to their circumstances--regardless of those circumstances. These families are continually faced with incidents that disrupt family life and make a mockery of previous adjustments. Events seem to occur regularly and prevent the family from staying one step ahead--they seem to consistently lag behind whatever is required of them.

Almost every parent in the epilogue interviews currently belongs in one of the two subgroups that continually face challenges. Two families encountered no untoward events in the postdischarge phase, by their own evaluation. One parent in this group described a marvelous post-hospitalization trajectory, and at 12 years of age, her children have a clean bill of health. She was told that it would probably take 7 years for her children to catch up with their peers. Another couple's child is currently 9 years of age and has been typically healthy. However, when details are sought, even some of these children had some health problems or needed special assistance in school, which parents seem to discount as relating to their precarious start in life. The remaining parents, whose lives have changed in a major way, fall into one or the other of the categories--most of these parents cycle through new challenges and modes of adaptation (or lack of) as they and their children live out their lives. Whether life is basically good or full of never-ending adversity would be their decision, not mine.

> I threw out all my baby books about the first year of life. I wouldn't even look at them because I knew that my child was never going to be able to do those things like he was supposed to. I had to change what I thought having a baby was going to be like, 'cause it wasn't anything like the book says.

Even though most families who have children will not confront situations involving unusual developmental passage, disability, and disruptions, such difficulties will still be the focus of the remaining discussion. As Howe (2001) defends his methodology of considering the "worst response parents can have to their children that can be imagined," so this discussion will remain true to its purpose of emphasizing those cases which seem to have negative outcomes and need to be addressed better in the future. Howe justifies his approach, which he calls the *magnified example*, by explaining that initial exploration of the worst-case scenarios allows extrapolating backwards from the worst case to easier situations, possibly revealing factors that may be invisible in less difficult situations. This enables us to "identify the factors care providers can change" in situations where we might otherwise not see a problem or a solution (p. 192).

Constructing a Life for the Family

Even 9 or more years later, families vividly remember feeling ill-prepared for life at home with a NICU graduate. A 180° repositioning in relation to control overwhelms many families upon discharge. Whatever the baby needs, parents now have to provide it or make sure that it is provided by the assigned agency or health professional. They face the usual tasks related to feeding, cleaning, and comforting, but also medications, oxygen, apnea monitors, NG tubes, special procedures and treatments (dialysis for example), and in some cases the management of complicated equipment such as ventilators. Even the usual tasks can create special demands on parents as infants may be tube fed or continue to receive IVs, require surgical dressings, and exhibit sensitive startle reflexes. Additionally, although parents attempt to feed, clean, and comfort, infants can vomit repeatedly, cry continuously, and simply fail to sleep in any regular fashion. One parent said she felt like a baseball player who was on both teams--there was no rest.

Despite warnings to many parents to keep the baby at home and to limit visitors, there were requirements to comply with physician office visits, follow-up clinic visits, and numerous other appointments for tests and treatments. Such segregation was taxing. One mother said, "It suddenly dawned on me. Although we were told not to take the children out in public and expose them to possible infections, here I was sitting with other very sick children in the pediatrician's office!" The children in the office waiting room were undoubtedly more sick than any child this mother felt she might encounter at the mall or would allow into her home. So that ended the imposed isolation and she started to expand her social life with the children.

Mental and Physical Challenges

Whether a baby stops eating, is unable to retain feedings, has breathing difficulties, gets a fever, or develops abnormal signs and symptoms, parents need to decide what to do: telephone for advice, get emergency assistance, or arrange yet another appointment.

Additionally, like parents in the original study, the epilogue mothers had not necessarily regained stable health status when the child or children were discharged. Some women's physical health was compromised by the demands of a high-risk pregnancy or birth, while others were burdened by psychological problems, including clinical depression.

Over the years of responsibility for their special child, parents learned numerous skills in many areas and certainly became informed about health care issues including the various conditions the infant had or developed, resources, and payment practices. One parent indicated that professionals generally talk to you as if you are an idiot. "Physicians spend 2 minutes with us and think they know exactly what we should do," one mother said, "but they are not the ones that go home with the kid. They don't have to do what they think parents should do. They think, it's no big deal. Well, it is."

Another mother described regular appointments with many specialists so that consulting with a doctor nearly became a way of life. When her child was 7 years old she finally became angry about the orthopaedic checkups. She felt they were rarely gaining anything from the daughter's visits. Although the surgeon was "supposed to be the ultimate guy," she concluded that the visits were more beneficial to his students and residents than to her daughter. Each visit meant repeating her history to a new assistant with little new information added about her own daughter's condition or progress, and nothing new in the way of recommendations. So she stopped those appointments and never looked back.

Another woman faced complex medical care focused on almost absent kidney functioning in her son. Given an estimate of about 10% kidney functioning, the child started dialysis at 10 months of age. Since the mother was quite young, questioning a physician's advice never occurred to her. Her change in demeanor and her metamorphosis into an advocate for her son evolved over time. Primarily because of her observations that her son suffered when the professionals did not listen to her, she began to change from an unquestioning, compliant parent to one who gradually placed value on her own judgment. When her son was about 4 years of age, bladder surgery was recommended. Instead of simply accepting the suggestion, she followed her intuitive feelings and sought some additional advice, prompted by the fact that the surgery would be irreversible. Most parents she consulted indicated that the surgery resulted in a nightmare for their children. So she went back to the nephrologist with her decision. She questioned the physician, and finally the physician looked at her and said, "The only way you can possibly understand this procedure and its outcome is to go to medical school and practice nephrology for 15 years." The mother said, "And that was her answer to my question. And I just said, 'excuse me!!' I was, well fine, I am not even going to be nice anymore. We went to another physician."

Eventually when the child was age 5, this mother donated her own kidney for her son. Over the years, all of the urology problems required decisions about where to live to accommodate the dialysis and regular follow-up; which transplant center to choose, what resources existed for auxiliary support related to medical, educational, and social needs for her son; where to locate other children with whom the child could identify and share experiences; who could provide support for her and her husband as parents, and how to plan for the future. These she learned to face with confidence.

One couple's child was plagued with respiratory difficulties, both RSV (respiratory syncytial virus) and flu, as well as some conditions whose etiologies were undetermined. These all compromised the child's health severely, and the couple was desperate to find something to prevent the respiratory complications. The mother heard about gamma globulin infusions (IV Ig) from a home health nurse whose own son was in a study using this substance. When the mother consulted the pediatrician, the physician said she did not think the child should receive IV Ig. However, the mother went ahead and contacted the researchers and had the child evaluated. The child was approved as a viable candidate after much pushing by her mother, and received the IV Ig for 4 years. The mother believes that it saved her child's life as the girl's lungs were able to grow and mature and heal. The child no longer succumbs to such overwhelming respiratory distress. Her mother confessed, "It was hard. Was it the right thing to do? It was going to save her life and I was going to do it."

One mother discussed the various therapies that had to be coordinated for her son. There was PT, OT, and speech therapy as well as appointments with a nutritionist and a home health care.[h] Such circumstances were difficult. She called herself a perfectionist and believed that it was hard not to be picky. She believed, quite correctly, that when some of the treatments were implemented incorrectly, her son's life would be at risk. She had difficulty trusting some professionals. When they did not do the procedures the way she believed that they ought to be done, it was arduous not to complain.

In addition to physical needs, parents faced developmental delays in language and communication skills. Twins in one family were delayed in verbal skills and, in order to communicate with them, their mother taught them sign language. At about 5 years of age, she and her husband both noticed that the boys did not ask questions. She was puzzled and did not know if they did not know how to ask questions or whether their lack of information processing skills prevented this form of communication. She partially attributes the language skill delay to their almost continuous ear infections and their inability to hear adequately. Infection haunted the twins for the first 6 years of their lives. She labeled the first 2 years the "lung years" and the following 4 years the "ear years." There were numerous rehospitalizations for both fungal and bacterial infections, and finally a need to move to the superantibiotics for treatment when the first level of antibiotics failed to successfully treat the children. This mother also put a sign on her front door advising visitors that they could not enter if they had a cold. If they did come in to visit, they had to wash their hands and be careful in their contact with her children.

One parent was concerned about the child's perception of pain and shared the following incident, which was relayed by the child's preschool teacher.[i] The teacher saw the child lying on the ground looking up at the sky and thought he was just looking at the clouds but decided that she ought to check on him. So she asked him, "What are you doing over here on the ground?" He pointed to the top of the slide and said that he fell, "from clear up there." It didn't register with him that if he was hurting, he should let someone know. He was 6 or 7 then, and he has had to learn to respond when he gets hurt. "I had to always check him to be sure he wasn't really hurt when he had an accident because he didn't cry," the mother said. He has gradually changed, noticeably so after he acquired a baby brother, and came to respond more normally to hurtful situations.

This was not the only parent to mention a child's insensitivity or conditioning related to pain. Another mother, whose children were prone to lung and ear infections, specifically indicated that she learned to look for other signs and symptoms of these infections in place of pain. She believes the children had so many painful experiences in the NICU that they simply learned they had to endure pain. She was alarmed by the daily eye examinations her children had in the NICU and gave that as an example of the cruelty inflicted upon the infants from which there was no relief.

Several diagnoses were not made until years after discharge, such as cerebral palsy, and some parents understand that other disabilities may still gradually surface. A number of parents were prepared to expect additional evaluations about special needs when their children started school. As the children were required to apply selected cognitive skills passing through various elementary grades, they were sometimes challenged by tasks that they had difficulty learning--more so than their peers. Other parents recognized that puberty is another landmark where developmental delays could negatively impact their children. On the other hand, one mother was amazed to discover that often puberty comes early to girls with developmental problems. She called this the "greatest joke in the world that anyone's ever played on me." Everything about the child is delayed, but at 10 years of age, she began menstruation and developed secondary sex characteristics while in a grade 2-3 class.

Some parents moved outside mainstream medical practice for solutions to their children's problems. Parents described alternative medication options and homeopathy as well as programs that promised a more holistic approach to improve the children's development. One mother described her children's diagnoses of central auditory processing disorder, dyspraxia, amblyopia, and poor gross and fine motor skills. She continually searches for and implements supplementary programs for her twins that target their neurological development. She has faith and hope that interventions implemented since discharge while their brains are still developing, will enable them to continually progress. She indicated that they are permanently delayed in their development, but does not view them as handicapped. This woman is fairly realistic in her expectations as she discussed the hyperbole accompanying various program advertisements. She explained that she is looking not for a cure but rather for steady improvement. If program advertisements promise an improvement in the child's abilities equal to 1 to 2 years, she is satisfied if her children show an improvement equivalent to a 10 to 11 month gain. For her, even a 10% achievement is worth the effort and money.

Emotional disabilities can also develop later. In one case, the consulting psychiatrist attributed the emotional instability of the child to the initial insult during birth and the early weeks of life, although it did not manifest itself until the child encountered more complex events in life. For this girl, treatment for her bipolar condition was not begun until the 7th grade, and the treatment has been successful. Social skills that should have been learned in the pre-puberty years were not learned and that also has negatively affected her relationships with both siblings and classmates.

A common theme among several families was their need to finally face the reality that their child was simply never going to "catch up." One mother confessed that she had finally comprehended that it was unrealistic to think that other children would stop developing and her child would then be more like others the same age. These children were always going to be different in one way or another. One father summarized his daughter's situation by saying that she has a great deal of trouble keeping up with the other kids but has to learn to live in a normal society. Parents did not necessarily agree on the best treatment for these children.

Ongoing Support and Resources

"We really didn't even know anything about babies, period" one mother said. "I lived in an apartment in which those that were close to my age, 20-24, didn't know a thing about disabled babies. How can a new mother get any support in a situation like that?" And so, life at home with the discharged, high-risk infant begins. Support is essential because, as parents of these disabled children, they are such a select group. They are surrounded by parents of normal children and yet need other adults to whom they can relate, who have similar problems with their children, who have similar needs. One father noted, "Resources are abominable, minimal when you go home and everyday without services and early intervention for the baby has its own consequences. What about towns that do not have these services, or families who do not qualify?"

Parents benefited from special programs and other offerings for children with disabilities or chronic conditions, when they were available and when the children were eligible. Some were able to locate day programs, respite care in the home, day camp, or extended summer camps that catered to such conditions as asthma, diabetes, autism, Down syndrome, and post-transplant needs. There were also some one-to-one or personal services where a volunteer regularly visited the child, or took on a Big Brother/Big Sister type of role. Whether or not such services are available depends upon the community, and often the size of the town severely limits such benefits. Some parents formed their own groups, becoming activists to meet their needs--such as the Parents Empowering Parents group in Massachusetts.

Finances were a critical element in relation to many aspects of life for the parents who were interviewed, whose financial status was better than that of many families in similar circumstances. More often than not, costs of alternative therapies were not reimbursed by insurance coverage, especially when they were self-prescribed. However, for one mother described earlier, the family's financial investment in alternative therapies was a priority because of the potential impact on her children's entire lives. She believes that children like hers should have optimal opportunity to benefit from any improvement such therapies offer. The challenge for her was that little data exists regarding to the possible benefits from such therapies for children who were as small as hers at birth. Besides the programs aimed at neurological development, she also uses nutritional therapy and vitamins to supplement traditional medical advice.

One mother discussed a complicating financial factor.

> We had to have a separate medical fund for [child] so that we didn't lose our SSI money.J My dad started the fund and he is really picky about how we use that money. I'm scared to death of him and afraid to ask most of the time. For example, our insurance doesn't cover all of [child's] medications but my dad won't let us use the money for that. You don't argue with my father. He tries but they (both of the mother's parents) just aren't always sure what to do--and we have to make do.

One mother discussed advocacy strategies that she took for her child. This woman relied on her reputation having grown up in her current place of residence. She believed she was supported in her activist role because everyone knew her. People felt some sort of accountability towards her. She thought that they viewed her as a fair person and as someone who did not speak when she was angry. She felt she knew how to make it easy for people to deal with her when she wanted to make a difference for her daughter--and in this she was successful.

Parents believed that in most cases they had to fight for what they got. Rarely does someone come by and say, "Oh, by the way, would you like $10,000 for your medical bills?" they observed. Parents noted the need to look, hunt, and find a resource. Then the paper work had to be completed in order for the agency to determine if you qualified. Families did not expect to have care provided free, nor did they expect to obtain funding and services without evidence but, sometimes the process was very frustrating for them.

Some parents used families as support, others reflected upon friendships. One woman mentioned her in-laws, who were overwhelmed at first, but as the children grew older "became just great with them." Another described her perception of her family relationships as *weird.* "We really don't talk about anything serious," she said. "My mom pretty much just listened to me. She'd take time off to come with me to the doctor's appointments and my parents let us borrow their car." All of these endeavors indicated support for parents.

One woman discussed support from friends in some detail.

> We received support from a number of people, but in some cases we didn't get the kind of support we needed. Friends changed. Some people came out of the woodwork that I would have never expected to see in a thousand lifetimes and provided us with many things we needed. Others simply disappeared.

One participant, a NICU nurse, had a unique view. Her nurse friends were very supportive while the baby was in the hospital. After the baby went home and the nurses saw what it was really like for these parents, the nurses did not understand all of the difficulties, and they were frightened. The baby's continuing problems were in stark contrast to the nurses' concept of life after discharge. This mother's friends had to face the evidence that their work did not always result in the outcomes they thought they produced, and they did not want to be reminded, so the support mostly ended.

Effect on Women and Their Vocations

All of the women who were interviewed were the primary caregivers for the children, including supervision of physician visits and other therapies on into high school. Most of these woman had had professional lives or paid employment prior to the pregnancy, birth, or subsequent hospitalization of the child. Some continued their employment, while others made it a point to work at home full-time. These are very individual decisions and each family had to weigh the risks and benefits. Only one woman admitted that she regretted the decision to remain at home full-time: "I became a stay-at-home mom and I would still say to stay away from full-time work. I regret not having the courage or whatever to at least work part-time." She believed that she might have gained a better perspective in raising her children if she had had the stimulus of work outside the home and other adult company.

How circumstances change over time for women is represented by one woman's story.

> I felt as if it took me 10 years to come out of the fog I went into when she came home from the hospital. I kept very busy--working with my daughter. I had two other children, I worked, and I went back to school and obtained my master's degree. In the meantime I self-destructed at one point and realized I had to change my life style. But I have managed and it's OK now.

One of the themes in this area was the conflict many woman faced, between being caregiver and mom--their differentiation. One woman noted her perception that she was the child's nurse for so many years, instead of her mom. Another discussed wanting to have "normal" time with her children and to not continually be their therapist. She did not want to always be engaged in therapeutic activities when she was with them. However, the caregiver role definitely has benefits. One mother described how she always sees herself as the hub of the wheel for issues related to her child's life. She wanted to maximize opportunities for the child in order for her to reach her fullest potential. As the individual in charge, the mother could do that. Part of her problem now that the child is 15 is relinquishing that coordinating role. The mother assumed that role fairly early and became very comfortable in it, but now feels that, given the maturity of her daughter, some changes ought to be made.

For some families, the absence of the woman's salary significantly impacted the family's financial status. One father saw the situation as an opportunity for his wife to quit a job she really did not like--to stay home with the child. He agreed with this at the time but would have preferred that she return to work later. Such an arrangement never materialized and they felt some financial loss over many years.

Survival of the Marital Relationship

The personal, intimate nature of this aspect of the parents' lives prevented some of them from revealing any detail about the exact effect of life with the high-risk infant on their marriage. A few parents acknowledged that the effects were not anything beyond simply becoming parents rather than being a couple. This was more likely in families whose children did not have serious sequelae.

The more common theme was an acknowledgment that the circumstances were a real strain on the marriage. As one father articulated, although divorce may not occur, many aspects of the relationship can falter. The needs of the infant, and later the child as it grows and develops, are critical. Such needs are right up front and in some respects the easiest to meet because they cannot be skipped or ignored. According to this father, it is the other things in life that should require attention that can slide by--such as the spouse. These needs are not so obvious and that is the risk, the danger. Marriage, other children, family members--these relationships can waver and fail; negligence can lead to their demise.

Often when husbands see the children's needs superseding their own, they can feel out of the loop. Men have a crucial role in caregiving, and they need to see that, one father noted. Women are very vulnerable when their children have special needs, but husbands can be the glue that holds everything together, surmised another father. One woman related that her husband thought she ought to get over their situation much better--"Suck it up a bit faster and get on with life," he told me. "But it was hard and I had no help in working it out."

As with other aspects of a relationship over the course of several years, the view of marriage changes. One mother noted,

> At first the challenge brought us closer, but now we're just like roommates rather than spouses. We've come close to leaving each other. Sometimes our child brings us close but at other times he's a wedge. We need to remember it's not the child's fault that he is so sick.

One divorce occurred in this group of families during postdischarge care of high-risk child. This woman subsequently entered a second marriage and had a second high-risk infant, as well. Details about the ex-husband are unknown, but he does remain in contact with his child.

Siblings and Additional Pregnancies

> On the one hand, if you don't have other children you focus all of your energy on this special needs child. The child can benefit from the extra effort. But if you are not careful, the child can be spoiled. But on the other hand, the child herself can be prevented from being exposed to a

> normal environment and dealing with social situations that all children need to face when raised with other siblings.

So begins one parent's examination of the effects of adding siblings to their family. When the disabled child is an only child, the parent can deny or avoid recognizing the profound delays the child is experiencing, some parents observed. This is not always helpful, either for the child or for the parent.

For some families, of course, whether or not to have additional children given the presence of a child with special needs was a moot point, as other children already existed. In some cases, the birth of the special needs child did end childbearing in the family, for various reasons. Some families were affected by the negative attitudes of friends relative to the risk of having a second disabled child. Other families were affected by the increased demands of the child, while some avoided childbearing because of an obvious possible risk to the woman's life. The same serious complications could occur in subsequent pregnancies and a few women were warned not to risk another pregnancy as their problems would assuredly reoccur. Other women knew they would be able to have successful medical interventions and go on to have uneventful pregnancies. Some parents wanted more children, but faced infertility problems when attempting to have those additional children.

Occasionally there simply was not any plan. One woman embellished that idea:

> I didn't mean to become pregnant. I applied for this job and I really wanted it. I knew that they couldn't refuse based on the pregnancy once they called me back with an offer, but we had to work it out. My husband and I were terrified how the whole thing would work out. Each subsequent pregnancy lowered my stress a little as we were able to have children who did not have any [genetic] difficulties. As soon as I saw my second child, I knew it was OK. I had amnios with each pregnancy. My husband and I never resolved the issue of prenatal testing--I wanted the testing just for the information. There was no way I would terminate a pregnancy. [Husband] was like, how could you possibly do this again!! The third pregnancy was even easier but it was still very, very unnerving. Having a disabled child flavors everything, forever. It is the ongoing sorrow. Even when I was with my sister after our third child was born, it was hard for me to see her not have her whole world fall apart when she had her baby--it makes me jealous. I

have to fight those feelings because they are so ugly. But, you must not let it define you.

When other children already are present in the family, parents must deal with the children's attitudes toward the new addition. Other children in the family can resent the additional attention a special needs child requires, but parents can initiate strategies that reduce this resentment. There can also be benefits for the "normal" siblings as well, one woman noted. Children can be taught many lessons related to diversity, dealing with adversity, accepting limitations, and other moral values without compromising their own development. Another woman warned parents of the need to carefully observe their children and work with them throughout all family relationships. Children can exert cruelty in subtle ways. Also children can appear to be dealing with the situation in a positive manner, yet later hard feelings can manifest in ugly ways when they are older, and perhaps away from parental supervision. She recalled her contrary relationship with her brother and believed that the same potential existed among her own children. Family relationships are an ongoing challenge, and the growing maturity of the children helps solve some of the problems.

Spirituality and Religious Faith

Parents have gone through profound changes in various directions--from coming to realize the essential nature of a spiritual life in order to cope with adversity, to completely rejecting any sort of religious faith. A few reject the formal aspects of religious faith and public worship but believe that their spiritual life is richer because of this experience. Some acknowledge that the NICU experience changed their spirituality from an insignificant element in their lives to one of importance. The degree of importance varied. Some thought that they could not have coped with their situation without believing in a greater power at work in their lives beyond human intervention. One mother responded, " I am more reflective now. There have been times when I felt hopeless but I would think, she's in my hands now, and that would get me through. This has strengthened my faith."

One mother shared a more detailed philosophy. She began with the story of her own childhood of despair. Her father was alcoholic and abusive to her mother. Just before she turned 15, her mother, who was severely depressed, committed suicide-and the girl found her afterward. By the time she reached her 20s, this woman believed that, perhaps,

> God had finally dished out everything He was going to dish out for me. Perhaps I had been through all the tough times that I was going to have in my life--but then this child was born. I searched so hard. Why would this happen to me? Why again, do I have to suffer like this?

She noted that some people had the audacity to suggest that the child had its tenuous hold on life to teach her a lesson.

She has "searched her soul" over the years to find a suitable explanation, to face the challenges her daughter presented and not lose hope. She has rejected organized religion, which, she says,

> ...makes me very angry. And that's what has changed for me. Before, I tried to be a part of it but now it is a turn-off. My husband is very much the same way. He feels deserted. So, this has changed my faith but it has made it stronger in a lot of ways--but very nontraditional. It works.

Educational Efforts

For all of the children who had on-going problems, education was a formidable experience.[k] One mother related her experience:

> Children have to be in the right place at the right time. Some locations do not have real options but there are times when the child needs to be in a "special ed" class, or a self-contained class for some educational opportunities and then with the other age-appropriate children at other times. When children are segregated, they miss out in terms of social mores. Also, I believe that we really give up on people's disabilities a little too early in terms of how much academically they can get. My daughter was in an 8th grade science class that originally was not thought to be appropriate for her level of ability, but she still remembers those concepts. She was exposed to a lot of things that she never would have been exposed to in the special education class. She also learned from the social experience of that class. It was immeasurably beneficial.

The children had special requirements in some areas; reading was difficult for a number of children, as was acquiring language skills. Early intervention programs are essential for such children, yet not all parents were informed by professionals about the available services. Parents discussed how they lost a year or more years of intervention when it would have been so important to initiate such interventions. Also, early intervention sometimes contains options and parents need essential information in order to make choices that would most benefit their child.

Educational needs are not always simple. For example, simply a lower grade may not be the answer. One mother of a 10-year old explained, " Developmentally he's at the 4-year level but in the 3rd grade in school. His language is really delayed and he is reading at the 1st grade level. He doesn't really fit anywhere so we are doing the best that we can." Another mother who had her child in an age-appropriate grade observed that he was much slower doing homework than her other children for the first few years. Then in the 4th grade, "something kicked in and things went better until the 6th grade." So circumstances can change.

An example of a particular cognitive skill deficit was described by one woman.

> School will always be a struggle for my daughter. Remembering things that are automatic for most of us are difficult for her. She needs to process things that are simple and that are done without thought by most other children.[1] It is not extreme but I notice it. Sometimes she doesn't get the concept of right and wrong correct. She requires a lot of explanations for things that other kids just pick up. Interacting with other children is difficult because several years were lost when she had to miss playing with other children.

Although we hear about the lack of common sense and difficulty in retaining such basic information in children with fetal alcohol syndrome, the absence of this characteristic seemed to be present in some of these children as well.

Birth Story

In our original conceptualization of this project, we planned to begin to interview the high-risk children themselves when they became verbal and could possibly relate some of their own stories. One special area of interest to us was the child's own version of the birth story. Although we did not have an opportunity to speak to the children during the epilogue interviews, we did ask the parents about the child's knowledge of the birth story. In a few cases, parents were very protective in relation to the knowledge to which their children were exposed. For example, one parent said that she would never allow interviewers like ourselves to discuss this topic with the child. A couple of other parents wanted to be sure to arrange their interview schedule so that the child was out of the house and could not accidentally overhear our conversation.

One obvious response from parents was simply that the child knew--no further detail. Others elaborated. "Yes, we told the children because we didn't want them hearing anything second-hand. We didn't want other members of the family bringing it up." Parents also indicated that they wanted to prevent neighbors, church members, or peers of their children from enlightening them, as well. They wanted to inform the children themselves. Some parents shared baby pictures, albums, and videos with the children. Most parents used the word "special" to convey the child's birth status to him or her. One parent took her son to the NICU to actually see and know what takes place there. She said, "He knows what a special kid he is and how much a part of his life those nurses were. He needs to appreciate what everyone has done." A less detailed approach was also taken. One father said, "She knows that she was born early but not the details. I don't even think she knows exactly what that means yet (9 years of age currently). She does take birth pictures to school and all that and probably plays up her small size a little bit to get some attention."

One mother has contemplated the situation in depth:

> She hears me talk all the time about her prematurity and she has been photographed on many occasions. She loved the limelight and the cameras, but as she gets older she is less enthusiastic about the attention. Recently she grabbed a picture of herself with her feeding tube in one hand and a cracker in the other. She was inquisitive and wanted to know if she had eaten the cracker. I think that she is at the developmental stage to begin to be able to cognitively process what has been only memories. I believe she has a memory of her experiences and they were very hard for her. They are stored in her body and in her mind but thus far she doesn't usually like to talk about it too much.

Finally, some parents admitted that they had not thought of this aspect. While discussing this question one mother contributed,

> I am disappointed now that I cannot remember this stuff any better than I do. I wish I would have written these stories down so that [child] would have had them. I began to write about our life with her, but I never got past age 3. So I don't have it for her.

However, such a record for the first 3 years of life is a significant accomplishment. She seemed to undervalue her effort. One woman explained that she did not know if this child knows or if any of her children know their birth story. But the question did catch her attention. She responded, " That's an interesting question. Maybe her understanding of the birth is a place to visit next year."

Given the difficulties and challenges encountered by these children, it might even seem unfair not to have told the children their birth stories. Perhaps if the child knew the circumstances of the birth, they would have a greater understanding of their present condition and a rationale for their troubles as opposed to their peers. Maybe this is one of those cases of denial in which everyone says the child does not know but in reality more fully understands her or his own history than we realize.

A Gaze into the Crystal Ball

A wide range of children's ages are represented by the parents, so that some are more circumscribed in the potential events they are facing with these children while others are very near to launching their children into adult life.[m] All parents sustain or at least depict a picture of hope as they envision a meaningful life for the child. One mother described her vision:

> It is hard to say. When I look at the last 10 years and see where she has come, I don't want to sell her short. When she was 5, I would have never thought we'd be where we are today. I'd like to see her live outside my home although she is going to need support 24 hours a day. I don't want any of my kids living with me after they are 20. She also needs to live her life and not order me around. But I am not happy with the options that are out there for her. I'd like her to have a meaningful job. But you know, you really should be asking her these things. I am not the person you should be talking to, because as these children mature, they must be able to speak for themselves, to the degree that they can.

Parents are ambivalent, as evidenced by such comments as, "I am trapped between thinking my child can grow up and be normal and having people bring me back to reality where he might never live alone." Another parent said,

> I hope my child can develop friendships and not be lonely as an adult. Her teachers praise her abilities and talents, but her peers are put off by her quirkiness and eccentricities. She is in counseling and I think it will be fine. I have seen a lot of improvement. I am looking forward to the time when she will be on her own. I wonder if she will fail and have to move back home. But then I guess every parent has some misgivings about that.

Making and keeping friends is a common concern, since many of these children were deprived of contact with other children for years. Some were at home for long periods of time because of illnesses or essential equipment. Others were in and out of the hospital many times. Prolonged adult contact rather than play with children also occurred. Parents acknowledged the need for their children to make friends first before they embark on a trail of crushes, dating, and courtship. One father observed,

> I basically believe some days that the child will have an unhappy life and never be able to live independently and then think on other days that she will find some kind of niche in society. I'm not sure that what she has learned will be conducive to getting a job and supporting herself.

And finally, one mother sees her child as an attractive spirit who magnetizes people. "She's beautiful," her mother goes on, "She's happy to be alive and she smiles all the time. These are qualities that people like." She later countered these observations with her conclusion that she really doesn't know, on balance, what the outcome might be. "Maybe she'll somehow carry out the teachings I've tried to do. It is not going to be easy for her I think, unless she works very hard at overcoming some of the obstacles she is going to have."

Some particular concerns include a parent's worry about her sons' social skills--for boys who are small this can be especially challenging. One mother mentioned that her son is now 12 and has yet to exceed the 50th percentile either in weight or height. Finding partners for life is another matter: developing meaningful relationships with the opposite sex or finding a significant other and getting married. Some parents, have not yet allowed themselves to go that far into the future, thinking of independence, college, and marriage.

Two mothers' thoughts about the future ranged beyond just their own children's prospects. First this mother:

> I am very protected--middle class and Caucasian. We need to understand a whole new world out there in terms of parents who are poor, are of different ethnic backgrounds, different races. We also need to better understand alternative modalities and healing for these infants. I wouldn't change what they did for my child, they kept my baby alive. But there is more out there and different ways of healing that may be more beneficial to these babies and their families.

Then another woman responded:

> We need more services and support for individuals and families with disabilities and to stop segregating and isolating them. We are all on this continuum and disability is part of it. As a white, middle class American--I had all the privileges basically, but because of my child's disability, I also know about discrimination, perhaps prejudice, or just being uncomfortable with it [disability]. There are really three kinds of people related to attitudes toward disability: those who have a family member and belong to "the club," those who somehow inherently understand and take the disabled for who they are, and those who only see tragedy. I cannot sustain people in my life who only see this as a tragedy.

Advice to the Uninitiated

Hope is the concept that transitions across the parents' own gaze into the future and their advice to other parents in similar situations. "Keep up hope. The hand you have been dealt is out of your control. Our child has problems but it hasn't been all that terrible," advised one parent. Some combined hope with love:

> Love your children--it is a medicine of its own. We could have been less intense as parents, but maybe that is why [child] developed the abilities she has. Do all that you can for the child. Have a 'can do' attitude but accept limitations.

However, these parents do not minimize the need for information and the role parents must acquire in relation to their child's needs. They go right to the beginning and plead that all parents should know about NICUs and the possibility for its use. Then parents ought to see the older NICU graduates. One parent went to a reunion and only two of the children were over 5 years of age. She wants her child's picture to continue to be posted on the preemie picture board in the NICU, because "if you hang in there, you can see success."

Advocacy is an important role. Several mothers admonished:

> You must be the child's advocate until you are able to teach them self-advocacy. You must believe in yourself, you know this child--better than doctors, better than teachers, better than social workers. It's OK to grieve. But question the doctors--nail them to the wall until they listen. You must become comfortable in this role and develop a hard shell. Otherwise decisions will not be made that are right for her/him or what's not, how things are going to go. There will be people at every stage of your life who think they know better. I had a physician who threatened that if the test got screwed up because of my demands, it would be my fault. But I knew what would be traumatizing for my child and what would not be a problem. We did it my way.

One father noted,

> Preemies have a different beginning, but that beginning could affect them for the rest of their lives. It may be minimal, but then again it may not. Parents need to be prepared for being different or being typical. Parents need to be advocates for the child, encourager and protector. There is nothing more important.

Parental support groups were another important element. A variation on this theme was express by one mother, who relayed:

> There was a support group in the nursery but mostly parents of prematures attended. Their children were not as sick as mine and I would suggest that not all parents in the NICU be lumped together. I even hated mothers who had sick children because I had this healthy looking baby that had all these life-threatening problems. I have finally met about 60 families who have a child like mine but it has taken years to do that [the child is now 10]. If only the social worker had found such families for me earlier.

Another mother explained:

> Parents need to connect to other parents--those who have lived what they are encountering.[n] My organization promotes talking to other parents. I know that physicians are often wary that parents or others who are consulted will provide medical advice. That simply is not true. Mostly people in our group just listen. We also connect parents to a whole bunch of different families, so they hear a whole bunch of different things. We do not promote anything. There are many ways in

> which solutions can be worked out. Talking to other parents should not be a threatening thing; it is an empowering thing. Parents have to live with the consequences of these decisions.[o]

Conclusion

One mother summarized her story,

> The experience of having a baby in the NICU becomes part of your family history, but you cannot really ever forget. It may not be on your mind every day. But it can quickly come back,

Another mother shared that 12 years later she thinks about the NICU experience constantly--from both good perspectives and bad ones. Her family now has a relative in the pediatric intensive care unit who is in a coma. She thinks about the progress her son has made and it gives her hope for her nephew. Raising a child who has had a high-risk experience is just as the opening to this section states; although you can plan to go to Italy, you arrive in Holland and that aspect of your destiny cannot be changed--the remainder of your life is different. Sometimes the experience is as wonderful as fields of tulips and displays of Rembrandts, but occasionally there is a leak in the dike and it takes extraordinary effort to prevent a complete flood.

Unfortunately the general public lacks a balanced perspective of NICU outcomes based on media coverage. The public sees the beautifully cultivated fields of tulips and does not necessarily appreciate the constant work and effort to prevent the sea water from flowing over the land and destroying its fertility. A recent story in a general magazine was another tale of the miracle baby, although the language was somewhat more tentative when the possible long-term outcomes were discussed (Gordon 2001). Data about long-term results is accumulating, however. Whether or not the professionals who first counsel the parents in the NICU are ready to acknowledge the meaning of that data is questionable from some perspectives. One parent in this group of interviews had the experience of being both a NICU nurse and a parent of a high-risk infant. She cautioned:

> When I started speaking out, it was really hard for my co-workers to hear what I have to say. Because it means that what they do isn't all peaches and cream. It's not the outcomes that they thought they were having. They thought they were keeping these babies alive so they'd go

> home and be normal and happy kids. And all of a sudden, this was in '93 so it just started coming out, the long-term effects. And so they, they were scared and they didn't really want to hear what I had to say. So they would turn away and try not to listen. Some, not all of them but the majority of them, would turn away. But I knew and I understood their side. I once had expected that too.

Many of these parents speak positively about their relationships to the special needs child described here. The word *gift* comes through as a descriptor for these children. Parents try to accept special needs children as a gift in their lives despite the changes initiated by the high-risk experiences. Since the risks for these children appear to be unavoidable as they grow up, then we need to continue to explore possible effective interventions that focus on outcomes related to personal and environmental factors in order to attain the highest levels of development (McCormick & Richardson 2002). These factors have not been the target of intense investigation. But such an approach brings us back then to the children's parents.

In many cases, however, parents are a *gift* to their children as they maximize their children's destiny. One mother emphasized not limiting one's hope. Parents must encourage their children and have the children themselves set goals, and not be afraid to try. As another mother explained, the self-advocacy movement, which in part supports adults with disabilities, has "nothing for us without us" as a mantra. These children must be part of such a movement. Our government is supposed to be representative, but until policy at every level is shaped by people who consult with the disabled, it is not truly representative of this group. The disabled must be empowered to effect the changes they require. Parents are these children's first line of support. But, such an effort also requires all of us. Hopefully, all of these family stories, as well as those in the original interviews will strengthen and expand the knowledge base related to the continuing interest in high-risk infants, their outcomes, and their parents.

Notes

[a] I am indebted to Anne Hurst, cofounder of Parents Empowering Parents (PEP), who alerted me to this essay. Together with Kelly Ouellet and Beth Pond, Ms. Hurst formed a support group for parents in order to provide a place for "parents and caregivers of children with special needs to go and be with

others who could share their feelings about having children who are 'different.'" Their website is at http://www.communitygateway.org/pep.

[b] The rationale for admission to the NICU varies. Approximately 11% of newborns in 1998 were premature (Grossman 2000) while in 2000 the rate was reported as 11.4% (Richardson 2001). Various reports in the 1990s showed that low birth weight affected 7% of infants and *very* low birth weight affected 1% (Hack et al. 1995). Another source set NICU admissions at 10% of births (Deacon & O'Neill 1999). Congenital problems and abnormal labor and delivery are also rationale for admission to the NICU although not every baby with these problems is necessarily admitted to a NICU. Physicians also consider infection, and problems with various body systems or processes: respiratory, cardiac, metabolic, and gastrointestional. Immediately following birth, life is risky. 40,000 babies die each year (Shiono & Behrman 1995). Neonatal mortality in the first month accounts for 75% of infant mortality in the first year of life (Paneth 1995).

[c] Although it was possible to locate those parents who participated in our original project, we did not want to use that option. We are hopeful that we will obtain funding in the future and have the opportunity to re-interview the original sample. If we had used them for the Epilogue, then our findings would have been contaminated in terms of any future research data. We did not want to take that risk. Given the possibilities of locating other families (see note below), we simply took another course of action to gather these perspectives.

[d] Families were accessed by several strategies. One was simply based on personal knowledge about the family history and those parents' willingness to voluntarily participate in an interview if they had not been in the original study. Second, advertisements were placed in the classified advertisement sections of metropolitan newspapers. The message called attention to parents of high-risk newborns with a specific birth date that would ensure accession of families with children more than 4 years postdischarge from the NICU. Both an email address and telephone number were provided for a response. A third strategy used the internet. Various websites were explored and contact was made with the webmaster or other identified individuals who had an email address. A fourth strategy developed out of the internet contacts. Dianne Maroney volunteered to take flyers to a meeting where parents of NICU graduates would be in attendance. Words are inadequate when attempting to express my thanks for such kindness like Dianne's. Together the strategies were successful and volunteers from each of these attempts were used. I would like to emphasize that this was **not** a research endeavor and thus differs from the information and presentation of parental perspectives reflected in all of the earlier portions of this book. Less rigorous strategies were appropriately used. However, the identities of the participants were promised the same confidentiality as those in the original project. Given that this was not a

research project, any parent who wanted to be named was offered that option. We would like to specifically thank Sheila Allen, Shelly Dowdle, Dianne Maroney, Jim Maroney, Anne Hurst, Stephanie Lerner-Ernsteen, and Carolyn Schimanski, who were among those volunteers. Words cannot express our appreciation for their sharing of such personal experiences with us. Undoubtedly they want to reach out to other parents and their participation is part of these parents' gift to others who face the same or similar situations. The information in this section is simply anecdotal and should be evaluated as such based on the selection process. Similarities among parents regardless of the method that was used to access them were interesting to us.

[e] Throughout this section, the new interviews will be designated "epilogue" interviews and the interviews from the earlier portion of the project will be the original interviews whenever the groups need to be distinguished from one another.

[f] As noted in Chapter 7, Catlin and Carter (1999-2000) completed a project wherein they created a neonatal end-of-life palliative-care protocol. At the time this manuscript was submitted, that protocol was not yet published but was scheduled for an issue of *Journal of Perinatology* entitled Creation of an end of life palliative care protocol. For an overview see Catlin and Carter (2001).

[g] The Rev. John Hanson in a sermon on January 6, 2002 at Presbyterian Church of the Master, Omaha, Nebraska, included some commentary on the ideal versus reality in various aspects of our lives including marriage, parenting, and work. He presented this particular set of statistics.

[h] Hack et al. (2002) reported on their longitudinal study of very-low-birth-weight infants which is an extension of earlier reports which ended at eight years of age. This report followed their cohort until 20 years of age. One of the findings related to neurosensory impairments which were higher than the control group. Also the VLBW infants were subnormal in height. Additional characteristics were also examined.

[i] Concurrent with these interviews and the development of the draft for this section of the book, one of my students, Donna Myers, investigated procedural pain in the neonate as a research utilization project. I am grateful to have been alerted to possible studies in this area. Various experiences during neonate hospitalization cause pain and at least two sources support the frequency of painful treatments and procedures (Porter, Wolf, & Miller 1999; Deacon & O'Neill 1999). The former study reported an average of 700 per infant (<28 weeks' gestation) while hospitalized. The latter source, noted that 3,000 procedures were performed on 54 infants during hospitalization. These procedures are often invasive and could be considered painful. Some believe that when painful procedures are regularly administered without pain control, infants become conditioned to the lack of either comfort or relief of pain, eventually failing to respond to such stimuli--such as by crying. This could

help explain the lack of response to pain in these children in later years. They simply have learned that crying will not alert others to their needs. As reported by Porter, Grunau, and Anand (1999), pain and stress in newborns can result in permanent structural and functional changes. Research results show that long-term effects on premature infants can be increased sensitivity or less sensitivity to noxious stimuli.

[j] Supplemental Security Income (SSI) is a federal program for the aged, blind, or disabled. To qualify, the individual must have limited income and resources and live in the United States. When eligible, the person receives monthly benefits (Information available at: http://www.state.sc.us/ddsn/pubs.now/gov.htm).

[k] Difficulties in the educational arena are supported by the long-term study by Hack et al. (2002). These investigators only reported on very-low-birth-weight infants however. They found that fewer of these infants when adults completed high school, enrolled in postsecondary study (men only), and had lower academic achievement scores.

[l] As I listened to this woman I was reminded of fetal alcohol syndrome, although there was no mention of such a possibility in any aspect of the parent's story. To get a fuller understanding of my comparison, you might read Michael Dorris's story of his son in *The Broken Cord* (published by HarperCollins in 1989).

[m] Hack et al.'s report (2002) despite the degree of morbidity in their group of VLBW infants, uncovered some positive outcomes as well. Their cohort reported less drug (including alcohol) use, less contact with the police, and lower rates of pregnancy. Although these children do not "outgrow" their vulnerability, as noted by McCormick and Richardson (2002) in an editorial comment on this report, differences in these children do not increase in adolescence. In fact, despite the formidable challenges, these children are able to overcome such barriers and in many cases depict their quality of life higher than their peers.

[n]The need for parental support is undeniable but as children with special needs grow and develop, they too need to connect with children who are like them. One mother explained how her son guarded the fact that he had a gastrostomy tube but once he met another boy with one, he acted less conscious about the device.

[o] The Summer 2001 volume of *Advances in family-centered care*, a publication of the Institute for Family-Centered Care in Bethesda, Maryland (7900 Wisconsin Avenue, Suite 405), includes an extensive description of "the ways in which family members are serving in volunteer and staff positions in NICUs in the United States and Canada" (p. 2). Such institutionalized roles for parents have been evolving, and the trend appears to be growing. Interestingly, listening to families is an important concept to these endeavors.

APPENDIX

The Research Enterprise

In general, because the literature contained minimal knowledge about parental perceptions of ethical decision-making related to their experiences with a high-risk newborn, this project was undertaken to expand the knowledge base (Benoliel 1984). The major purpose was to explore and describe the ethical dimensions of the NICU experience from the parents' perspective at each of three points in time: predischarge, 6 months postdischarge, and 4 years postdischarge (Artinian 1988). During that process, it was anticipated that the moral orientations of the parents would also be identified. We (as principal investigator and research assistant) anticipated the delineation of major themes at each phase that would represent the families' ethical viewpoints (Knafl & Howard 1984). Similar procedures were followed for each phase of the project. After the interviews were completed for each phase, a primary analysis of the data was implemented, focusing on the identification of ethical issues and the parental perception of the decision-making process and their current situation. A secondary analysis utilizing each participant's set of interviews was conducted after completion of all phases, including interviewing, analyzing, and presentation of the results. The purpose of the secondary analysis was to identify and describe the moral orientation of the participants as they discussed the NICU experience or some ethical conflict they encountered. Later, as a result of the secondary analysis, a more thorough examination of the interview data by gender was conducted, leading to a formulation of a feminist analysis (theoretical) and a separate description of themes from the fathers' perspectives.[a]

The Research Design

A qualitative, exploratory, descriptive research design was used to investigate the parents' perceptions of their actual and/or potential ethical decision-making experiences. Ethical theory itself cannot be *tested* in the sense that the concepts and theoretical relationships can be subjected to empiric investigation. However, research can be used to increase understanding of the knowledge and processes related to the ethical domain. As posited by Chinn and Kramer (1991), the critical ethical questions are "Is this right? For whom? Is this responsible?" and the appropriate interactive process for eliciting such information is through dialogue.

In-depth interviewing, a type of dialogue, has long been a staple research device for social scientists (Berg 1989; Gilchrist 1992; Taylor & Bodgon 1984). As a qualitative method, Taylor and Bodgan described the in-depth interview as a face-to-face encounter between interviewer and participant in which the informant's perspective on life, experiences, or circumstances is explored. This is a dynamic process whereby the investigator is the research tool, posing the initial questions but also, in the process of the dialogue, learning what additional questions to ask. Specifically, in-depth interviewing is most useful when one wants to learn about events not directly observable. The knowledge that individuals bring to ethical decision-making and their processes of determining right action or good behavior are not completely discernible through observation, but are revealed only through interaction with those individuals.

Sampling Plan and Setting

Sample size in qualitative approaches is usually determined by examining the resulting data (Parse et al. 1985). The process of accessing new informants ceases when no new information is acquired, sometimes referred to as the *saturation of the data*. For the initial phase, we anticipated that 8-12 participants would be necessary (Field & Morse 1985). However, since this project was planned as a longitudinal investigation, some attrition in the sample was inevitable. Therefore accessing participants continued beyond the point of saturation. In addition, we had some concern about the composition of the sample early in the study. Although this is explained later in the section on Procedure, it affected sample size by providing some impetus for continuing to interview parents after data became repetitious. The final sample was more than double the originally planned minimum of 8-12; actually, 32 families participated in Phase I. Phase II included 28 families and, in Phase III, while 24 families were located, only 23 were willing to participate. All potential participants were English speaking and able to hear a normal tone of voice.

Parents of high-risk neonates were the target population. Based on their infants' status, parents were selected for possible inclusion in the study by the NICU staff. The head nurse was the major person responsible for family contact. Merenstein and Gardner's (1985) criteria for a high-risk newborn were used: birth weight less than 2500 grams, gestational age less than 37 weeks, Apgar[b] scores less than 5 at 1 minute and 5 minutes, bilirubin[c] above 15 ml/dl, or need for surgical interventions and/or presence of birth anomalies.[d] Only one criterion was necessary for inclusion in the study.

Personnel at a Level III neonatal nursery, in the Mid-west were contacted after a pilot study was completed but prior to development of the grant proposals which were submitted to fund the project. Relevant medical and nursing staffs agreed to the implementation of the project in their unit. The NICU consisted of about 16 isolettes in a large teaching hospital. The unit served not only the metropolitan area in which it was located but also the surrounding geographic region extending into several states. Approximately 30 nurses staffed the unit, including a discharge-planning nurse. Five neonatologists were associated with the unit (full-time and part-time) and a complement of residents was present during each of their rotations. Others in attendance included one social worker, and personnel such as respiratory therapists, laboratory persons, pastoral care staff, medical students, and students of nursing who provided care or observed in the unit on a regular basis.

Instruments

In the naturalistic paradigm, the investigator is the instrument (Lipson 1991). Neither of us had any NICU clinical experience although the research assistant was a pediatric nurse and coordinator of a parent-child course in a baccalaureate nursing education program when the project began. She later retired from her faculty position but continued in her role as a research assistant throughout the remainder of the project. As principal investigator, I was also a faculty member in the same program and taught several courses at the graduate level. My clinical area was community health and I had a long time interest in and study of bioethics.

As strangers to the clinical area of the NICU, we believed that we were in an advantageous position, especially given the focus of the project on understanding the parents' perspectives of ethical decision-making (Pinch 1993). With our background, it was not possible to predict in any detail information about the neonates, their status, progress, or the usual parental responses. Field (1989) discussed both advantages and disadvantages of conducting qualitative research in one's own culture. As nurses, we were both members of the culture of health care. Our clinical expertise was not directly related to neonatal intensive care although we both possessed some knowledge relative to our roles in various types of follow-up care. We concluded that our lack of detailed knowledge was an advantage. The discussion of infant status in Chapter 2 embellishes this idea and explicates its fuller meaning.

A modification of a semi-structured interview guide devised by Lyons provided the framework for each interview (1983). Table A.1 reproduces an outline of the original general interview guide. Lyons's guide was based on the combined work of Kohlberg (1958, 1973, 1975, 1981, 1984; Kohlberg et al. 1983) and Gilligan (1977, 1979, 1982a. 1982b) both of whom pioneered psychological research related to moral development. (See Table A.2 for a schematic representation of their theories).

As theoretical background related to the interview guide, Kohlberg's earliest research was conducted with boys and men and resulted in the positing of a universal theory of moral reasoning (1958). Building on the accomplishments of Piaget (1932), Kohlberg posited a cognitive-developmental, universal theory.

Briefly, Kohlberg's theory represents a paradigm wherein moral development consists of six stages, two at each of three levels beginning with a preconventional level in which obedience to moral rules is fear or ego-motivated (1975). The second or conventional level is formed out of mutually determined rules based on interactions with others individually or from an understanding of social systems in general. The postconventional level is an understanding of moral obligations from outside one's place in society. The third level most emphasizes the ability to determine universal rules from an autonomous, rational, logical, objective, and abstract position--the ideal decision-maker. Kohlberg's theory is commonly referred to as one with a justice orientation.

Table A.1 *Original Basic Interview Guide*

1. Looking back over the hospitalization of your infant(s), what stands out for you?
2. In your situation, was there ever a time when you weren't sure what was the right thing to do?
    Describe it.
    What would you identify as the conflict for you?
    What did you do?
    Do you think it was the right thing to do?
    How did you know it was the right thing to do?
3. How would you describe yourself? (Alternatively: How do you see yourself?)
    Is the way you see yourself now different from the way you saw yourself in the past?
    What led to these changes?
4. What does morality mean to you?
    What makes a moral problem for you?
    What does responsibility mean to you?
    When responsibility to self and others conflict, how do you choose?
5. Closure: Is there anything you would like to add, based on the interview we've just completed?
    Are there any questions you have of me?

Gilligan eventually questioned the exclusion of women from Kohlberg's psychological research and a marginalization of women's perspectives (1982a). Gilligan's theory emphasizes connections with others by an individual who is situated and embedded in culture, language, discourse, and history (Hekman 1995). Broadly speaking, Gilligan's theory can also be divided into three levels: a most basic level focusing on survival; a second level exemplified by selfless, maternal caring; and a third level of interdependency in which self-valuing is included in decision-making (Miller 1984). Gilligan's theory is said to have a caring orientation in moral development. More details about these theories are included in Chapter 5.

Although Lyons was primarily interested in exploring the moral orientation of her subjects, the questions of the interview guide elicited information that could be analyzed to identify ethical dilemmas

Table A.2 *Theories of Moral Development*

A THEORY OF JUSTICE[a]

Preconventional Level

Punishment and obedience orientation

The instrumental-relativist orientation

Conventional Level

The interpersonal concordance or "good boy - nice girl" orientation

The "law and order" orientation

Postconventional Level

The social-contract, legalistic orientation

The universal-ethical-principle orientation

A THEORY OF CARING[b]

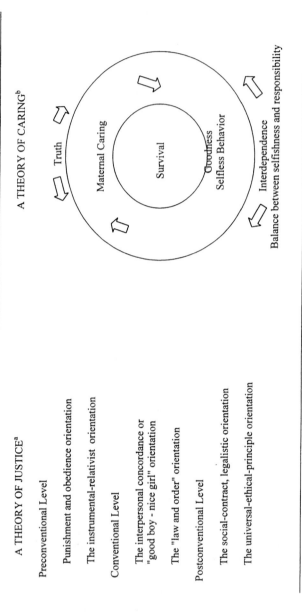

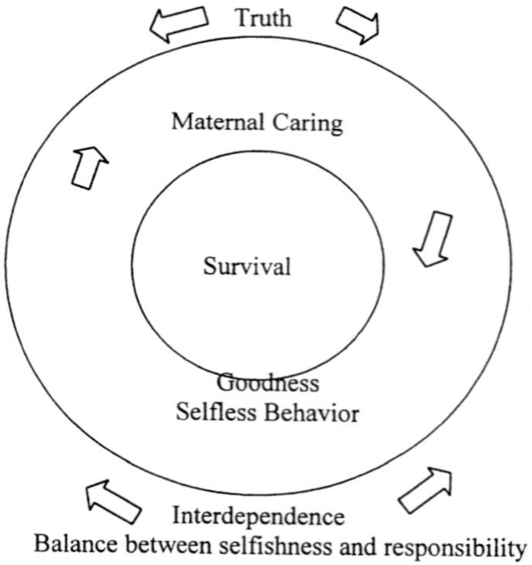

[a] Based on: Kohlberg, L. 1975. The cognitive-developmental approach to moral education. *Phi Delta Kappan, 61*, 670-677.
[b] Based on: Gilligan, C. 1982. *In a different voice*. Cambridge, MA: Harvard University Press.

and more detailed material relative to perceptions of the decision-making process, as well as moral orientation. Additionally, the informant could be led to focus on any situation including health care of high-risk neonates, such as this project required. I conducted a pilot study, which affirmed the possibility of fruitful discussions and productive analysis using a modified version of Lyons' guide (Pinch 1990).

Phase I interviews began with a request for parents to look back over the hospitalization of their baby in the NICU and to describe the event that was most outstanding. Building on the parental description, the experience was explored for any sense of conflict, for the presence of a struggle between right and wrong or good and bad, and for possible decision-making. If parents did not use the NICU as a basis for their outstanding event, they were eventually led to discuss their perceptions of the NICU experience. Regardless of when the sense of conflict occurred, it was probed in terms of when it arose, what they thought, what they did, how it was resolved, and their rationale for the decision. Careful and detailed probing was used especially to examine the NICU circumstances for possible conflict or its absence.

As more and more interviews were completed, probes were revised, added, and subtracted. My research assistant and I worked closely together, conferring after each interview to evaluate the effectiveness of the questions and probes. Both the audiotape of the interview and the hard copy of the transcript were reviewed to further refine the interview process and maximize its effectiveness (Berger & Kellner 1981). For example, the term *morality* used in the later portion of the interview did not seem to be understood by the informants. Substitutes were developed and the question was revised. Much later it seemed that the word *morality* was not itself a problem but rather the connection of morality with the NICU experience.

In subsequent interviews the initial question was varied. Parents were more globally instructed to simply tell the interviewer the story of their experience in the NICU. In addition questions were initially posed to reflect a more value free direction.[e] For example, decision-making was explored in general rather than by first directly asking parents to think about a conflict or a time when they weren't sure what was *the right thing to do*. After the parents completed their own stories through open discourse, if they had not mentioned ethical conflicts or dilemmas, more pointed questions were asked. The bioethical literature was replete with dilemmas about many treatments including the use of ventilators, ECMO, surgery, and drugs. The bioethical debate entailed controversy about starting and stopping treatments, quality of life of the infant, iatrogenic effects of treatment, negative outcomes for the infant, experimental treatment, and who should ultimately make these decisions. When these concerns had not been addressed, we introduced them into the discussion.

The interview concluded with opportunities for parents to add anything they wanted that might not have been covered by the questioning and subsequent dialogue and for them to ask us any questions. This frequently became a prolonged process. Sometimes parents began another topic as the interviewer was leaving, but more often they simply emphasized points already shared during the interview.

One decision we had to make early in the study related to the conflict created by the dual roles of nurse as clinician and nurse as researcher. Neither of us was ever responsible for providing health care services to these participants or their children. However, as clinicians, it was apparent during various interviews that some of these families continued to need assistance or services that they were not getting. Occasionally parents directly asked our advice. They had already identified a concern but wanted reassurance or support in bringing this issue to the attention of their providers. Teaching and referral were not roles we had planned to implement, hence the ethical dilemma of what steps to take and what steps not to take. While we did not want to compromise the research design and mix intervention with interview dialogue, we did not believe it was ethical to ignore the needs of these parents. We realized that our purpose was not to provide nursing services and any intervention no matter how minimal, could theoretically forever change the subsequent data we gathered.

We decided upon a strategy of refraining from any response (assessment, gathering more data) and/or intervention during the interview if the parents noted a problem. Then, when the research session was concluded and the tape recorder turned off, we would pursue the possible problem and make recommendations as necessary. We were careful to explain that providing clinical services was not our purpose, but they might find (whatever seemed to fit their need) helpful. Sometimes, of course, we did not have a solution. In those instances we shared our concern and recommended that they bring the issue to the attention of the individuals who were currently providing them with other health services. In fact, communication with their primary care provider was always stressed.

Interviews also included the collection of demographic data about the parents, such as marital status, occupation, education, religious preference, family size, financial status,[f] health insurance coverage (including Medicaid or Medicare or other community services), and ethnic identification. Using selected demographic data, chi squares were calculated for parental characteristics comparing the later phases with the data from Phase I. Despite a 13% attrition rate, the results indicated no statistically significant changes in the composition of the group at different phases except for financial status of the family and working status of the mother between Phase I and Phase II. Therefore, this procedure affirmed the similar configuration of the group from phase to phase. Attrition did not significantly alter the group continuing in the study from those originally participating. When a child had died, parents were no longer interviewed. The project did not examine parent experiences with or adjustment to the death of a child. A specific question about their infant's status closed the demographic data section.

Phase II interviews continued to utilize a basic format grounded in an investigation of moral conflict, augmented by sample probes and queries formulated during the Phase I experience. At this point, 6 months postdischarge, parents were first asked to look back over the past 6 months and describe "What stands out for you?" Their description was surveyed for possible conflict and any identified conflict was explored in terms of its meaning for the parents, alternative actions they considered, action taken (if any), rationale for this choice, and other relevant details.

Parents were then led to re-examine their experience in the NICU from the 6 month postdischarge viewpoint by telling us their story of the NICU experience. Specific probes were again used to identify possible conflict, a choice between right and wrong or good and bad. Particular ethical dilemmas as described above from the bioethical literature once more formed a basis from which we probed parental experience relative to these issues if informants did not specifically name them. Demographic data were updated, and the interview concluded with an opportunity for parents to add comments they felt would more completely represent their experiences.

In the pilot study, Phase I, and Phase II, parents were interviewed separately or together as best met their needs and schedule. As suggested by a consultant, for Phase III we attempted to interview all participants separately. The consultant suggested that separate interviews would facilitate the expression of independent stories and ideas about the NICU experience, which may have been masked by the previous discussions with both parents present. This was not an attempt to get the participants to make contradictory statements but to more readily get at individual perceptions, avoid one individual dominating the conversation, or get into a situation wherein the participants would correct one another. The consultant did not believe this change would compromise the project in any way. In fact she strongly believed that it would enrich the data by adding a dimension not included in the previous phases (Morse 1991).

In Phase III the wording and possible probes of Brown and associates were also utilized to shape the interview (Brown, Argyris et al., 1988; Gilligan 1987; Gilligan, Ward et al. 1988). The first item for this phase of the project asked each parent to tell the story of her/his experiences in the NICU. If no decision-making situation was spontaneously recalled and discussed, then the parent was asked, "Was there ever a time when you were not sure about the right thing to do?" The intervening time since the previous interview was also specifically reviewed. Parents were asked how they might want to change the NICU experience in light of their present situation, and the rationale for their suggestions was elicited. Since so little moral responsibility was associated with decision-making in the NICU or for their infant in subsequent circumstances, parents were pointedly asked for an example of a moral dilemma. And, as in both previous interviews, parents were able to voice any concerns or add any information not addressed during the dialogue.

Procedures

Common to all portions of the study was the Institutional Review Board (IRB) process and approval. The pilot study and the first phase required separate IRB reviews. The informed consent form was reviewed at Phases II and III, and a copy was offered to the informants if they had lost their first copy. The original informed consent provided authorization for the entire longitudinal project, so a new document was not used in the later phases.

Names, addresses, and telephone numbers were kept in a secure area to protect the confidentiality of the participants. All identifying material was removed from computer files and hard copies. Each family was assigned a code which remained the same for the entire project. Identification of their data including transcripts of interviews and summaries of demographic information was always recorded by the code number.

Confidentiality was discussed with each transcribing service where the risk of disclosure was possible. Confidentiality was a familiar concept for each agency, as they frequently had other contracts involving health care services, medical records, and personal information. All demographic data on the audiotapes were recorded on a master form by family code number and then erased from the tapes before delivery to the transcription service. However, it was impossible to remove all identifying information from the audiotapes especially when participants named health care providers, other specific individuals, and institutions or agencies.

Much of the presentation, publication, and product construction involved the use of quotations. This could provide a possible compromise to confidentiality, although we labored to remove identifying material. No family member who assessed these materials ever indicated a lack of confidentiality. For example, almost the entire scripts for both videotapes of the predischarge phase were composed of quotes from the informants. The first videotape production was a short (7 minutes) product which included still photographs of the NICU setting and the infants in the study with an audio overlay of selected quotes from the pilot study and Phase I interviews. The second videotape product (full-length, 28 minutes) utilized an original script based on Phase I interviews. The script writer developed a story about one couple's experiences, as portrayed in the videotape, that represented the major themes from the research results. The actors' lines encompassed many direct quotes from the participants.

All parents who participated in the study were invited to the premier showing of the full-length videotape. At that public event, neither of us acknowledged the presence of research participants in the audience. However, some parents chose to reveal their identity and discuss their responses to the video. Some parents claimed to recognize their own remarks in the video dialogue when they discussed their responses during the post-premier open forum. But most statements were common to a number of people in terms of the concept or issue addressed, particularly if the idea was incorporated into the video dialogue. We are certain that parents were not necessarily correct in attributing these quotes specifically to themselves. Overall, there was neither negative criticism nor vocalized objection regarding the use of the quotes. Several families requested copies of written material produced after the various phases were completed. Reprints of journal articles were sent to these families and no objections were voiced about accuracy or confidentiality. Several families borrowed the video to privately view in their homes if they had been unable to attend the premier performance.

Pilot Study

Five families from my community health case load or acquaintance volunteers comprised the sample for the pilot study. Interest in the topic was activated through interaction with families in my case load, so five families similar to those who earlier had spontaneously voiced concerns about the NICU experience, their subsequent adjustment to life with the baby, or decision-making in general participated in systematic, semi-structured interviews. A purposely selected sample represented contrasting and diverse characteristics of parents with high-risk infants. The children varied in age at the time of the interview from newly discharged from the NICU to 3 years of age. Also, one infant died shortly before one parent's interview.

The pilot study provided an opportunity to evaluate the selected interview guide and decide whether or not the anticipated project was feasible. As a direct result of the pilot study, a decision was made to conduct Phase I prior to the infant's discharge from the NICU. Interest in the topic of ethical decision-making in the NICU was sparked by my community health experience. A greater understanding of the family's perceptions of ethical dilemmas at this particular time was an important purpose for a study, based my observations of these families in the community health practice arena. However, when the families were interviewed. a question was raised about whether the recall of experiences from the NICU was affected by the passage of time. With this consideration and after consultation with colleagues about the memory/recall dimension, the decision was made to shift the first phase of the study to the earlier predischarge situation. The changed schedule would create a knowledge base with which to contrast and/or compare the six-month postdischarge data. This strategy was a very important outcome of the pilot study.

The completion of the pilot study also enhanced the prospects of acquiring funding for the more extensive phases of the project. Results of the pilot study were incorporated into grant proposals. Funding was not immediately forthcoming and several versions of the proposal for Phases I and II were rejected before acceptance by an internal funding source at my place of employment.[8] In turn, completion of Phases I and II and subsequent publication strengthened the proposal for Phase III and resulted in funding through the special call for research grant proposals from the National Center for Nursing Research on Bioethics and Clinical Practice.[h]

Major Phases

Prior to funding, hospital administration granted permission to conduct the study in the targeted Level III nursery. After discussions with the nursing supervisor, the NICU head nurse, chief neonatologist, and a hospital physician/administrator, the procedure for contacting prospective participants while protecting confidentiality was determined. Unit nursing personnel initiated contact with prospective participants as requested by the hospital physician/administrator and approved by the Institutional Review Board. Information sessions were provided for the NICU staff in order to familiarize them with the project and admission criteria for participants, to give them a written handout summarizing the project for parents, and to request that they ask parents to consider participating in the interviews. We then met with families who expressed an interest in participating in our project. A convenience sample resulted.

Arrangements were made to use a lounge area near the NICU as one setting choice for the interviews. Other choices included my office, the family's own home, or other quiet facilities in the community. A chart review was scheduled after the completion of the interviews for Phase I. We wanted to hear the parental perspective only through their stories, not combined with any other viewpoint such as the staff's, or from specific data about the infant as recorded in the chart.

We were totally dependent upon the screening and selection decision-making of the head nurse and her staff. There was no reason to doubt the staff's understanding of the project's admission criteria. However, telephone contact with the head nurse was initiated periodically when referrals slowed or interviews failed to elicit serious bioethical issues as described in the literature. I did not seek specific data about the infant or its situation at this point nor did the head nurse volunteer any information about infants or parents. On occasion I pressed my case to make sure that infants did in fact meet the admission criteria. Additionally, a direct request for families whose babies were *really* sick was also made. The results of Phase I explain our frustration, but in relation to the research procedure it is simply necessary to know that the head nurse was *not* contacting families of marginally sick newborns (Pinch 1993). She was doing exactly what she had been asked to do and she appropriately refrained from telling us anything beyond specific families' interest in discussing the project with us.

In practice, the head nurse actually made most of the parental contacts based on input from her staff, rather than a variety of staff members directly calling us. Parents were provided with a descriptive handout about the project and, if they agreed to meet with one of us, a means for parent contact was arranged. Telephone contact was frequently utilized, but when this was not possible, we went to the unit to meet parents during an anticipated visit to the infant. The latter arrangement was necessary when families did not have a telephone in the home.

We made appointments with prospective participants and described the project. We obtained informed consent and conducted interviews at a time and place mutually agreeable for the participants and ourselves. We reviewed informed consent at all subsequent interviews. In most cases during Phases I and II, we interviewed both parents together. This strategy was efficient, as parents often had limited time in which to schedule an interview. Approximately half of the sample lived outside the major metropolitan area and time was a precious commodity for these individuals. Interviews were often combined with visits to the nursery or, after discharge, were scheduled when follow-up visits for the baby correlated with the second phase of the project.

As previously noted, one of the project consultants strongly suggested interviewing parents separately for Phase III.[i] We employed this strategy throughout the last phase. Although this was a change, it was not viewed as compromising either the method or the results but rather as enhancing the findings. Parents could not hear what their partners said and thus might feel greater freedom to express a separate or perhaps different perspective. Conducting interviews with both parents present, allowed individuals to discuss the event or idea with each other or to simply agree with the first speaker rather than devise an original response. Each strategy has both positive and negative features. Separate interviews prevent arguments between parents during the session which can be embarrassing and challenge the interviewer to keep the discussion on target.

Most Phase I interviews were conducted in a private hospital lounge where it was possible to minimize disturbances and interruptions. A few parents asked to be interviewed in their home or my office. Phases II and III were usually conducted in the participants' homes with a small number at the participant's place of business, at some public facility (restaurant, motel), or over the telephone using a jack device in order to tape record the discussion. The latter choice resulted from the long distances between locations, some caused by family moves after discharge of the infants from the NICU. Although most interviews could be conducted in person, travel to some locations would have been unreasonable given the limited research funds and our own time restrictions.

Telephone interviewing versus face-to-face dialogue may have some advantages as well as limitations, although little background material was located relative to this strategy for qualitative research.[j] It is especially necessary to consider the elements of quiet and distraction while interviewing in the participant's home. With telephone interviews, it seemed less likely the interviewer or the participant would be distracted by other events nearby. This presumes the interviewer has carefully chosen a quiet, relatively isolated place to conduct the telephone interview. But with prospective arrangements, such things as children playing or otherwise making noise, cats climbing up curtains, or interruptions by other members in the household seem to be less apt to occur with the interviewee on the telephone. Our telephone interviews were in fact trouble-free.

Nonverbal communication cannot be noted on the telephone, but this can be a benefit as well as a limitation. With only verbal information to focus upon, the words gain importance, as sensory input is more restricted. In face-to-face interviews, concentration is required to really hear what the participant is saying and subsequently to follow-up on what is said, not what is perceived by the combination of non-verbal and verbal cues. Some nonverbal cues reinforced by sounds like crying, laughing, snorting, or others can be recognized over the telephone, of course. But the interviewer is less likely to ignore, repress, or simply not recognize the importance of the participant's statements in a telephone conversation. In any situation, some very important information can be missed during an interview. The following example, only one of several incidents that occurred, will illustrate this point.

The research assistant conducted an interview and returned the tape for my review prior to transcription as planned. During the review, I noted some especially heart-wrenching episodes in this family's life. I was also somewhat puzzled, since not much probing had been used relative to at least one of the stories, which involved a painful rejection of the parents by other relatives. I called the research assistant to convey my observations and offer encouragement because of the emotional tone of the interview. The research assistant was unable to identify the participant's story as part of the interview she had conducted. In fact, she claimed some sort of mix-up and thought that perhaps I had heard the story directly from a participant or somewhere else. We both then listened to the tape of what was clearly her interview, and she found it difficult to believe that these participants had told such a devastating story but she did not remember it. We decided that it was such an excruciating tale, and the experience of telling it had been so emotionally wrenching for the couple, that the research assistant immediately repressed the incident. There were a few probes and the story itself was quite complete, but the incident was an interesting turn of events.[k] It gave us both a lesson in how, as interviewers, we can tend to want to either move quickly away from negative responses or ignore them. Or we can be distracted by the emotional response and not follow through as thoroughly as we might otherwise when we are not watching someone share such devastation. We found support can be conveyed over the telephone, so distance need not be a limitation in this regard. In fact, some individuals may find it easier to let their emotions through when the interviewer cannot actually see them. In certain sensitive situations, such as research involving experiences with rape or domestic violence, telephone interviewing may enhance assurances of anonymity. If the interviewer never sees the participant, there can be little or no possible accidental recognition if the two meet in a post-interview circumstance.

Another example of the distraction of nonverbal communication involved a somewhat different element. In this circumstance, we labeled the phenomenon *hearing what you see*. One of our observations when discussing infant status with the participants in the six-month postdischarge interview was the subtle disparity between what parents were saying and their nonverbal cues. The parents were friendly and sociable. Their facial expressions were pleasant as they began to describe the infant, its development over the 6 months, and its present status. What was surprising was that the congenial expressions in many cases never left their faces even as they shared serious turns of events and, in a few situations, grim outcomes. Their presentation of themselves seemed to be continuing evidence of a need or desire to be perceived as mature adults, in control of themselves, adjusting to their circumstances. However, the risk as an interviewer is to get caught up in the nonverbal cues and not pursue these issues because, as bad or important as they might be, they do not seem to be as significant from the participants' perspective as they really were. Some parents did become quite emotional during the interview, and such a response must be acknowledged to give a balanced description of the interviews. But the interviewer needs to be alert to any contrasts between what is nonverbally expressed and what is said and, most of all, must not be swayed by facies or body language.

All interviews were recorded on audiotape. The importance of this strategy cannot be overemphasized. The example above shows not only the possible advantages of telephone interviewing, but also the risk of losing data if the interview is not recorded verbatim. When dialogue is repressed or ignored, it may not be reconstructed in post-interview, process-recording notes. Data are permanently lost. Training and experience do enhance interviewing skills, but there is always the chance of a lapse due to a variety of reasons. We had few experiences in which the participant was averse to audiotaping. On one occasion a woman participant seemed to try to avoid speaking so that the discussion could be easily recorded. First she seated herself on the sofa with her back against the arm. The tape recorder had been placed on the end table next to the sofa arm so her chosen position directed her voice away from the recorder. Her action was not explored and she did not object when the interviewer moved the recorder to her own chair in order to increase the quality of the recording. No one actually refused when the informed consent item about tape recording was reviewed. Once interviewing actually began, most participants forgot the tape recorder was working.

Immediately after each interview, the interviewer added field notes directly onto the audiotape. Any dialogue that had ensued after the tape recorder was turned off was summarized. Recall that some parents renewed the conversation as we went out the door or got into our cars. As soon as possible after the interview, the interviewer reviewed the audiotape before the second investigator listened to it. Then the audiotape was transcribed verbatim on computer diskettes by a contracted service and hard copies were printed for analyses after the transcription was corrected. The interview text was printed only on the left half of the paper. The right half was left blank for us to add notes and codes.

In the meantime, we could confer, critique the interview, and make any necessary changes or corrections in our approach before the next interview was conducted (May 1989). Details of data analyses are discussed below. After the analysis was completed, various summaries were created. Material was synthesized until a concise, descriptive version was formulated. Later complete reports summarizing the total phase of the project, the results, and interpretation of the data were prepared. The results were shared with the unit personnel where the participants' infants were hospitalized. Other presentations and publications were prepared to reach broader audiences (See Table P.2).

To begin Phase II and Phase III, participants were contacted at the address on file for them. A letter was sent explaining the project again and asking if they were still willing to participate in the next phase. The letter indicated that a follow-up telephone call would be made to ascertain their decision. In some cases, families had moved. We were fortunate when forwarding addresses were available, but for some, their whereabouts were unknown.

We became very creative in our attempts to locate the missing families. We continued to be cognizant of our ethical responsibilities related to confidentiality and believe we balanced these needs appropriately. In contacting any agency where we thought a family might be receiving services, we said only that we would like to contact a parent whose child might be a patient. We told the agency that we had had contact with the family at an earlier point and our current information for follow-up was incorrect. We did not specifically mention the project, so participation remained confidential. We did not ask the agency to verify our supposition about their possible contact with the family. Rather we simply asked the agency to forward our letters to parents in their case load as appropriate. This was successful in some situations. Actually, parents who had been somewhat difficult to locate but were eventually found expressed admiration for our efforts and a positive feeling about our making such an attempt to find them. To them, our endeavors represented how much we cared and they felt important relative to the project. The remainder of the procedure for the data collection was then implemented in a fashion similar to earlier phases. Additional research activities including and following the analysis were also comparable.

Professional consultants were utilized throughout all phases of the project. Additional expertise in qualitative methodologies,[l] and NICU clinical practice[m] were sought to augment our own education and background. Some of the consultants were faculty members as well and also brought these skills to the consulting process. At each phase consultants reviewed the grant proposal prior to the implementation of the study and made many valuable suggestions. Selected consultants, depending upon the planned strategies for maintaining scientific rigor, reviewed the description of the results. All professional consultants provided constructive feedback for us as well as suggestions for additional references. Parent consultants were also included as a verification strategy.[n]

Participants were paid for each interview. The payment was quite small and more symbolic of our gratitude than possessing any monetary significance. During Phases I and II, each family received $10.00. In Phase III, each parent received $25.00.

Participants

The sample of parents for this project was relatively heterogeneous. Table A.3 is a summary of the parents' characteristics as collected in Phase I (32 mothers, 19 fathers). In addition, 2 grandmother caregivers who were primary providers of child care, were interviewed. In Phase II, 28 families were represented in the interviews (28 mothers, 1 caregiver grandmother, and 17 fathers) while 23 mothers and 15 fathers were located and willing to be interviewed for Phase III. Although 2 fathers discontinued participation in the project at Phase II, 1 father who had not participated in Phase I joined the study in Phase II, for a total of 17 men. Two fathers discontinued participation in Phase III.

Infant data were gathered through a chart review conducted after the primary analysis of the data was completed. Table A.4 is a summary of the characteristics for the 42 infants (6 sets of twins, 2 sets of triplets, 24 single births). The discharge summary of the chart was a key source of information. The remainder of the chart was reviewed for several factors including general information about meetings with parents, arrangements for parental education, and the provision of news about the infant to parents from the staff.

At the Phase II interview, 34 infants were included in the 28 families. These children varied in their degree of recovery since discharge from the NICU. Twelve of the children had serious problems, which could be categorized as requiring long-term intervention. Thirteen infants had a questionable status in that parents indicated follow-up was requested so additional tests or procedures might be performed at a later time. Eleven children had no apparent residual problems. These latter children were no longer followed at the high-risk clinic.

At the time of the Phase III interviews, 32 children were represented by the willing parent participants. Although most parents initially stated that their child(ren) was good and progressing mentally and physically, only 1 child was actually found to have had no problems in its current status. Serious problems were the situation for 6

Table A.3 *Summary of Parent Characteristics*

Informants	
Mothers	32
Fathers	19
Grandmothers	2

Marital Status	
Married	26
Single	6

Age in years	Mothers	Fathers[a]
20 and under	4	0
21-25	4	2
26-29	9	7
30-39	15	10

Ethnic identification	Mothers	Fathers
Caucasian	24	17
African-American	5	2
Blend	1	0
Oriental	1	0
Hispanic	1	0

Educational level	Mothers	Fathers
<High School	5	0
High School	9	4
>High School	14	12
College (graduated)	3	2
>College	1	1

Occupation[b]	Mothers	Fathers
Blue-collar	5	10
White-collar	14	8
Professional/ Business	4	1
None	9	0

Religious preference	Mothers	Fathers
Roman Catholic	10	7
Protestant	19	10
Buddhist	1	0
None	2	2

Financial status[c]	
Adequate	18
Inadequate	8
Missing data	6

Health care benefits	
Had policy	21
No policy	5
Missing data	6

[a] Fathers: data only from those interviewed
[b] Categories based on Warner in Friedman (1981)
[c] Categories based on Geismar & LaSorte (1964)

of the children. All of the remaining 25 children had delays in growth and development, or significant problems requiring ongoing interventions, or both delays and the need for continuing treatment.

Data Analysis

Two totally different data analysis procedures were used, one for the primary content analysis and later, another for the secondary analysis for moral orientation. The primary content analysis will be described first. This analysis occurred during each phase. The secondary analysis was made after all three phases were completed.

Table A.4 *Summary of Infant Characteristics*

Days in NICU	**Birth Weight**	**Gestational Age**
1 day (expired) = 1	540 g = 1	Low is 24 weeks
<30 days = 18	600-999 g = 15	24-26 weeks = 7
30-60 days = 8	1000-1599 g = 8	27-30 weeks = 14
61-90 days = 5	1600-2099 g = 7	31-34 weeks = 15
91-120 days = 7	2100-2499 g = 4	35-37 weeks = 4
>120 days = 3	------------[a]	------------[a]
Highest stay = 235	>2500 g = 6	>37 weeks = 2
	Missing = 1	
APGAR Score	**Diagnoses and Treatments**	**Bilirubin High**
0 (1"), 1 (5") = 1	Criteria = presence of	3ml/dl = 3
Below 5 at 5" = 21	surgical interventions	------------[a]
-----------[a]	and/or birth anomalies[a]	Above 15 ml/dl = 3
Above 5 at 5" = 18	Different diagnoses = 90	High, 25.9 ml/dl = 1
Missing = 2	Different procedures = 61	Missing = 1

[a] Cut-off in criteria for high-risk status as defined by Merenstein and Gardner[62]

Primary Analysis

Interviewing and primary content analysis for all three phases occurred concurrently, with the two researchers working closely together (Manning & Cullum-Sawan 1994; Weber 1985). Phases I and II were conducted over a period of 12 months beginning with the infants' hospitalization in the NICU and continuing with the second interview 6 months after discharge. Phase III interviews, funded separately, were implemented over an 8-month period when the children were about 4 years of age. Working alone, I completed the pilot study analysis and the secondary analysis for moral orientation.

For the pilot study, I transcribed the audio-recorded interviews verbatim into computer files and completed the content analysis myself. The analysis began with the first interview and consisted of several readings of the raw data (hard copy of the transcript). I completed the first reading while simultaneously listening to the audiotape so I could make notes about the affective or nonverbal dimensions of the interview. Codes were created for the issues identified in the interview. Codes were applied to various groups of data: words, sentences, and even complete paragraphs (Patton 1980;

Weber 1985). Memos and theoretical notes were generated as well, to record the ongoing impressions and meanings of the verbatim data (Corbin 1986). Multiple copies of the transcripts could be printed so that clean copies were available to cut, collect, merge, and paste as needed during the analysis process. Themes were named as codes were categorized; descriptive summaries were devised. Only one simple procedure was instituted to establish some validity during the pilot phase. A parent-child expert reviewed the final description of the results. Although presentations of the pilot were scheduled shortly after this step of the project was completed, no publication occurred until significantly later (Pinch 1990).

As the interviews were conducted, reviewed, and refined for Phases I and II, the research assistant and I worked separately to begin to code the corrected, hard copy of the verbatim transcripts. The process of analysis duplicated that of the pilot study, except that the two of us met to discuss the coding of each interview after it was completed. The outcome of these discussions represented a blending of both of our analyses. Since the hard copies had been generated from computer files, printouts of data by specific question, code, or other category could be utilized to examine and re-examine data and reduce it. In Phase III, Ethnograph (version 3.0) was used to assist in the management of the data (Seidel et al. 1988; Tesch 1990). Themes, categories, and subcategories were inductively derived and a unifying principle was named for each phase (Corbin 1986; Field & Morse 1985; Knafl & Howard 1984; Strauss & Corbin 1990). The literature review served as an information base for bracketing during the analysis of the data (Berger & Kellner 1981). This body of knowledge functioned as the source of prevailing norms or previous approaches to this topic in bioethics and health care, while the interviews were analyzed.

Several strategies to test the rigor of the investigation were implemented during the three major phases (Kirk & Miller 1986; Krippendorff 1980; Sandelowski 1986). These varied a little as new suggestions appeared in the literature, but the basic goal remained the same: to continue faithfulness to our goals and to leave an obvious paper trail of our work (Hinds et al. 1990; Sandelowski 1993). An experienced qualitative researcher examined randomly selected interviews and compared our description of the results with the raw data. The results included the themes, categories, and subcategories and their summaries. We developed a guide for these reviews. The report included the reviewer's decisions relative to the match between raw data and description, justification for these decisions, and any notation about major flaws, omissions, or redundancies, for example. Another reviewer, a nurse clinician who was an experienced NICU nurse as well as a community health nurse following high-risk infants postdischarge, reviewed randomly selected interviews and the same description of the results. She also addressed these issues in terms of her own clinical experience. The resulting affirmation represented credibility (confidence in the meaning of the results as determined by participants and others), fittingness (congruence with an acceptable explanation of reality), auditability (the process for decision-making during data collection and analysis, described and located), and confirmability (agreement between two or more independent reviewers regarding the credibility, fittingness, and auditability of the study) (Lincoln & Guba 1985; Sandelowski 1986). Finally, parents, similar to the sample but not in the study were utilized as reviewers to provide another measure of validity (Knafl & Webster 1988; Swanson-Kauffman 1986). The consultant reports were either written or audiotaped and then transcribed. Both of us reviewed these reports carefully and followed up on suggestions by revising research report drafts to better explain our results or provide additional rationale for our decisions.

Formal research presentations and publications were planned as a peer review strategy for the results of both the primary (for each phase) and secondary analysis (Field & Morse 1985). Abstracts of each phase including the pilot study were accepted for presentations and posters at a variety of local, national, and international conferences and meetings. Additionally, research reports of all phases of the project were peer reviewed and published in prestigious journals.°

Secondary Analysis

In order for me to examine the interviews, interpret the results, and identify the moral orientation of each informant in this project, clean copies of all interviews were made. Each individual's interviews were then clustered together for the subsequent tasks of the analysis process. A total of 52 sets resulted (mothers n = 32; fathers n = 20). Although three phases of the research had been completed, a few individuals had fewer than three interviews (mothers n = 9; fathers n = 4). In all of these cases it was thought that the existing interviews contained sufficient data to conduct the analysis.

The selected approach to the secondary analysis was categorized as a hermeneutical strategy by Gilligan and her associates in their research on moral development (Brown, Argyris et al., 1988; Brown, Debold et al., 1991; Brown, Tappan et al., 1989). This developmental psychological method is directed by a detailed reading guide generated by scholars at the Center for the Study of Gender, Education, and Human Development at Harvard University.

Each set of interviews was read at least four times as suggested by the reading guide in order to determine whether an interviewee was caring oriented, justice oriented, or a mix, when discussing a moral dilemma. Each reading of the interviews had a different focus.

1. first reading to understand the story of the participant.
2. second reading to locate those portions of the interview most closely connected to the self (*I*, *me*, or *myself* statements).
3. third reading to identify evidence of a caring orientation.
4. fourth reading to mark instances where a justice orientation was present.

Each reading was summarized, and after the entire procedure was completed, a final overall evaluation was completed for each participant, which included an explanation of the relative use of caring and justice orientations. Color coding of each reading was used to facilitate the interpretation (yellow highlighting to capture the major items of the story, green underlining for discussions of self, red underlining for care statements, and blue underlining for justice discussions).

Based on these readings four interpretive decisions were made for each participant (Brown, Argyris et al., 1988):

1. Presence of voice--whether caring and/or justice was present in the discussion.
2. Predominance of voice--which of the voices (or both or neither) was dominant; that is, more frequently present during the entire interview.
3. Alignment of voice--which of voices the respondent preferred (which one was more frequently selected for self or the voice an individual emphasized).
4. Relationship of voice--the relationship of the self to others in the described conflict (unequal/equal as in a hierarchical structure; attachment/detachment).

Through the use of the conclusions drawn from these interpretations, the results were categorized according to the coding guide and quantitatively summarized for a concise overview of narrative types represented by the participants. The resulting typology used in this process is presented in Table A.5.

It is critical to note that the results using this method are reached on the basis of a subjective, highly interpretative process. Using a hermeneutical, psychological procedure depends upon the reader's vision and organizing framework. The resulting numerical calculations of various elements of moral orientation are many steps from the actual words of the participants. Using these simple statistics is a very liberal strategy that quickly summarizes the results but risks compromising the naturalistic perspective upon which the research is based. Small differences in percentages across elements should not be focused upon too closely. The more global meaning, such as which voices were iden-

Table A.5 *Abbreviated Typology for Coding Moral Orientation Data During Secondary Analysis*

A. Presence of Paradigm
- ____ 1 - Both justice and care
- ____ 2 - Only care
- ____ 3 - Only justice
- ____ 4 - Neither justice nor care

B. Predominance of Paradigm
- ____ 1 - Justice
- ____ 2 - Care
- ____ 3 - Neither

C. Alignment of Self and Paradigm
- ____ 1 - Justice
- ____ 2 - Care
- ____ 3 - Both
- ____ 4 - Neither

D. Organizing Framework
- ____ Inequality/Equality (I/E)
- ____ Attachment/Detachment (A/D)
- ____ Both (B)
- ____ Neither (N)

Narrative Type ____

Note. This format was devised by us, based on the work of Brown, Argyris et al., 1988

tified in these interviews across genders and within each gender, is a more significant conclusion than the exact percentage reported by gender or small differences between the genders.

Although a common subsequent step with quantitative data, might be the calculation of a chi-square statistic, using the cross-tabulation data in the contingency tables to test the significance of different proportions, this step is not used in work based on the method described by Brown and associates. No hypotheses were posited; results were quantified only to describe the characteristic moral voices of the sample, not to conduct statistical analyses (Brown, Argyris et al. 1988; Polit & Hungler 1995).

A common criticism of Brown and associates' method (1988) is that some reviewers are not able to examine isolated quotes in publications and subsequently categorize them according to the designated moral orientation. That is, using publications by Gilligan and her associates specifically, quotes presented as examples of justice or care voices are not categorized by blinded readers with those labels chosen by the researchers. For example, if a group of sentences or even a paragraph quote is removed from the research report and given to a reader, there can be a high degree of error in that reader's blinded labeling of the quote as representing justice or care. However, since the significance of the researcher's holistic understanding of the interview is indispensable to the method, it is likely that individual sentences or even a paragraph could be misleading or insufficient to fully represent the orientation of the participant. Such a limitation applies to this research project as well, and the reader needs to bear this in mind when reading the results of the secondary analysis (Chapter 5).

Additional Analysis

Given my feminist interests, I found it strikingly apparent during this project that some type of commentary was required relative to the feminist dimension. The analysis for this additional element was more theoretically centered than data-dependent; however, the exercise was strongly motivated by the results of the study and concurrent exposure to feminist thought.

Initially I critically examined various narrative sources from several disciplines relative to their treatment of motherhood. The resulting summary was organized historically. Second, the numerous research studies addressing caregiving and neonates were scrutinized for their presentation of women's roles in caregiving versus discussions of men alone or parents together as caregivers. Family research was also surveyed for its portrayal of women's roles as mothers. From the studies I drew some general conclusions about the situation for women as mothers. When the information from the studies was combined with selected results from the moral orientation analyses of the women's interviews in the project, implications for ethical decision-making in the NICU were posed. The resulting paper was presented at a national conference and expanded for the presentation in Chapter 6.

When an opportunity arose to present a paper about fathers' perceptions of the NICU experience, the interviews of the 20 fathers from the entire project were utilized to summarize paternal perspectives separately. For this endeavor a less rigorous process than the previously described content analysis was applied. All of the fathers' interviews from each phase were read and highlights of each interview were recorded. In addition, the summaries from the secondary analysis for the fathers were read and again, highlights were recorded. The notes were all combined and a conceptualization of the comments was initiated. Both interviews and secondary analysis summaries were re-examined as necessary and the conceptualization was completed.

Commonalties among the fathers were identified to illustrate the major themes among this cohort. Outlier examples were selected when the issues they represented seemed important in understanding the breadth of possible responses. Some comparison with the general results of the primary analysis was completed, as were a number of comparisons with examples from mothers in the study when feasible.

General Limitations

The interpretation of qualitative data, regardless of the strategies implemented to introduce a degree of scientific rigor, is highly dependent upon the individual(s) conducting the analysis. The resulting data are also subject to the purpose of the researcher. In this project, ethical decision-making was the phenomenon under investigation. The very outcomes of two analysis procedures in this project, using the same data, are testimony to the possible variations in interpretation. That does not imply the data are not useful or dependable (in the *truth* sense of dependable). Rather, the reader should understand that an investigator's different approaches to the analysis and organization of results will produce different outcomes, instead of concluding that the investigator made an erroneous explication of the results.

Yet another example of the use of data and interpretation might help to clarify the situation. By the end of the project (all three phases), the value of communication to the parents was quite clear. At one conference rather than present the resulting themes and unifying concept from each phase of the research, I organized the various communication implications of the themes and concepts for the presentation within a model of communication theory. This approach utilized the same data, but selected portions to emphasize communication, the phenomenon of interest for that moment.

As the research assistant and I worked on the primary analysis, each of our perspectives was broadened by the other's viewpoint. Many of our observations and notes about the interviews overlapped; in fact, most of the elements we targeted were the same. There were a few instances, however, when one of our perspectives informed the other's viewpoint. It would be dishonest not to admit that if a third person had been included in the analyses procedures, a somewhat different slant might have been introduced at times. But the major themes would remain and, given the study's purpose, ethical decision-making would still be targeted for discussion and analysis of results.

Although generalization of this study's results is limited, cognitive utilization is an appropriate step in exploring the application of qualitative data to clinical situations (Stetler 1994). Results of qualitative studies are usually not directly applied to patients (or in this case the families of patients). New information gained through a project such as this one focusing on the high-risk neonate and parental ethical decision-making can, however, influence a health professional's thinking in the clinical context. This is a more diffuse but still important aspect of knowledge building and research utilization in professional practice.

A descriptive article or book may motivate professionals to be more observant the next time they are in situations similar to those described in the project's reports. Reading the reports may raise questions about the behavior of individuals or outcomes in selected situations compared to the description of the research results. Professionals may note similarities or differences between the project reports and their own clinical circumstances. Another research study may germinate as an outcome of an *ah-hah* experience emanating from the new knowledge gained in this study, combined with the next analogous experience. Certainly as a researcher, I hope so.

Future Studies

The last chapter of this book details the implications of this work or the future in the area of neonatal care and beyond as families integrate NICU graduates into their lives. A few words will be said here about future research to bring closure to this technical aspect of the project. First, every researcher wants her or his work to be enlightening and useful to other practitioners. The interest in the project documented by invitations to share this work at conferences and requests for copies of either present work or information about work in progress has been constant over the entire implementation of the project. Numerous requests for assistance have come from graduate students. The implications of all these requests are difficult to track, but some additional research has emanated from this project (Brinchmann 2000a; Brinchmann & Nortvedt 2001; Currier 2001; Davis 1994; Kirschbaum 1994; Martin 1990; Overbay 1996; Raines 1998, 1999; Scharer & Brooks 1994; Schlomann & Fister 1995; Swigart et al. 1996) including work that specifically affirms our results (Sudia-Robinson & Freeman 2000). This work has been theoretically influential as well in a wide variety of discussions (Harms & Giordano 1990; Jameton 1994; Mellien 1993; Penticuff 1992, 1994; Scharer & Brooks 1994; Schlomann 1992; Schlomann & Fister 1995; Zaner & Bilton 1991).

I anticipate that my own future research projects will continue in this area. The exact nature of those enterprises is unknown at this point. As I write, this book is as yet unfinished. That particular milestone must be reached before I contemplate new work. Some kind of work will go on, however, as anticipated in previous grant proposals. The focus of the next activity will depend partially upon the latest developments in the area of bioethics and neonates.

As a final element of our research process, the results of the pilot study will be summarized. Since the pilot work was preliminary to determining the need for a full project, the results of that preparatory activity and its analysis will be reviewed.

Pilot Study Results

One couple (married) and 4 women (3 single, 1 married) participated in the pilot study. The women ranged in age from 16 to 36; the man was 36. The couple was Jewish, one woman was Roman Catholic, and the remaining individuals were Protestant. The 16-year-old was a student, 1 woman was unemployed, 1 woman was a blue-collar worker, and the remaining participants were business personnel or professionals. Ethnic identification included 1 African-American, 1 Mexican-American, and 3 Caucasians. This was the first pregnancy for 3 of the women.[p] Two women had caesarian sections, one for a prolapsed cord and the other because of her own escalating complex, multiple, physiological problems. Three women had preterm labor, which could not be stopped. One woman was hospitalized 6 weeks prior to delivery.

All of these parents experienced an infant's stay in the NICU for periods that varied from 2 weeks to approximately 12 weeks. The shortest stay was that of an infant who died. Only one woman had a multiple gestation (twins) although a second participant had had a previous twin pregnancy. However, only one fetus had lived through the previous pregnancy.

Three major themes were identified during the analysis of the results of the interviews with these five families: *presence of conflicts in the NICU, feelings of stress, and doing the right thing for the baby.* All acknowledged that their experiences in the NICU had indeed included not just one conflict, but in some cases many conflicts. The way these individuals perceived the conflicts and the context of the assorted situations varied. In general, the level of stress created by enduring the baby's residence in a NICU was a common thread among the various specific conflicts. All parents felt vastly unprepared for this high level of stress. Although all parents felt intense stress, the actual conflicts they named were more or less infant-centered. But their own level of stress made it difficult to deal with a baby's need for intensive care.

One mother was not sure that she should keep her baby. She felt pressured by her mother to keep it. She frequently reviewed all of the arguments and examined them as she struggled to make this decision. The baby's precarious status and her own feelings of inadequacy were most prominent in her consideration of her future.

The baby's tenacious hold on life and need to gain strength were articulated by several women. One interview was intensely emotional as the woman sobbed and showered herself with guilt and blame for the infant's precarious status and later death from multisystem failure. Although she was offered the opportunity to close the interview on several occasions, given her obvious emotional distress, she insisted that she needed to tell the whole story. She clearly indicated her need to talk, as well as her need later to terminate the interview. The self-blame for the baby's condition rested on her disregard for her own health status, which in turn compromised the infant's prenatal development. She had ignored both her diabetic condition and hypertensive state.

For one woman, Cynthia, this was not her first high-risk infant experience. She focused on the stigma attached to infants with birth defects. Previously she had given birth to an infant with Trisomy-13.[q] During that earlier experience, she was concerned about the negative attitudes of the staff toward her infant and its possible differential treatment. The baby with Trisomy-13 lived for about 2 weeks but the parents were able to bring him home from the hospital before he died. The woman and her husband were both skilled in resuscitation procedures as they had decided to institute these for respiratory problems should the infant have an arrest at home. But when the baby's heart failed, then they were going to stop any treatment. Their baby died at home in the caring environment his mother wanted for him.

In the more recent pregnancy, this same woman was expecting twins. One of the twins was diagnosed with anencephaly but died in utero.[r] She expressed great comfort in the circumstances of this infant's death.[s] This is her story:

> *Death with dignity*. Cynthia was invited to participate in the pilot study because she had given birth to a 30-week neonate, one of a set of twins. This was Cynthia's second experience with a baby in the NICU. Cynthia also talked about events during an earlier pregnancy when they had an infant with Trisomy 13. A diagnosis of anencephaly was made by ultrasound in the most recent pregnancy. Additionally, an amniocentesis was completed due to the obstetrician's concern that there might be another chromosomal disorder, although Cynthia had had a normal pregnancy and birth (girl) several years previously. Cynthia was told she was expecting a boy and a girl. So, when the physician said, "the chromosomes are fine and it is a girl," she and her husband concluded that the male was the anencephalic twin. The anencephalic baby subsequently died. When Cynthia finally gave birth to the boy, she first thought the healthy baby had died in utero. Her confusion was eventually cleared and she was able to rejoice in the boy's birth. As it turned out, the girl-twin was the one with anencephaly, and had died in utero.
>
> Cynthia wanted to tell how important it was for a baby to die with dignity. Cynthia said,
>
>> ...had she lived, from what we had been told, they would have put her in a regular nursery and they would have kept her back out of the way so that other parents would not have to look at her. I don't know the morality of that and if that was just...I was very comforted in the fact that she died the way she did [in

> utero]. It was good for the baby to die before she was born. I felt that that gave her some dignity. Because she didn't have to put up with being that baby in the back of the nursery. Kind of not wanting to look at her. So for her, that was good.
>
> The death in utero from Cynthia's perspective gave the baby dignity, surrounded by her mother's body, and grieved for by both parents. Cynthia went on to express that this was a very personal opinion which she would not force on anyone else. Other parents may not have been able to tolerate such circumstances--having a baby die in utero. Some may have wanted to end such a pregnancy early; "I could not have done that," Cynthia concluded.
>
> The second twin delivered at 30 weeks and his tenure in the NICU was actually the rationale for her inclusion in the pilot study but we were grateful that Cynthia was willing to share both of her experiences with us. Her conflicts about the more recent infant's hospitalization arose from her knowledge of potential infant problems based on her friendship with a neonatal nurse. She worried about the infant's status and whether or not he could survive a ventricular bleed, bronchopulmonary dysplasia, infection, and other crises.

Doing the right thing for the baby, the second theme of the pilot study, was also central to these parents' concerns. Parents realized that decisions had to be made for the infant almost constantly due to its condition and the need for treatment. They acknowledged that they had been informed about these decisions, but no family felt that their permission was sought for the treatments to be initiated. Families did not have the responsibility for decision-making, they explained, while the infant was in the NICU. Parents recalled signing informed consent documents, many in fact, but the process was a perfunctory one. Participants assured me that they never refused the request for their signatures but they knew whatever was requested would be done regardless of their preference. Nevertheless, families were not unhappy with these particular circumstances. The parents did not view decisions for the infants negatively; in that they did not disagree with the proposed treatments and procedures.

One family was especially articulate about their role in ethical decision-making. First they said that they had never connected the treatment of their child and ethical decision-making until they were prompted to think about their experience in such a manner during the interview with me. They then recalled an incident several months after the discharge of their daughter from the NICU. When they were at home watching a television program about a NICU, they could not believe the program actually reflected their experiences--yet, given the scenes, the infants, and the stories of the professionals and parents, it had to be similar. They had been so caught up in the swirl of events, the *extraordinariness* of it. They were unable to process much of their experience when they were actually living it. They described their lives as having a dream-like quality as they moved from work, to the hospital, to home for sleep, and then back into the same cycle again. Day after day this cycle continued until they were finally able to bring the infant home. They could not imagine doing anything more than they had done. They were stressed; they were exhausted. The father shared this opinion:

> There was a physician who oversees the entire program. I thought I'd never forget her name. She was excellent. Again, she didn't give us any choice, but she was real aggressive. She didn't pull any punches, she was pretty blunt about how slim her chances were in the first place...we didn't find out until just a few days ago that she [physician] did consult the pulmonary specialist [infant is now 1½ years old]. We just took her back for a check-up and he [pulmonologist] remembered her. The baby was such a tough case. Three preemies were born at the same time as our daughter. They basically all had the same treatment. The same decisions were made right down the line to be completely aggressive. And all sets of parents feel the right thing was done, although the outcomes have been very, very different. One has died and the other child has severe cerebral palsy.

One participant, a nurse, recalled the NICU experience in light of her present position.

> I think a lot about these things [the NICU] now. I have always thought... about how much resources you expend on a critically ill person. Is because technology is available, does that mean you use it? Should you use it? I have always thought, no. Just because it is available doesn't mean you have to use it. But since working in ICU...the respirator is pretty common now. And in our daughter's case, that is all they did. They didn't have to do much else. She developed a stress ulcer...she was on hyperal...but no surgeries. On some of the other kids they had to do surgery, lots of it.

The father continued:

> I look at the child that died that had multiple anomalies as well as respiratory failure, and I wonder if I would have wanted them to

> continue that for her. And so I still ponder this. I think about it from time to time. It wasn't a decision we had to make. And based on my own personal values, I don't know if I could have called it off. They thought that there was a reasonable chance that she could live. That...what if she was going to be retarded as a result of her treatment? Is that a reason to stop? Some pretty frightening things to think about and I'm...and we asked them. Because of her treatments, what will her intelligence be? And we don't know, they said. We just don't know. Not that they offered us any chance to do anything different. They were going to go on but if they told us she is going to be profoundly retarded, what would I have done? What is it that I wanted done? I don't think we ever really talked about this. We talked about her mental state, what she'd be like but not *ever* what we wanted them to do about it. Could we have stopped them?

One parent asked whether or not it would be appropriate to have the responsibility to make treatment decisions. The experience was so overwhelming. The mothers may not yet have recovered from a high-risk pregnancy or birth experience.

> It might be immoral to push you to make a decision... you were too tired to make. I was aware of what was going on and everything but I never gave it much thought. Maybe 6 months later there is a kind of sobering-up process. Maybe if she were still in that situation, critical, being sustained like that with maybe no hope or little hope. Maybe I would start to think differently.

Communication issues are a natural dimension of a decision-making discussion. Parents shared their common belief that they could call the nursery at any time to check on the status of their baby. Families also were comforted by their experiences with the nurses as a source of information and as a link with their child when they were away from the NICU. The staff did call parents when significant events occurred, whether they were moments for celebration or concern. The woman whose baby died explained that the nurses called her when they thought the baby was in the final crisis. "When the baby got worse, [the nurses] called me so I could come and hold her."

Possible lack of knowledge and understanding was a critical part of the parents' perception of their role in decision-making. The NICU was perceived as a foreign place even for those who had a health care background. Indeed, if some of the technology was familiar, these infants as the nurses' own children were a different category of patients and it changed the whole tenor of the environment for them. The intensity of the work setting and the apparent high level of skill required to deliver adequate care to the infants made parents feel quite inadequate. Paradoxically they also were impressed with the routine of the nursery. Here the care was not special but something the health professionals did every day, all week long, for months at a time. This created a calm and implicit minimization of risk that seemed to stifle ethical concern and any moral imperative related to the interventions.

Medical terminology, so easily voiced by the professionals, was frequently not understood by parents. Consent requires being informed, but these individuals described assimilating information as troublesome. Making one decision can be difficult enough, but then progress or setbacks require another decision and yet dozens more. As one parent discussed possible surgery for the infant, the dilemma was not simply contained in this one decision to have or not have surgery. Either way it entailed making additional decisions in the future, which generally parents could not envision. With only a partial understanding of the information, it became an impossible task. One parent related her observation that the second experience in the NICU was easier because they knew what to expect and they were acquainted with the personnel in the unit and the unit itself. She also voiced her perception that they received more attention from the nurses because as parents they were already familiar individuals.

Although parents did not uniformly connect ethics or morality to decision-making in the NICU, they were able to address issues of morality in related circumstances. Both women whose own prenatal health had adversely affected the infant's outcome specifically said they were bad. They knew, but felt helpless in their situations, to change their lifestyle to optimize the pregnancy. One woman simply said, "I killed the baby." The other woman said that she never realized the possible direct effect of her behavior on the fetus and its outcome.

Two women discussed being able to do the right thing as their definition of morality, although this was not connected with treatment for their infants. One woman enlarged upon this idea by describing how one should treat others as you would want to be treated. The other emphasized doing the best you could do under the circumstances. Context was quite important for her. Being forced to agree to another person's decision was also included in these ideas about right actions and behavior. A final notion was the relationship of values and standards to morality, but again, not initially connected with neonatal care. Love and commitment were important components of these values and standards for one individual. Religious traditions were also noted.

Conclusion

Based on the experience with the pilot study, additional research seemed warranted. A decision to move forward was made and implemented through writing grant proposals to obtain funding. Several factors informed the decision. The lack of an active role in ethical decision-making in the NICU was a surprise in light of the body of literature attesting to the fact that parents are involved in decisions for their infants. These parents all volunteered various reasons for their belief that they had not been involved in decision-making. One obvious explanation is that parents do not remember their participation. They certainly affirmed their fatigue, stress, recovery status, and other contributing factors. The participants did recall communication and information sharing, however. They also cited requests to sign informed consent documents. They did not perceive these activities as decision-making, nonetheless. Informed consent is the gold standard of voluntary, knowledgeable participation in treatment decision-making. But that was not the impression parents gave as they looked back over their experiences in the NICU.

Looking back, of course, may not give as accurate a perception of events as discussing them closer to the moment they occurred. Although insight gained from interviews conducted after the infant has been discharged is both interesting and useful, it seemed necessary to set the base line for gathering data at an earlier point. That point might better be the period when the infant was still in the NICU, not yet discharged, but with a sufficient history to allow decision-making opportunities to arise in the course of events.

Ultimately parents will be the caregivers for their infant (or infants). Ethical questions can be raised about the a nominal role in decision-making as evidenced by this group of parents, given most of their children's minimal compromise in growth and development and the parents' relatively short experience with child-rearing since discharge. Understandably in some cases, caregiving may extend to adult years or in extreme cases may include life-long responsibility of the parent for the child. Are there any ramifications when parental responsibility in decision-making for their infant is compromised or absent? Should parents be relieved of their moral obligations at the point in the child's life when the use of technology is sophisticated and the treatment regime quite complex? What exactly is the ideal situation for which we should strive? Based on the incongruency between the discussion in general bioethical literature and this group of participants, further investigation appears to be required.

Notes

[a] Material from this analysis is included in Chapter 7.

[b] Apgar scores are based on evaluations of the infant taken immediately after birth. The test is named for Virginia Apgar, an anesthesiologist, who devised it. Each of five physical dimensions is measured and scored from 0 and 2: heart rate, respiratory effort, muscle tone, response to stimulation, and skin color. A total score of 10 is the best possible.

[c] Bilirubin is a waste product that comes from the destruction of red blood cells. When present in large amounts it causes the skin and white portion of the eye to take on a yellow color. If too much bilirubin accumulates in the body, it can cause brain damage which can result in retardation, cerebral palsy, and hearing loss.

[d] Merenstein and Gardner's 1985 edition of the *Handbook of Neonatal Intensive Care* was the current edition available at the time of the project's inception. Since no new families were added in Phases II and III, newer editions were not required.

[e] Revisions were based on a meeting with Janice M. Morse, RN, PhD (Nursing), PhD (Anthropology) consultant to the project in Phase III.

[f] For Phases I and II financial status was designated by a simple *adequate* or *inadequate* choice with a separate question about health insurance. Dollar amounts of family income were never requested. In Phase III, a more nuanced approach was utilized in which income was probed for relative adequacy (more than adequate, adequate, less than adequate, or not at all) on 6 dimensions: meeting daily living needs, rent or mortgage payments, food bills, health care needs, participation in recreation, and other (with a request to specify item). This format was developed by Marie L. Lobo, PhD, then at The Ohio State University, College of Nursing, Columbus, Ohio and shared with a group of researchers at the Midwest Nursing Research Society Meeting, in April 1989.

[g] Health Future Foundation, Omaha, NE, provided funds for Phases I and II.

[h] The National Center for Nursing Research (NCNR) became the National Institute for Nursing Research (NINR) in 1993. This placed nursing research more in line with the other health disciplines at the National Institutes of Health, Washington, DC.

[i] Janice M. Morse, RN, PhD (Nursing), PhD (Anthropology) suggested interviewing parents separately on a pre-project consultation. This was extremely helpful for the principal investigator but Dr. Morse is not responsible for the

implementation of Phase III nor any limitations that resulted.

[j] Telephone interviewing is discussed at great length relative to quantitative approaches such as survey research. See Dillman (1978), a classic in the field, and Fontana and Frey (1994).

[k] This incident is included in the discussion of the results. The story is labeled *Thanksgiving Holiday* and can be found in Chapter 3.

[l] In Phase I and II, Patricia Nilsson, RN, MS, served as a methods consultant; for Phase III, Dr. J. Morse (1991) served.

[m] For Phases I and II, Susan E. Reinarz, MSN, RN, served as an expert clinical consultant; for Phase III, Dr. J. H. Penticuff (1993) served.

[n] Parents of high-risk neonates who served in various consultant capacities throughout the project were: Sheri Lyons, RN; Karen Graalfs, LuAnn Peters; and Kim Gardner.

[o] See Table P.2 for specific presentations and publications.

[p] See Figure 1 in Pinch (1990) for a more specific description of the demographic information by individual.

[q] Trisomy-13 is a congenital condition in which there is an extra chromosome instead of the usual pair. It is one of several syndromes caused by various abnormalities of the chromosomes. This particular defect results in many signs including but not limited to mental retardation, malformed ears, cleft palate or lip, small mandible, cardiac defects, convulsions, renal anomalies, umbilical hernia, and malrotation of the intestines. If these infants survive the pregnancy and birth, they do not usually live more than 2 years. This participant's baby had cleft palate and lip, fused eyelids, blind, open ductus, and severe stenosis. The mother refused to give permission for an autopsy so the full extent of his defects were not ascertained. She objected to the autopsy because she did not want any more abuse to his body; his condition at birth was more than anyone should have to bear.

[r] Anencephaly is a condition wherein there is markedly defective development of the brain. Cranial bones are also absent. Usually the cerebral and cerebellar hemispheres are absent and only a rudimentary brain stem develops. The condition is incompatible with life although infants may live for some days. They are especially prone to infection due to the exposed cranial tissue.

[s] The preference for the death in utero rather than after birth is in direct contrast to the featured case study in an article by Holzman (1999). A couple in their early 40s were expecting twins and a multiple gestation pregnancy was *medically ill advised* for the woman. The decision facing them was the possible use of selective reduction for the pregnancy. Conflicting interests in the case were hard to balance and while attempting to determine the best possible outcome for all involved, the parents had reached an impasse. So to overcome this hurdle, Holzman suggested the parents rethink the situation in terms of "What would cause the most long-term pain?" Instead of maximizing happiness or analyzing the situation in terms of beneficence, the concept of nonmaleficence was

introduced into the discussion. How could these parents avoid harm? For the woman, the worst possible outcome was carrying a dead fetus for any period of time, the precise result of a pregnancy reduction. As Holzman stated, "...expecting a mother to live with her dead baby...inside of her was the ultimate unethical request" (p. 484) from this woman's perspective. Although Holzman's lesson for us is to introduce the possibility of asking our patients not only what would be best but also what choice would be worst, there is another lesson here. Given the contrast with the story of Cynthia, we should expect wide variety in values, traditions, and beliefs that individuals bring to decision-making.

GLOSSARY

Definitions in philosophy and ethics are especially open to debate. However, when reading this book, it may be helpful to refer to some basic ideas about terminology incorporated in various bioethical discussions. In many cases these terms are further elaborated in the bioethical literature as they themselves become the focus of debate.

Advance Directives Instructions related to individual choices about future health care, especially for situations in which the individual patient her/himself is no longer able to articulate those choices. One type of written form is a living will, another is a durable power of attorney for health care whereby another individual is vested with the authority to make health care decisions when the originator of the directive is unconscious or incompetent.

Aesthetics_As a philosophical concept, the study of the nature, types, and criteria of values and values judgments related to the beautiful, the artistic, or material objects.

Antiprinciplism A general movement in bioethics begun in the late 80s in which the widespread use of ethical principles (autonomy, beneficence, nonmaleficence, justice) as a foundation for decision making is critically examined.

Autonomy The ethical principle in which freedom or the liberty to act on personally chosen plans is central. This includes the respect for persons and their dignity, values, beliefs, and traditions.

Axiology The study of the nature, types, and criteria of values and value judgments in philosophy. Axiology consists of two areas: aesthetics and ethics.

Beneficence The ethical principle in which doing good is central. Sometimes this is expanded to include preventing harm or removing/ preventing harms. Whether or not this is beneficence or nonmaleficence is debated by some.

Bioethics The general body of principles and values of a particular culture or group as they relate to life. This has come to be associated most closely with ethics in health care. That is *bios* is more narrowly focused to mean life as affected by health, sickness, illness, disease, or trauma.
Casuistry A method of analysis based on the use of individual cases or situations. A paradigm case is often used to begin this process followed by modifications of the case to determine whether or not the ethical principle or theory which supports a decision in the paradigm case continues to sustain the recommended moral action.
Clinical Ethics A normative type of ethics in which principles and values are used to determine morally acceptable decisions in health care practice including medicine, nursing, pharmacology, dentistry, and the allied health professions.
Consequentialism A theoretical perspective in which the outcomes or results (consequences) are of primary importance for the decision making process. One kind of consequentialism is utilitarianism.
Cosmology branch of philosophy dealing with the origin and structure of the universe as well as its characteristics: time, space, causality, freedom.
Deontology A philosophical theory in which rules and guides for behavior, or decisions regarding moral action are formulated based on a search for the definition of duty. Decisions and rules are determined irrespective of the outcomes or consequences. Sometimes called nonconsequentialist in orientation.
Epistemology The study of or theory about the nature, limits, and foundation of knowledge.
Ethics The study of the nature, types, and criteria of values and value judgments related to persons and their relationships with other individuals, their characteristics, actions, conduct, and behaviors.
Extraordinary treatment Interventions or actions that are not morally obligated to be implemented or accepted by patients, as determined by the person who is the object of the treatment.
Feminism The theory of the political, psychological, sociological, and economic status of gender with special emphasis on the understanding of women's roles, perspectives, and possible oppression, suppression, and repression.
Ideology A systematic body of concepts about human life, culture, and society.

Justice The ethical principle in which fairness and equality are central. This can encompass material resources (distributive justice) or fair treatment of individuals, groups, and communities (psychological, legal, political, social).

Medical Ethics The study of ethics with a special emphasis on the practice of medicine. The physician's perspective and her/his relationship to the patient, community, or nation is of central concern.

Metaethics The philosophical division of ethics focusing on the meaning of moral terms, the nature of moral discourse, and the foundations for moral principles (Flexner, 1987).

Metaphysics A division of philosophy that includes ontology (being, existence), epistemology (knowledge), and cosmology (the universe as an orderly system; space-time relationships).

Morality Right or wrong conduct; ability to determine the rules of such conduct. As opposed to ethics where right and wrong are studied, this refers to the decisions of conscience one makes and the subsequent action taken based on that decision.

Nonconsequentialism A theoretical perspective which minimizes or discounts consideration of the potential outcome as a focus in ethical decision making.

Nonmaleficence The ethical principle in which avoiding harm is central. Sometimes this is expanded to mean prevention of harm as well. Whether or not the latter is beneficence can be a matter of debate and disagreement in ethics.

Normative ethics A division of ethics in which an inquiry is made about which guides, rules, laws, theories, and principles best meet our moral needs. **Applied** normative ethics is the use of such standards to understand and solve moral or ethical dilemmas.

Ontology A division of metaphysics in which the nature and relations of being or existence are central.

Ordinary treatment Those interventions or actions which are morally obligated as determined by the person who will receive them.

Paradigm A pattern, example, or model.

Phenomenology Philosophical study and description of observable events, objects, facts, or circumstances. Also means the study of the mind, its development and functioning.

Philosophy Discipline in which the search for truth or wisdom through logical reasoning is central. An analysis of fundamental beliefs about life. The discipline or field of study includes areas such as logic, axiology, metaphysics, ontology, epistemology, and phenomenology.

prima facie "At first sight" or "on the surface." An obligation, what one ought to do, a duty.

Principles Abstract concepts such as autonomy and beneficence that serve as comprehensive or fundamental rules, laws, or codes of conduct. The use of these principles in bioethics was a dominant influence during the first decade.

Teleological A theoretical perspective which focuses on the outcome or goal, not the means to get there. The ends are justified regardless of the means.

Theology Discipline in which the rational interpretation of religious faith, practice, and experience are central to the theories, systems, and opinions which are studied and used.

Utilitarianism A philosophical theory in which rules and guides for behavior, or decisions regarding moral action are formulated based on a determination of the manner in which the greatest possible happiness, pleasure, or good can be created. The outcome or the consequence is central to these considerations. Sometimes called a teleological theory or consequentialism.

Virtue Character traits of the individual. In ethics, attributes usually related to morality or aspects of conscience. Examples of virtues include integrity, fidelity, veracity, charity, and caring.

REFERENCES

Abandonment case draws mixed reaction. 2000. Retrieved January 11, 2000 from http://www.msnbc.com/news/354738.asp

Abel, E.K., & Nelson, M.K. 1990. *Circles of care: Work and identity in women's lives*. Albany: State University of New York Press.

Able-Boone, H., Dokecki, P, R., & Smith, M. S. 1989. Parent and health care provider communication and decision making in the intensive care nursery. *Children's Health Care*, 18(3), 133-141.

Achtenberg, B., & Sawyer, J. (Producers). 1983. *Nursing ethics: Code Gray* (28"). Boston: Fanlight Productions.

Adler, J. 1987. Every parent's nightmare. *Newsweek*, 109(11), 56-60.

Adler, J. 1988. What if your worst nightmare came true? A father's tale. *Esquire*, 109(6), 147-150.

Affleck, G., Tennen, H., & Rowe, J. 1990. Mothers, fathers, and the crisis of newborn intensive care. *Infant Mental Health Journal*, 11(1), 12-25.

Alecson, D.G. 1995. *Lost lullaby*. Berkeley, CA: University of California Press.

Amato, M., & Schneider, H. 1991. Survival of a 390 grams Swiss infant. *Journal of Perinatal Medicine*, 19(4), 313-315.

American Hospital Association, 1988. *Hospital statistics*. Chicago, IL: The Association.

American Hospital Association. 1992. *AHA hospital statistics*. Chicago, IL: The Association.

American Hospital Association. 1994-1995. *Hospital statistics: The AHA profile of United States Hospitals*. Chicago, IL: The Association.

American Medical Association. 1994. *Physician characteristics and distribution in the U.S.* Chicago, IL: The Association, Department of Data Services.

American Society for Reproductive Medicine. 2000. Frequently asked questions. Retrieved February 8, 2001 from http://www.asrm.org/Patients/faqs.html

Anderson, B., & Hall, B. 1995. Parents' perceptions of decision making for children. *Journal of Law, Medicine & Ethics*, 23, 15-19.

Annas, G. J. 1983. Disconnecting the Baby Doe hotline. *Hastings Center Report*, 13(3), 14-16.

Anner, J. 1994. Kangaroo care: A father's story of caring for his premature daughter. *Childbirth Instructor Magazine*, 4(2), 12-14, 16-17.

Anspach, R. R. 1993. *Deciding who lives: Fateful choices in the intensive-care nursery*. Berkeley: University of California Press.

Ariès, P. 1962. *Centuries of Childhood: A social history of family life*. New York: Knopf.

Arras, J. D., Asch, A., Macklin, R., O'Connell, L., Rhoden, N. K., & Weisbard, A. J. 1987. Standards of judgment for treatment. *Hastings Center Report*, 17(6), 13-16.

Arras, J.D., Coulter, D., Fleischman, A.R., Macklin, R., Rhoden, N.K., & Weil, B. 1987. The effect of new pediatric capabilities and the problem of uncertainty. *Hastings Center Report*, 17(6), 10-13.

Artinian, B.A. 1988. Qualitative modes of inquiry. *Western Journal of Nursing Research*, 10(2), 138-149.

Asch, A., Cohen, C. B., Edgar, H., & Weisbard, A. 1987. Who Should Decide. *The Hastings Center Report*, 17(6), 17-21.

Asch, A, & Geller G. 1996. Feminism, bioethics, and genetics. In S.M. Wolf (Ed.). *Feminism & bioethics: Beyond reproduction* (pp. 318-350). New York: Oxford University Press.

Assisted reproductive technology success rates-1997. National summary and fertility clinic reports. 1999. U.S. Department of Health and Human Services and Centers for Disease Control and Prevention. Retrieved February 8, 2001 from: http://chc.gov/nccdphp/drh/art97/pdf/art97.pdf.

Aumann, G. M-E. 1988. New chances, new choices: Problems with perinatal technology. *Journal of Perinatal and Neonatal Nursing*, 1(3), 1-9.

Avery, M.E. 1994. Changes in care of the newborn: Personal reflections over forty years. *Neonatal Network*, 13(6), 13-14.

Avery, G.B. 1998. Futility considerations in the neonatal intensive care unit. *Seminars in Perinatology*, 22(3), 216-222.

Babies and technology. 21 August 2000. *Nightline* (transcript). Retrieved August 24, 2000 from http://abcnews.go.com/onair/nightline/transcripts/n1000821_trans.html.

Bailey, C.F. 1986. Withholding or withdrawing treatment on handicapped newborns. *Pediatric Nursing*, 12(6), 413-416.

Baker, J.P. 1996. *The machine in the nursery: Incubator technology and the origins of newborn intensive care*. Baltimore, MD: The John Hopkins University Press.

Baldwin, D.C., Daugherty, S.R., & Self, D.J. 1991. Changes in moral reasoning during medical school. *Academic Medicine*, 66(9), S1-S3.

Barber, P.A., Marquis, J.G., & Turnbull III, H.R. 1992. Parental perspectives on treatment-nontreatment decisions involving newborns with spina bifida. In A.L. Caplan, R.H. Blank, & J.C. Merrick (Eds.). *Compelled compassion* (pp. 123-153). Totowa, NJ: The Humana Press Inc.

Bard, B., & Fletcher, J. 1968. The right to die: A father speaks; A theologian comments. *The Atlantic*, 221, 59-64.

Barker, K.K. 1998. A ship upon a stormy sea: The medicalization of pregnancy. *Social Science and Medicine*, 47(8), 1067-1076.

Barr, J.M. 1998. Understanding pediatric intestinal pseudo-obstruction: Implications for nurses. *Gastroenterology Nursing*, 21(1), 11-13.

Barthel, J. 1985. His name is Jimmy. Should he have been allowed to live? *McCall's*, 113(2), 109-111, 156-158, 160-161.

Bartholome, W.G. 1988, December 7. Withholding/withdrawing life-sustaining treatment and the pediatric patient. Pediatric Grand Rounds, Creighton University Medical Center, Department of Pediatrics.

Bartrick, S., 1983. A world of kindness: A patient's view: The father of two prematurely born children describes his personal experiences. *Nursing Times*, 79(33), 70.

Basinger, K.S., Gibbs, J.C., & Fuller, D. 1995. Context and the measurement of moral judgement. *International Journal of Behavioral Development*, 18(3), 537-556.

Bass, L. S. 1991. What do parents need when their infant is a patient in the NICU? *Neonatal Network*, 10(4), 25-33.

Bauman, Z. 1993. *Postmodern ethics*. Cambridge, MA: Blackwell.

Baxley, N., & Associates (Producer). 1983. *Born dying* (20 minutes, color). Available from Carle Medical Communications, Urban, IL.

Becker, P.H., & Burke, S. 1988. Neonatal drug addiction: An analysis from two moral orientations. *Holistic Nursing Practice*, 2(4), 20-27.

Bedrick, A.D. 1992. Driving home at 5 AM (editorial). *American Journal of Diseases of Children*, 146, 281-282.

Belkin, L. 1993. *First, do no harm*. New York: Simon & Schuster.

Benfield, D.G., Leib, S.A., & Reuter, J. 1976. Grief response of parents after referral of the critically ill newborn to a regional center. *New England Journal of Medicine*, 294(18), 975-978.

Benfield, D.G., Leib, S.A., & Vollman, J.H. 1978. Grief response of parents to neonatal death and parent participation in deciding care. *Pediatrics*, 62(2), 171-177.

Benko, L.B. 2001, April 16. Chipping away at SCHIP. *Modern Healthcare*, n.p.

Benoliel J.Q. 1984 Advancing nursing science: Qualitative approaches. *Western Journal of Nursing Research*, 6(3), 1-9.

Berg, B.F. 1995. Listening to the voices of the infertile. In J.C. Callahan (Ed.). *Reproduction, ethics, and the law* (pp. 80-108). Bloomington: Indiana University Press.

Berg, B.L. 1989. *Qualitative research methods for the social sciences*. Boston: Allyn and Bacon.

Berger, P., & Kellner, H. 1981. *Sociology reinterpreted*. Garden City, NJ: Anchor Press/Doubleday.

Bernard, J.S. 1975. *The future of motherhood*. New York: Penguin Books Inc.

Berseth, C.L. 1987. Ethical dilemmas in the neonatal intensive care unit. *Mayo Clinical Proceedings*, 62, 67-72.

Berseth, C.L., Kenny, J.D., & Durand, R. 1984. Newborn ethical dilemmas: Intensive care and intermediate care nursing attitudes. *Critical Care Medicine*, 12(6), 508-11.

Between twins [On-line]. 2000. Retrieved January 12, 2000 from http://www. msnbc.com/news/204464.asp

Births [On-line]. 1998. Retrieved July 11, 2000 from http://www.cdc. gov/nchs/faq/birthsl.htm..

Blackburn, S., & Lowen, L. 1986. Impact of an infant's premature birth on the grandparents and parents. *JOGNN*, 15(2), 173-178.

Blackburne-Stover, G., Belenky, M.F., & Gilligan, C. 1982. Moral development and reconstructive memory: Recalling a decision to terminate an unplanned pregnancy. *Developmental Psychology*, 18(6), 862-870.

Blackington, S.M., & McLauchlan, T. 1995. Continuous quality improvement in the neonatal intensive care unit: Evaluating parent satisfaction. *Journal of Nursing Care Quality*, 9(4), 78-85.

Blakemore, B. [on-line] 2000. An ethical dilemma: Who should decide whether premature babies live or die? Retrieved September 1, 2000 from http://abcnews.go.com/onair.CloserLook/wnt000705_preemie_feature.html

Blatt, M., & Kohlberg, L. 1975. The effects of classroom moral discussion upon children's level of moral judgment. *Journal of Moral Education*, 4, 129-161.

Blaustein, M., & Kassell, D. (Co-Producers). 1999. *For love of Julian.* Available from Winstar Cinema, New York.

Blustein, J. 1989. The rights approach and the intimacy approach: Family suffering and care of defective newborns. *Mount Sinai Journal of Medicine*, 56(3), 164-167.

Boardman, C.H. 1995. NICU treatment team function and its effect on parental stress. *Occupational Therapy in Health Care*, 9(2/3), 17-50.

Bogdan, R., Brown, M.A., & Foster, S.B. 1982. Be honest but not cruel: Staff/parent communication on a neonatal unit. *Human Organization*, 41(1), 19-37.

Born too soon. 2000, May. *Life, Collector's edition.* 48-62.

Bradford, J., & Sartwell, C. 1997. Addiction and knowledge; Epistemic disease and the hegemonic family. In H.L. Nelson (Ed.). *Feminism and families* (pp. 116-127). New York: Routledge.

Bridge, P, & Bridge, M. 1981. The brief life and death of Christopher Bridge. *Hastings Center Report*, 11(6) 17-19.

Brinchmann, B.S. 1999. When the home becomes a prison: Living with a severely disabled child. *Nursing Ethics,* 6(2), 137-143.

Brinchmann, B.S. 2000a. *"Protecting" the parents? A qualitative study of parental participation in life-and-death decision-making concerning their premature children.* Unpublished paper.

Brinchmann, B.S. 2000b. "They have to show that they can make it;" Vitality as a criterion for the prognosis of premature infants. *Nursing Ethics*, 7(2), 141-147.

Brinchmann, B.S., & Nortvedt, P. 2001. Ethical decision making in neonatal units: The normative significance of vitality. *Medicine, Health Care and Philosophy,* 4, 193-200

Brody, H. 1981. *Ethical decisions in medicine* (2nd ed.). Boston: Little, Brown and Company.

Brody, H. 1989. Transparency: Informed consent in primary care. *Hastings Center Report*, 19(5), 5-9.

Brody, J.K. 1988. Virtue ethics, caring and nursing. *Scholarly Inquiry for Nursing Practice*, 2(2), 87-101.

Brooten, D., Kumar, S., Brown, L.P., Butts, P., Finkler, S.A. Bakewell-Sachs, S., Gibbons, A., & Delivoria-Papadopoulos, M. 1986. A randomized clinical trial of early hospital discharge and home follow-up of very-low-birth-weight infants. *The New England Journal of Medicine*, 315, 934-939.

Brown, L. 1991. A problem of vision: The development voice and relational knowledge in girls ages 7 to 16. *Women's Studies Quarterly*, 19(1/2), 52-71.

Brown, L., Argyris, D., Attanucci, J., Bardige, B., Gilligan, C., Johnston, K., Miller, B., Osborne, D., Ward, J., Wiggins, G., & Wilcox, D. 1988. *A guide to reading narratives of conflict and choice for self and Moral voice* (Monograph #1). Cambridge, MA: Center for the Study of Gender, Education and Human Development, Harvard University, Graduate School of Education.

Brown, L.M., Debold, E., Tappan, M., & Gilligan, C. 1991. Reading narratives of conflict and choice for self and moral voices: A relational method. In W.M. Kurtines & J.L. Gewirtz (Eds.). *Handbook of moral behavior and development: Theory, research, and application* (pp. 25-61). Hillsdale, NJ: Lawrence Erlbaum.

Brown, L.M., Tappan, M.B., Gilligan, C., Miller, B.A., & Argyris, D.E. 1989. Reading for self and moral voice: A method for interpreting narratives of real-life moral conflict and choice. In M.J. Packer & R.B. Addison (Eds.). *Entering the circle: Hermeneutic investigation in psychology* (pp. 141-164, 306-309). New York: State University of New York Press.

Brown, L.P., York, R., Jacobsen, B., Gennaro, S., & Brooten, D. 1989. Very low birth-weight infants: Parental visiting and telephoning during initial infant hospitalization. *Nursing Research*, 38, 233-236.

Brown, P.A.L. 1987. *Paternal role acquisition: A comparison of fathers of high risk newborns and fathers of healthy newborns.* Unpublished master's thesis, University of Nebraska Medical Center, Omaha, NE.

Brown, P., Rustia, J., & Schappert, P. 1991. A comparison of fathers of high-risk newborns and fathers of healthy newborns. *Journal of Pediatric Nursing - Nursing Care of Children and Families*, 6(4), 269-273.

Broyles, R.S., Tyson, J.E., Heyne, E.T., Heyne, R.J., Hickman, J.F., Swint, M., Adams, S.S., West, L.A., Pomeroy, N., Hicks, P.J., & Ahn, C. 2000. Comprehensive follow-up care and life-threatening illnesses among high-risk infants: A randomized controlled trial [Electronic version]. *JAMA*, 284(16). Retrieved March 26, 2001 from: http://jama.ama-assn.org/issues/v284n16/rfull/joc00849.html

Bucciarelli, R.L. (1994). Neonatology in the United States: Scope and organization. In G. B. Avery, M. A. Fletcher, & M. G. MacDonald (Eds.). *Neonatology: Pathophysiology and management of the newborn* (pp. 12-31). Philadelphia: J. B. Lippincott Co.

Buchanan, R.C. 1986. 77 days: A father's journal. *Second Opinion*, 2, 64-91.

Bunker, J.P. 1995. Artificial organs and life-support systems. In W.T. Reich (Ed.). *Encyclopedia of bioethics* (pp. 198-206). New York: Simon & Schuster Macmillan.

Butler, N. C. 1989. Infants, pain and what health care professionals should want to know now - an issue of epistemology and ethics. *Bioethics*, 3(3), 181-199.

Calhoun, C. 1997. Family outlaws: Rethinking the connections between feminism, lesbianism, and the family. In H.L. Nelson (Ed.). *Feminism and families* (pp. 131-150). New York: Routledge.

Callahan, D. 1984. The Hastings Center: A short and long 15 years [Special supplement]. *Hastings Center Report*, 14(2), 1-16.

Callahan, D. 1986. How technology is shaping the abortion debate. *Hastings Center Report*, 16(1), 33-42.

Callahan, J.C. (Ed.). 1995. *Reproduction, ethics and the law: Feminist perspectives*. Bloomington, IN: Indiana University Press.

Callahan S. 1979. An ethical analysis of responsible parenthood. *Birth Defects: Original Article Series*, 15(2), 217-238.

Callahan, S. 1988. The role of emotion in decisionmaking. *The Hastings Center Report*, 18(3), 9-14.

Candee, D., Sheehan, T.J., Cook, C.D., Husted, S.D.R., & Bargen, M. 1982. Moral reasoning and decisions in dilemmas of neonatal care. *Pediatric Research*, 16, 846-850.

Cantor, N.L. 1995. Life, quality of: Quality of life in legal perspective. In W.T. Reich (Ed.). *Encyclopedia of Bioethics* (pp. 1361-1366). New York: Simon & Schuster Macmillan.

Caplan, A. 1987. Conclusion. In A. Caplan & C.B. Cohen (Eds.). Imperiled newborns (Special Report; pp. 30-31). *Hastings Center Report*, 17(6), 5-32.

Caplan, A.L., Blank, R.H., & Merrick, J.C. 1992. *Compelled compassion: Government, intervention in the treatment of critically ill newborns*. Totowa, NJ: Humana Press.

Caplan, A., Capron, A.M., Murray, T.H., & Penticuff, J. 1987. Deciding not to employ aggressive measures. *Hastings Center Report*, 17(6), 22-25.

Caplan, A., & Cohen, C.B. (Eds.). 1987. Imperiled newborns: A special study, introduction. *Hastings Center Report*, 17(6), 5-6.

Caplan, G. 1960. Patterns of parental response to the crisis of premature birth: A Preliminary approach to modifying the mental-health outcomes. *Psychiatry*, 23, 365-374.

Caplan, G., Mason, E.A., & Kaplan, D.M. 1965. Four studies of crisis in parents of prematures. *Community Mental Health Journal*, 1(2), 149-161.

Capron, A.M. 1987. Anencephalic donors: Separate the dead from the dying. *Hastings Center Report*, 17(1), 5-8.

Cardwell, M.M. 1993. Family nursing research: A feminist critique. In S.L. Feetham, S.B., Meister, J.M. Bell, & C.I. Gillis (Eds.). *The nursing of families: Theory/research/education /practice* (pp. 200-210). Newbury Park, CA: Sage Publications.

Carol Gilligan presents the Virginia and Leonard Marx Lecture. 1997, December 16. *News Bureau*, Teachers College, Columbia University. Retrieved March 11, 2001 from http://www.tc.columbia.edu/~news bureau/InsideTC/archive/InsideTC971216.htm

Carper, B. 1978. Fundamental patterns of knowing in nursing. *Advances in Nursing Science*, 1(1), 13-23.

Carper, B. 1979. The ethics of caring. *Advances in Nursing Science*, 1(3), 11-19.

Carr, M.W. 1989. To treat or not to treat: The controversy of handicapped newborns. *Critical Care Nurse*, 9(8), 73-78.

Carter, S.L. 1998. Developmental follow-up of infants at high risk for delays. Retrieved March 26, 2001from http://www.comeunity.com/premature/followup.html.

Cassani, V.L. 1994. We've come a long way baby! Mechanical ventilation of the newborn. *Neonatal Network*, 13(6), 63-68.

Catlin, A.J. 1997, December. Listening to the voices of mothers of imperiled children. Unpublished paper presented at the 34th Biennial Convention-Scientific Sessions, Sigma Theta Tau International, Indianapolis, IN.

Catlin, A.J. 1998. *Physicians' perceptions of the dilemma of neonatal resuscitation for extremely low birth weight preterm infants*.

(Doctoral dissertation, Rush University College of Nursing). UMI #9826246.

Catlin, A. (Primary Investigator), & Carter, B. (Co-Investigator). 1999-2001. Neonatal comfort care protocol study. Retrieved January 7, 2000 from http://www.campus.nvc.cc.ca.us/nenoatal.

Catlin, A., & Carter, B.S. 2001. Creation of a neonatal end-of-life palliative-care protocol. *The Journal of Clinical Ethics, 12*(3), 316-318.

Catlin, A., & Carter, B.S. (in press). Creation of an end of life palliative care protocol for dying newborns. *Journal of Perinatology.*

Cerase, P.A. 1988. Ethical dilemmas in resuscitation of the very-low-birth-weight infant. *Journal of Perinatal and Neonatal Nursing*, 1(3), 69-76.

Chadorow, N. 1978. *The reproduction of mothering: Psychoanalysis and the sociology of gender*. Berkeley, CA: The University of California Press.

Chally, P.S. 1992. Moral decision making in neonatal intensive care. *JOGNN*, 21(6), 475-482.

Chan L. (2000, March). An evidence-based assessment: Strategies to shift cost from neonatal intensive care units (NICUs) to after care while preserving quality of neonatal care. Retrieved June 7, 2000 from http://www.usc.edu/hsc/research/cphor/cphor5h.html.

Chaney, E.A. 1986. The rights of disabled infants. *Journal of Pediatric Nursing*, 1, 409-411.

Chang, H.K. 1984. Mechanisms of gas transport during ventilation by high frequency-oscillation. *Journal of Applied Physiology*, 56(3), 553-563.

Chap, J.B. 1985-86. Moral judgment in middle and late adulthood: The effects of age-appropriate moral dilemmas and spontaneous role taking. *International Journal of Aging and Human Development*, 22(3), 161-172.

Chesler, P. 1972. *Women and madness*. San Diego: Harcourt Brace Jovanovich, Publisher.

Children's Defense Fund. 1994. One day in the life of American children. *Hastings Center Report*, 24(4), 3.

Chinn, P.L., & Kramer, M.K. 1991. *Theory and nursing: A systematic approach* (3rd ed.). St. Louis: Mosby Year Book.

Claiborne, W. 2001, July 14. Other couples cope with 7 kids. *The Washington Post*. Retrieved July 17, 2001 from http://www.washingtonpost.com/wp-dyn/articles/A60559-2001Jul13.html.

Clancy, G.T., Anand, K.J.S., & Lally, P. 1992. Neonatal pain management. *Critical Care Nursing Clinics of North America*, 4(3), 527-535

Clark, G. 1996. Neonatal intensive care: Life-saver or no life at all? *AAP News*, 12(7), 1, 6-8.

Clark, R.H. 1996. The safe introduction of new technologies into neonatal medicine. *Clinics in Perinatology*, 23(3), 519-527.

Clubb, R.L. 1991. Chronic sorrow: Adaptation patterns of parents with chronically ill children. *Pediatric Nursing*, 17(5), 461-466.

Cohen, C.B., Levin, B., & Powderly, K. 1987. Section 1: A history of neonatal intensive care and decisionmaking. *The Hastings Center Report*, 17(6), 7-9.

Cohen, M.A. 1976. Ethical issues in neonatal intensive care: Familial concerns. In A.R. Jonsen & M.J. Garland (Eds.) *Ethics of newborn intensive care* (pp. 54-63), Berkeley, CA: University of California.

Cohen, M.H. 1999. The technology-dependent child and the socially marginalized family: A provisional framework. *Qualitative Health Research*, 9(5), 654-668.

Conley, D., & Bennett, N.G. 2000. Is biology destiny? Birthweight and life chances. *American Sociological Review*, 65, 458-467.

Conner, G.K., & Denson, V. 1990. Expectant fathers' response to pregnancy: Review of literature and implications for research in high-risk pregnancy. *Journal of Perinatal and Neonatal Nursing*, 4(2), 33-42.

Contrattio, S. 1984. Mother. In M. Lewin (Ed.), *In the shadow of the past: Psychology portrays the sexes* (pp. 226-255). New York: Columbia University Press.

Cooke, R. E. 1973. Ethics and law on behalf of the mentally retarded. *Pediatric Clinics of North America*, 20(1), 259-268.

Coontz, S. 1992. *The way we never were: American families and the nostalgia trap*. New York: BasicBooks, HarperCollins Publishers, Inc.

Corbin, J. 1986. Coding, writing memos, and diagramming. In W.C. Chenitz & J.M. Swanson (Eds.). *From practice to grounded theory* (pp. 102-120). Menlo Park, CA: Addison-Wesley Publishing Company.

Crigger, N.J. 1997. The trouble with caring: A review of eight arguments against an ethic of care. *Journal of Professional Nursing*, 13(4), 217-221.

Crisham, P. 1981. Measuring moral judgment in nursing dilemmas. *Nursing Research*, 30, 104-110.

Cuming, B. 1988. My sorrow, my joy. *Ladies' Home Journal*, 105(8), 22, 24, 166.

Cummins, J. 2000, January 5. Abandoned babies, a new crisis? Aired on NBC Nightly News with Tom Brokaw. Retrieved January 6, 2000 from http://www.msnbc.com

Curran, C.E. 1970. *Contemporary problems in moral theology*. Notre Dame, IN: Fides Publishing.

Currier, S. 2001, January 15. Life-sustaining treatment decisions for critically ill infants. Presentation for the School of Nursing, Creighton University, Omaha, NE.

Curry, R.L. 1995. The exceptional family: Walking the edge of tragedy and transformation. In S.K. Toombs, D. Barnard, & R.A. Carson (Eds.). *Chronic illness: From experience to policy* (pp. 24-37). Bloomington: Indiana University Press.

Cuttini, M, & the EURONIC Study Group. 2001. The European Union Collaborative Project on Ethical Decision Making in Neonatal Intensive Care (EURONIC): Findings from 11 countries. *The Journal of Clinical Ethics*, 12(3), 290-296.

Davis, D.S. 1991. Rich cases: The ethics of thick descriptions. *Hastings Center Report*, 21(4), 12-17.

Davis, M.M. 1994. A history of neonatal ethical dilemmas from 1966 to 1985 (Doctoral dissertation, The Catholic University of America). *Dissertation Abstracts International*, 55(02B), 0364.

Deacon, J., & O'Neill, P. 1999. *Core curriculum for neonatal intensive care nursing* (2nd ed.). Philadelphia: W.B. Saunders Company.

De Pree, M. 1996. *Dear Zoe*. New York: HarperSanFrancisco Publishers.

Dillman, D.A. 1978. *Mail and telephone surveys: The total design method.* New York: John Wiley & Sons.

Doering, L.V., Dracup, K., & Moser, D. 1999. Comparison of psychosocial adjustment of mothers and fathers of high-risk infants in the neonatal intensive care unit. *Journal of Perinatology*, 19(2), 132-137.

Donley, C. & Buckley, S. (Eds.). 1996. *The tyranny of the normal: An anthology*. Kent, OH: The Kent State University Press.

Dougherty, C.J. 1995. Joining in life and death: On separating the Lakeberg twins. *Bioethics Forum*, 11(1), 9-16.

Drew, N. 1989. The interviewer's experience as data in phenomenological research. *Western Journal of Nursing Research*, 11(4), 431-439.

Duff, R. S., & Campbell, A.G.M. 1973. Moral and ethical dilemmas in the special-care nursery. *New England Journal of Medicine*, 289, 885-890.

Duff, R. S., & Campbell, A.G.M. 1976. On deciding the care of severely handicapped or dying persons: With particular reference to infants. *Pediatrics*, 57(4), 487-493.

Dunn, P.M. 1993. Appropriate care of the newborn: Ethical dilemma. *Journal of Medical Ethics*, 19, 82-84.

Dworkin, A. 1974. *Woman hating*. New York: Penguin.

Dyck, A. J. 1974. An alternative to the ethic of euthanasia. In R.H. Williams (Ed.). *To live and to die: When, why and how?* (pp. 98-112). New York: Springer-Verlag.

Eakes, G.G., Burke, M.L., & Hainsworth, M.A. 1998. Theory. Middle-range theory of chronic sorrow. *Image: The Journal of Nursing Scholarship*, 30(2), 179-184.

Ellis, R. 1984. Philosophic inquiry. In H.H. Werley & J.J. Fitzpatrick (Eds.). *Annual Review of Nursing Research* (pp. 211-227). New York: Springer.

Ellison, P., & Walwork, E. 1986. Withdrawing mechanical support from the brain-damaged neonate. *Dimensions of Critical Care Nursing*, 5(5), 284-293.

Engelhardt, H.T. 1978. Medicine and the concept of person. In T.L. Beauchamp & S. Perlin (Eds.). *Ethical issues in death and dying* (pp. 271-284). Englewood Cliffs, NJ: Prentice-Hall, Inc.

Ehrenreich, B., & English, D. 1978. *For her own good.* New York: Dell Publishing Co.

Erlen, J.A. 1994. Ethical dilemmas in the high-risk nursery: Wilderness experiences. *Journal of Pediatric Nursing*, 9(1), 21-26.

Evans, D. 1989. The psychological impact of disability and illness of medical treatment decisionmaking. *Issues in Law and Medicine*, 5(3), 277-299.

Evans, M.I., Robertson, J.A., & Fletcher, J.C. 1993. Legal and ethical issues in fetal therapy. In C-C.Lin, M.S. Verp, & R.E. Sabbagha (Eds.). *The high-risk-fetus: Pathophysiology, diagnosis and management* (pp. 627-639). New York: Springer-Verlag.

Evans, R. 1987, May 24. Someday they'll have a ward and no one will come. American Association for Children's Health Annual Conference, Halifax, Nova Scotia (unpublished presentation; audiotaped).

FAQs. [On-line]. 1997, updated 1999, May 23. Retrieved July 18, 2000 from http://fetalsurgery.ucsf.edu

Fenton, E. 1976. Moral education. *Social Education*, 40(4), 188-193.
Fernadez-Serrats, A.A., Guthkelch, A.N., & Parker, S.A. 1968. Ethical and social aspects of treatment of spina bifida. *Lancet*, 2(572), 827.
Ferrara, T.B., Hoekstra, R.E., Gaziano, E., Knox, G.E., Couser, R.J. & Fangman, J.J. 1989. Changing outcome of extremely premature infants (≤26 weeks' gestation and ≤ 750 gm): Survival and follow-up at a tertiary center. *American Journal of Obstetrics and Gynecology*, 161(5), 1114-1118.
Fertility and pregnancy abnormalities [On-line]. 1999, July 7. Retrieved June 5, 2000 from http://www.cdc.gov/niosh/psfpa.html
Fetal firsts [On-line]. 1997, updated 1999, May 23. Retrieved July 18, 2000 from http://fetalsurgery.ucsf.edu
Fewell, R.R., & Vadasy, P.F. 1986. *Families of handicapped children: Needs and supports across the lifespan.* Austin, TX: PRO-ED.
Fiedler, L.A. 1984. The tyranny of the normal. *Hastings Center Report*, 14(2), 40-42.
Field, P.A. 1989. Doing fieldwork in your own culture. In J.M. Morse (Ed.). *Qualitative nursing research: A contemporary dialogue* (pp. 79-91). Rockville, MD: Aspen Publishers, Inc.
Field, P.A., & Morse, J.M. 1985. *Nursing research: The application of qualitative approaches*. Rockville, MD: Aspen Publishers, Inc.
Figlio, K. 1977. The historiography of scientific medicine: An invitation to the human sciences. *Comparative Studies in Society and History*, 19(3), 262-286.
Fischbach, F. 1984. *A manual of laboratory diagnostic tests.* Philadelphia: Lippincott.
Fischer, A.F., & Stevenson, D.K. 1987. The consequences of uncertainty: An empirical approach to medical decision making in neonatal intensive care. *JAMA*, 258(14), 1929-1931.
Fisher, B., & Tronto, J. 1990. Toward a feminist theory of caring. In E.K. Abel & M.K. Nelson (Eds.). *Circles of care: Work and identity in women's lives* (pp. 35-62). Albany: State University of New York Press.
Fisher, J.A. 1992. *℞ 2000*. New York: Simon & Schuster.
Fisher, S. 1988. *In the best interest of the patient: Women and the politics of medical decisions*. New Brunswick, NJ: Rutgers University Press.
Fitzgerald, J.M., & Hyland, D.T. 1980. Perceptions of development: A comparison of role-taking and attitudinal measures. *Research on Aging*, 2(3), 351-366.

Fleischman, A.R. 1990. Parental responsibility and the infant bioethics committee. *Hastings Center Report*, 20(2), 31-32.

Fleishman, J.A. 1984. Personality characteristics and coping patterns. *Journal of Health and Social Behavior*, 25, 229-244.

Fletcher, J. 1972. Indicators of humanhood: A tentative profile of man. *Hastings Center Report*, 2(5), 1-4.

Fletcher, J. 1979. Prenatal diagnosis, selective abortion, and the ethics of withholding treatment from the defective newborn. In A.M. Capron, M. Lappe, R.F. Murry, T.M. Powledge, S.B. Twiss, & D. Bergema (Eds.). *Genetic counseling: Facts, values, and norms* (pp. 239-254). New York: Alan R. Liss.

Fletcher, J.C. 1986. Drawing moral lines in fetal therapy. *Clinical Obstetrics and Gynecology*, 29(3), 595-602.

Fletcher, J.C., & Jonsen, A.R. 1984. Ethical considerations. In M.R. Harrison, M.S. Golbus, & R.A. Filly (Eds.). *The unborn patient*. Orlando, FL: Grune & Stratton, Inc.

Flexner, S.B. (1987). *Random house dictionary of the English language* (2nd ed., unabridged). New York: Random House.

Fontana, A., & Frey, J. H. 1994. Interviewing: The art of science. In N.K. Denzin & Y.S. Lincoln (Eds.). *Handbook of qualitative research* (pp. 361-376). Thousand Oaks, CA: Sage Publications.

Fost, N. 1981. Ethical issues in the treatment of critically ill newborns. *Pediatric Annals*, 10, 16-22.

Fost, N. 1999. Decisions regarding treatment of seriously ill newborns. *JAMA*, 281(21), 2041-2043.

Francis, G.R., & Nosek, J.A. 1988. Ethical considerations in contemporary reproductive technologies. *Journal of Perinatal and Neonatal Nursing*, 1, 37-48.

Fraley, A.M. 1986. Chronic sorrow in parents of premature children. *Children's Health Care*, 15(2), 114-118.

Franck, L. S. 1992. The influence of sociopolitical, scientific, and technologic forces on the study and treatment of pain. *Advances in Nursing Science*, 15(1), 11-20.

Frazer, E., Hornsby, J., & Lovibond, S. 1992. *Ethics: A feminist reader*. Cambridge, MA: Blackwell.

Friedman, M. 1981. *Family nursing: Theory and assessment*. New York: Appleton-Century-Crofts.

Frigoletto, F.D., & Little, G.A. (Eds). 1988. *Guidelines for perinatal care* (2nd ed.). Elk Grove Village, IL: American Academy of Pediatrics Committee.

Frohock, F.M. 1986. *Special care: Medical decisions at the beginning of life*. Chicago: The University of Chicago Press.
Frontline: Making babies. 1999a. Retrieved June 12, 1999 from: http://www.pbs.org/wgbh/pages/frontline/shows/fertility/html
Frontline: Making babies. Frontline examines booming infertility business. 1999b. PBS Home Video (60 minutes). D. Hamilton & S. Spinks, Producers.
Fruend, P. 1971. Mongoloids and "mercy killing." Presentation at International Symposium on Human Rights, Retardation, and Research, Washington, DC.[reprinted in J. Reiser, A.J. Dyck, & W.J. Curran (Eds.).1977. *Ethics in medicine: Historical and contemporary concerns*. Cambridge, MA: MIT.]
Fry, S.T. 1989. Toward a theory of nursing ethics. *Advances in Nursing Science*, 11(4), 9-22.
Gadow, S. 1980. Existential advocacy: Philosophical foundation of nursing. In S.F. Spicker & S. Gadow (Eds.). *Nursing: Images & ideals* (pp. 79-101). New York Springer Publishing.
Gadow, S. 1990. A model for ethical decision making. In T. Pence & J. Cantrall (Eds.). *Ethics in nursing: An anthology* (pp. 52-55). NY: National League for Nursing.
Gaines, P. 1997, November 22. Iowa miracle brings help for D.C. sextuplets. *The Washington Post*. Retrieved July 17, 2001 from http://www.stepshow.com/news/sextuplet.shtml.
Garcia, W., & Schultz, C. (Producers). 1992. *A day at a time* (58"). Available from Filmakers Library, New York, NY.
Gardner, S. L. 1994. Perinatal outreach education: The beginning. *Neonatal Network*, 13(6), 49-50.
Gartner, A., Lipsky, D.K., & Turnbull, A.P. 1990. *Supporting families with a child with a disability*. Baltimore, MD: Paul H. Brookes Pub., Co.
Geismar, L.L., & LaSorte, B. 1964. *Understanding the multiproblem family*. New York: Association Press.
Gibbs, J.C., Arnold, K.D., Morgan, R.L., Schwartz, E.S., Gavaghan, M.P., & Tappan, M.R. 1984. Construction and validation of a multiple-choice measure of moral reasoning. *Child Development*, 55, 527-536.
Gilchrist, V.J. 1992. Key informant interviews. In B.F. Crabtree & W.L. Miller (Eds.). *Doing qualitative research* (pp. 70-89). Newbury Park, CA: Sage Publications, Inc.
Gilligan, C.F. 1964. *Responses to temptation: An analysis of motives*. (Doctoral dissertation, Harvard University). Abstract from:

Dissertation Abstracts Online: Dissertation Abstracts Item: AAG0258209.

Gilligan C. 1977. In a different voice: Women's conceptions of self and of morality. *Harvard Educational Review*, 47(4), 481-517.

Gilligan C. 1979. Woman's place in men's life cycle. *Harvard Educational Review*, 49(4), 431-446.

Gilligan, C. 1982a. *In a different voice*. Cambridge: Harvard University Press.

Gilligan, C. 1982b. New maps of development: New visions of maturity. *American Journal of Orthopsychiatry*, 52(2), 199-212.

Gilligan, C. 1987. Moral orientation and moral development. In E. Kittay, & D. Meyers (Eds.). *Women and moral theory* (pp. 19-33). New York: Rowman & Littlefield.

Gilligan, C. 1988. Remapping the moral domain: New images of self in relationship. In C. Gilligan, J.V. Ward, & J. M. Taylor (Eds.). *Mapping the moral domain: A contribution of women's thinking to psychological theory and education* (pp. 3-19). Cambridge, MA: Harvard University Press.

Gillligan, C., & Allanucci, J. 1988. Two moral orientations: Gender differences and similarities. In C. Gilligan, J.V. Ward, & J. M. Taylor (Eds.). *Mapping the moral domain: A contribution of women's thinking to psychological theory and education* (pp. 73-86). Cambridge, MA: Harvard University Press.

Gilligan, C., Kohlberg, L., Lerner, J., & Belenky, M. 1971. Moral reasoning about sexual dilemmas. Technical Report of the Commission on Obscenity and Pornography, Vol. 1 (No. 52560010). Washington, DC: U.S. Government Printing Office.

Gilligan, C., Ward, J.V., & Taylor, J.McL. (Eds.). 1988. *Mapping the moral domain. Cambridge*. MA: Harvard University Press.

Goldberg, G.L., & Runowicz, C.D. 1992. Ovarian carcinoma of low malignant potential, infertility and induction of ovulation: Is there a link? *American Journal of Obstetrics and Gynecology*, 166, 853-854.

Goldberg, S. 1990. Chronic illness and early development: Parent-child relationships. *Pediatric Annals*, 19(1), 35, 39-41.

Goldworth, A., Silverman, W., Stevenson, D.K., Young, E.W.D., & Rivers, R. (Eds.). 1994. *Ethics and perinatology*. New York: Oxford University Press Inc.

Gortner, S.R. 1985. Ethical inquiry. In H.H. Werley & J.J. Fitzpatrick (Eds.). *Annual Review of Nursing Research* (pp. 193-214). New York: Springer.

Gottlieb, M.C. 1998. Ethical issues in the treatment of families with chronically ill members - Part 1. *Marriage and Family Practice*, 1(21). Retrieved November 12, 1999 from http:www.counseling.org/enews/volume_1/0121b.htm.

Gordon, D. (2001). From the heart: Saving Melissa. *Family Circle,* 114(14), 74-77.

Griffin, T., Kavanaugh, K., Soto, C.F., & White, M. 1997. Parental evaluation of a tour of the neonatal intensive care unit during a high-risk pregnancy. *JOGNN*, 26, 59-65.

Grossman, K.N. 2000. Preemies prove resilient. Retrieved September 1, 2000 from: http://more.abcnews.go.com/sections/living/DailyNews/birth_premature0502.html.

Guillemin, J.H., & Holmstrom, L.L. 1986. *Mixed blessings: Intensive care for newborns*. New York: Oxford University Press.

Gustafson, J.M. 1973. Mongolism, parental desires, and the right to life. *Perspectives in Biology and Medicine*, 16, 529-559.

Gustaitis, R., & Young, E.W.D. 1986. *A time to be born, a time to die.* Reading, MA: Addison-Wesley.

Hack, M., & Fanaroff, A.A. 1986. Changes in the delivery room care of the extremely small infant (<750g): Effects on morbidity and outcome. *New England Journal of Medicine*, 314(10), 660-664.

Hack, M., & Fanaroff, A.A. 1989. Outcomes of extremely-low-birth-weight infants between 1982 and 1988. *New England Journal of Medicine*, 321(24), 1642-1647.

Hack, M., Flannery, D.J., Schluchter, M., Cartar, L., Borawski, E., & Klein, N. 2002. Outcomes in young adulthood for very-low-birth-weight infants. *New England Journal of Medicine*, 346(3), 149-157.

Hack, M., Klein, N.K., & Taylor, H.G. 1995. Long-term developmental outcomes of low birth weight infants [Electronic version]. *The Future of Children*, 5(1). Retrieved March 27, 2001 from http://www.futureofchildren.org/LBW/12LBWHAC.htm.

Hack, M., Taylor, H. G., Klein, N., Eiben, R., Schatschneider, C., & Mercuri-Minich, N. 1994. School-age outcomes in children with birth weights under 750 g. *The New England Journal of Medicine*, 331(12), 753-759.

Hall, S. 1996. An exploration of parental perception of the nature and level of support needed to care for their child with special needs. *Journal of Advanced Nursing*, 24(3), 512-521.

Hamelin, K., Saydak, M.I., & Bramadat, I.A. 1997. Interviewing mothers of high-risk infants: What are their support needs? *The Canadian Nurse*, 93(6), 35-38.

Hammerman, C., Lavie, O., Kornbluth, E., Rabinson, J., Schimmel, M.S., & Eidelman, A.I. 1998. Does pregnancy affect medical ethical decision making? *Journal of Medical Ethics*, 24, 409-413.

Haney, R.P. 1987, December 2. Human choices and the technological imperative: Values in conflict. Unpublished manuscript, Dean's Distinguished Lecture, University of Pennsylvania School of Nursing.

Hardwig, J. 1990. What about the family? *Hastings Center Report*, 20(2), 5-10.

Häring, B. 1968. *Shalom: Peace--the sacrament of reconciliation*. New York: Farrar, Straus and Giroux.

Harms, D.L., & Giordano, J. 1990. Ethical issues in high-risk infant care. *Issues in Comprehensive Pediatric Nursing*, 13, 1-14.

Harris, C. H. 1995. High risk infants: Thirty years of intensive care. *Bioethics Forum*, 11(1), 23-28.

Harrison, H. 1983. Parents and handicapped infants. *New England Journal of Medicine*, 309(11), 664-665.

Harrison, H. 1984a. The parents' role in ethical decision making. Paper presentation at the First Annual Conference of Parents of Premature and High Risk Infants International, Inc. Salt Lake City, Utah.

Harrison, H. 1984b. Premature care: Past and present. *Support Lines*, 2(1), 1, 5-7, 13.

Harrison, H. 1986. Neonatal intensive care: Parent's role in ethical decision making. *Birth*, 13, 165-175.

Harrison, H. 1992. Medical miracle or pyrrhic victory? *Birth*, 19(3), 157-158.

Harrison, H. 1993. Special article: The principles for family-centered neonatal care. *Pediatrics*, 92(5), 643-650.

Harrison, H. 1996. Include parents in NICU decisions. *AAP News*, 9(12), 24-25.

Harrison, H. 1997. Ethical issues in family-centered neonatal care. In A.H. Widerstrom, B.A. Mowder, & S.R. Sandall (Eds.). *Infant development and risk* (pp.175-195). Baltimore, MD: Paul H. Brooks Pub. Co.

Harrison, H. 2001. Making lemonade: A parent's view of "Quality of life" studies. *The Journal of Clinical Ethics, 12*(3), 239-250.

Harrison, H., & Kositsky, A., 1983. *The premature baby book: A parents' guide to coping and caring in the first years*. New York: St. Martin's Press.

Harrison, L.L., & Woods, S. 1991. Early parental touch and preterm infants. *JOGNN*, 20(4), 299-306.

Harrison, M.R., Golbus, M.S., Filly, R.A., Nakayama, D.K., Callen, P.W., deLorimier, A.A., & Hricak, H. 1982. Management of the fetus with congenital hydronephrosis. *Journal of Pediatric Surgery*, 17, 728-742.

Hauerwas, S. 1975. The demands and limits of care--ethical reflections on the moral dilemma of neonatal intensive care. *American Journal of the Medical Sciences*, 269(2), 222-236.

Harvey, B. 1994. Financing perinatal health care in the US. In A. Goldworth, W. Silverman, D.K. Stevenson, E.W.D. Young, R. Rivers, and Contributors (Eds.). *Ethics in perinatology* (pp. 341-354) New York: Oxford University Press.

Hawkins-Walsh, E. 1980. Diminishing anxiety in parents of sick newborns. *MCN*, 5, 30-45.

Heaman, D.J. 1995. Perceived stressor and coping strategies of parent who have children with developmental disabilities: A comparison of mothers with fathers. *Journal of Pediatric Nursing: Nursing Care of Children and Families*, 10(5), 311-320.

Hefferman, P., & Heilig, S. 1999. Giving "moral distress" a voice: Ethical concerns among neonatal intensive care unit personnel. *Cambridge Quarterly of Healthcare Ethics*, 8(2), 173-178.

Hekman, S.J. 1995. *Moral voices, moral selves: Carol Gilligan and Feminist moral theory*. University Park: The Pennsylvania State University Press.

Herman, R., & Mehes, K. 1996. Physicians' attitudes regarding Down syndrome. *Journal of Child Neurology*, 11(1), 66-69.

Herschl, R.B., & Bartlett, R.H. 1998. Extracorporeal life support in cardiopulmonary failure. In J.S. O'Neill, M.I. Rowe, J.L. Grosfeld, E.W. Fonkalsrud, & A.G. Coran (Eds.). *Pediatric surgery* (5th Ed; p. 89). St. Louis: Mosby-Year Book.

Hinds, P.R., Scandrett-Hibden, S., & McAuley, L.S. 1990. Further assessment of a method to estimate reliability and validity of qualitative research findings. *Journal of Advanced Nursing*, 15(4), 430-435.

Historical resources. n.d.. The NIH Institutes, Center and Offices. DeWitt Stetten Jr. Museum of Medical Resources. Retrieved June 12, 2001 from http://www.nih.gov/od/museum/history/nih-ico. html

Hoffnung, M. 1989. Motherhood: Contemporary conflict for women. In J. Freeman (Ed.). *Women: A feminist perspective* (4th ed.; pp. 157-175). Mountain View, CA: Mayfield Publishing Co.

Holding hands. 1999 October 30. *Irish Independent* [On-line]. Retrieved March 29, 2000 from: http://www.independent.ie/1999/302.d20a.shtml.

Holditch-Davis, D., & Miles, M. S. 1997. Parenting the prematurely born child. In J.J. Fitzpatrick & J. Norbeck (Eds.). *Annual Review of Nursing Research* (pp. 3-34), 15.

Holstein, C.B. 1976. Irreversible, stepwise sequence in the development of moral judgment: A longitudinal study of males and females. *Child Development*, 47(1), 51-61.

Holzman, I.R. 1999. The horns of the dilemma are sharp. *Cambridge Quarterly of Healthcare Ethics*, 8, 480-484.

Hopkins, P.D. 1997. Why does removing machines count as "passive" euthanasia? *Hastings Center Report*, 27(3), 29-37.

Horbar, J.D., & Lucey, J.F. 1995. Evaluation of neonatal intensive care technologies [Electronic version]. *The Future of Children*, 5(1). Retrieved March 26, 2001 from http://www.futureofchildren.org/LBW/11LBWHOR.htm

Hospers, J. 1972. *Human conduct: Problems of ethics*. New York: Harcourt Brace and Jovanovich, Inc.

Howe, E.G. 1998. Treating infants who may die. *Journal of Clinical Ethics*, 9(3), 215-224.

Howe, E.G. 2001. Helping infants by seeing the invisible. *Journal of Clinical Ethics, 12*(3). 191-204.

Hughes, M., McCollum, J., Sheftel, D., & Sanchez, G. 1994. How parents cope with the experience of neonatal intensive care. *Children's Health Care*, 23(1), 1-14.

Humes, E. 2000, October. Baby ER. *Readers' Digest*. 174-211.

Hummel, P.A., & Eastman, D.L. 1991. Do parents of preterm infants suffer chronic sorrow? *Neonatal Network*, 10(4), 59-65.

Hurt, H. 1984. Continuing care of the high-risk infant. *Clinics in Perinatology*, 11(1), 3-17.

Illich, I. 1975. *Medical nemesis: The expropriation of health*. New York: Bantam.

Imershein, A.W., Turner, C., Wells, J.G., & Pearman, A. 1992. Covering the costs of care in neonatal intensive care units. *Pediatrics*, 89(1), 56-61.

Inglis,, A.D. 1994. NANN's tenth anniversary: Getting experience together. *Neonatal Network*, 13(6), 89-90.

Isham, N. 1992. Name: Baby Sophia; Born: 2 mos. premature; Weight: 1½ pounds; Condition: Critical. *Family Circle*, 105(7), 100-102, 178-179.

Jack, D., & Jack, R. 1988. Women lawyers: Archetype and alternatives. In C. Gilligan, J.V. Ward, & J.McL. Taylor (Eds.). *Mapping the moral domain*. Cambridge, MA: Harvard University Press.

Jacobs, C. 1990. My baby has suffered enough. *Women's Day*, 53(4), 76-77, 128-130.

Jameton, A. 1994. Pediatric nursing ethics. In A. Goldworth, W. Silverman, D.K. Stevenson, W.E.D. Young, & R. Rivers (Eds.). *Ethics and perinatology* (pp. 427-443). New York: Oxford University Press Inc.

Jecker, N.S., & Reich, W.T. 1995. Care: Contemporary ethics of care. In W.T. Reich (Ed.). *The encyclopedia of bioethics* (pp. 336-344). New York: Simon & Schuster Macmillan.

Jeffcoate, J.A., Humphrey, M.E., & Lloyd, J.K. 1979. Role perception and response to stress in fathers and mothers following pre-term delivery. *Social Science and Medicine*, 13A(2), 177-185.

Jellinek, M.S., Catlin, E.A., Todres, I.D., & Cassem, E.H. 1992. Facing tragic decisions with parents in the neonatal intensive care unit: Clinical perspectives. *Pediatrics*, 89(1), 119-122.

Jennings, B. 1988. Ethics and ethnography in neonatal intensive care. In G. Weisz (Ed.). *Social Science Perspectives on Medical Ethics* (pp. 261-272). Dordrecht, Netherlands: Kluwer Academic Publishers.

Jerome, R., Harrison, M., Kellar, M., Pawlyna, A. & Sandler. 1997. Up Front: Cast away. *People*, 48(5), 40-45.

Johnson, J., & Mitchell, C. 2000. Responding to parental requests to forgo pediatric nutrition and hydration. *Journal of Clinical Ethics*, 11(2), 128-135.

Jones, M. 2001, July 15. Fetal surgery is a complicated procedure, getting more so. *The New York Times*. Retrieved July 17, 2001 from http://www.nytimes.com/2001/07/15/magazine/15FETAL.html

Jonsen, A. R. 1991, March 27. History of ethics in neonatal care. Lecture at Peter Kiewit Center, Omaha, NE.

Jonsen, A.R., & Garland, M.J. (Eds.) 1976. *Ethics of newborn intensive care*. San Francisco: Health Policy Program, School of Medicine, University of California; Berkeley: Institute of Governmental Studies, University of California.

Jonsen, A.R., & Lister, G. 1978. Newborn intensive care: The ethical problems. *Hastings Center Report*, 8(1), 15-18.

Kahn, J.P. 1999. The littlest patients. Retrieved May 12, 2000 from http://cnn.com/HEALTH/bioethics/9909/fetal.surgery/

Kahn, R. (Producer). 1998. *Dreams and dilemmas* (58 minutes). Boston: Fanlight Productions.

Kantrowitz, B., Wingert, P., & Hager, M. 1988. Preemies. *Newsweek*, 111(20), 62-67.

Kaplan, E.A. 1992. *Motherhood and representation: The mother in popular culture and melodrama.* New York: Routledge.

Katz, J. 1995. Informed consent: Legal and ethical issues of consent in health care. In W.T. Reich (Ed.). *The encyclopedia of bioethics* (pp. 1256-1263). New York: Simon & Schuster Macmillan.

Kaufman, F. 1990. The fetus's mother. *The Hastings Center Report*, 20(3), 3-4.

Keefe, M. 1987, April 1. Viewpoints: Family portrait. *Omaha World Herald.* p. 3

Kelly, G.A. 1958. *Medico-moral problems.* St. Louis, MO: The Catholic Hospital Association of the United States and Canada.

Ketefian, S. 1981. Moral reasoning and moral behavior among selected groups of practicing nurses. *Nursing Research*, 30, 171-176.

Ketefian, S. 1988. *Moral reasoning and ethical practice in nursing: An integrative review.* New York: National League of Nursing.

Kett, J.F. 1984. The search for a science of infancy. *The Hastings Center Report*, 14(2), 34-39.

Kirk, J., & Miller, M.L. 1986. *Reliability and validity in qualitative research.* Beverly Hills, CA: Sage Publications, Inc.

King, N.M.P. 1992. Transparency in neonatal intensive care. *Hastings Center Report*, 22(3), 18-25.

Kingsley, E.P. (1987). Welcome to Holland. Retrieved October 3, 2001 from http://www.nas.com/downsyn/holland.html

Kinlaw, K. 1996. The changing nature of neonatal ethics in practice. *Clinics in Perinatology*, 23(3), 417-428.

Kirschbaum, M.S. 1994. Deciding to authorize, forego, or withdraw life-sustaining treatment: The meaning for parents (decision-making, quality of life). (Doctoral Dissertation. University of Minnesota). *Dissertation Abstracts International*, 54(12B), 6135.

Kirschbaum, M.S. 1996. Life support decisions for children: What do parents value? *Advances in Nursing Science*, 19(1), 51-71.

Klaus, M.H. 1986. Ethical decision making in neonatal intensive care: Communication with parents. *Birth*, 13(3), 175.

Klaus, M.H., & Kennel, J.H. 1982. *Parent-infant bonding*. St. Louis, MO: Mosby.

Kleiver, L.D. 1989. Dax and Job: The refusal of redemptive suffering. In L.D. Kleiver (Ed.). *Dax's case: Essays in medical ethics and human meaning (*pp. 187-211). Dallas, TX: Southern Methodist University Press.

Kleiver, L.D. 1995. Rage and grief: Another look at Dax's case. In S. K. Toombs, D. Barnard, & R. A. Carson (Eds.). *Chronic illness: From experience to policy* (pp. 58-76). Bloomington: Indiana University Press.

Klitsch, M. 1983. Mercy or murder? Ethical dilemmas in newborn care. *Family Planning Perspective*, 15, 143-146.

Klotzko, A.J. 1998. Medical miracle or medical mischief? The saga of the McCaughey septuplets. *Hastings Center Report*, 28(3), 5-8.

Knafl, K.A. & Howard, M.J. 1984. Interpreting and reporting qualitative research. *Research in Nursing and Health*, 7, 17-24.

Knafl K.A. & Webster D.C. 1988 Managing and analyzing qualitative data: A description of tasks, techniques, and materials. *Western Journal of Nursing Research*, 10(2), 195-210.

Knief, A. 1998, July 12. How to advice from four parents of four quads or quints, full house takes work. *Omaha World Herald*, 1B.

Koch, T. 1999. Does the "Sanctity of Human Life" doctrine sanctify humanness, of life? *Cambridge Quarterly of Healthcare ethics*, 8, 557-560.

Kohl, M. (Ed.). 1978. *Infanticide and the value of life*. Buffalo, NY: Prometheus.

Kohlberg L. 1958. The development of modes of moral thinking and choice in the years ten to sixteen (Unpublished Doctoral dissertation, The University of Chicago, 1959). *Abstracts of Doctoral Dissertations*, X1959. 1959, 0140.

Kohlberg, L. 1968. Moral development. In *International Encyclopedia of the Social Sciences* (pp. 483-494). New York: Crowell, Collier and MacMillan, Inc.

Kohlberg, L. 1973. *Collected papers on moral development and moral education*. Cambridge, MA: Moral Research Education Foundation, Harvard University.

Kohlberg, L. 1975. The cognitive development approach to moral education. *Phi Delta Kappan*, 61, 670-677.

Kohlberg, L. 1981. *The philosophy of moral development: Moral stages and the idea of justice*. San Francisco: Harper & Row.

Kohlberg, L. 1984. *The psychology of moral development: The nature and validity of moral stages*. San Francisco: Harper & Row.

Kohlberg, L. 1987. *Child psychology and childhood education: A cognitive-developmental approach*. New York: Longman.

Kohlberg, L., Levin, C., & Hewer, A. 1983. *Moral stages: A current formulation and a response to critics*. Basel, Switzerland: S. Karger AG.

Kolbenschlag, M. 1979. *Kiss sleeping beauty good-bye: Breaking the spell of feminine myths and models*. Garden City, NY: Doubleday & Company.

Kopelman, L.M. 1995. Children: Health care and research issues. In W.T. Reich (Ed.). *Encyclopedia of bioethics* (pp. 357-368). New York: Simon & Schuster Macmillan.

Kopelman, L.M., Irons, T.G., & Kopelman, A.E. 1988. Neonatologists judge the "Baby Doe" regulations. *New England Journal of Medicine*, 318(11), 677-683.

Korones, S. B. 1976. *High-risk newborn infants*. Saint Louis, MO: The C.V. Mosby Company.

Kottow, M.H. 1998. Decision making in the critically ill neonate [letter to the editor]. *Journal of Medical Ethics*, 24(4), 280.

Kovaleski, S.F., & Goldstein, A. 2001, July 15. Septuplets make history and headway. *The Washington Post*. Retrieved July 17, 2001 from http:www.washingtonpost.com/wp-dyn/articles/ A62817-2001Jul14.html

Kratochvil, M.S., Robertson, C.M.T., & Kyle, J.M. 1991. Parents' view of parent-child relationship eight years after neonatal intensive care. *Social Work in Health Care*, 16(1), 95-118

Krawczyk, R., & Kudzma, E. 1978. Ethics: A matter of moral development. *Nursing Outlook*, 26, 254-258.

Krippendorff, K. 1980. *Content analysis: An introduction to its methodology*. Beverly Hill, CA: Sage.

Krollmann, B., Brock, D. A., Nader, P. M., Neiheisel, P. W., & Wissman, C. S. 1994. Neonatal transformation: Thirty years. *Neonatal Network*, 13(6), 17-20.

Kuhse, H., & Singer P. 1987. Debate: Severely handicapped newborns: For sometimes letting-and helping-die. *Law, Medicine & Health Care*, 14(3-4), 149-154.

Kupfer, F. 1982. *Before and after Zachariah: A family story about a different kind of courage*. New York: Delacorte Press.

Lantos, J. 1987. Baby Doe five years later: Implications for child health. *New England Journal of Medicine*, 317(7), 444-447.

Lantos, J.D., Miles, S.H., Silverstein, M.D., & Stocking, C.B. 1988. Survival after cardiopulmonary resuscitation in babies of very low birth weight: Is CPR futile therapy? *The New England Journal of Medicine*, 318(2), 91-95.

La Puma, J. 1999, July. Ethics: When ethics leans on jargon patients often denied choices [On-line]. Retrieved August 11, 1999 from http:// www.managedcaremag.com/archiveMC/9907/9907. ethics.html.

Lau, R., & Morse, C. 1998. Experiences of parents with premature infants hospitalized in neonatal intensive care units: A literature review. *Journal of Neonatal Nursing*, 4(6), 23-29.

Layne, L.L. 1996. "How's the baby doing?" Struggling with narratives of progress in a neonatal intensive care unit. *Medical Anthropology Quarterly*, 10(4), 624-656.

Lee, S.K., Penner, P.L., & Cox, M. 1991. Impact of very low birth weight infants on the family and its relationship to parental attitudes. *Pediatrics*, 88(1), 105-109.

Leininger, M.M. 1985. Transcultural care: Diversity and universality: A theory of nursing. *Nursing and Health Care*, 6(4), 209-212.

Leininger, M. 1981. *Caring: An essential human Need. Proceedings from the first three national caring research conference*. Thorofare, NJ: Charles B. Slack Publishing Co.

Lemburg, P. 1997, November. From the very beginning. History of ventilation in paediatric medicine [Electronic version]. Retrieved July 10, 2000 from http://www.dwhl.de/german/mt/mt-p/nb/ history/ANFANG0.htm

Levin, B.W. 1986. Caring choices: Decision making about treatment for catastrophically ill newborns (Doctoral dissertation, Columbia University). *Dissertation Abstracts International*, 47(11A), 4202.

Levin, B.W. 1990. International perspectives on treatment choice in neonatal intensive care units. *Social Science and Medicine*, 30(8), 901-912.

Lewit, E.M., Baker, L.S., Corman, H., & Shiono, P H. 1995. The direct cost of low birth weight [Electronic version]. *The Future of Children*, 5(1). Retrieved March 26, 2001 from http://www.futureofchildren.org/ LBW/04LBWLEW.htm

Lincoln, Y.S., & Guba, E.G., 1985. *Naturalistic inquiry*. Newbury Park, CA: Sage Publications.

Lipson, J.G. 1991. The use of self in ethnographic research. In J.M. Morse (Ed.). *Qualitative nursing research* (pp.73-89). Newbury Park, CA: Sage Publications.

Little, G.L., & Robinson, K.D. 1989a. Effects of moral reconation therapy upon moral reasoning, life purpose, and recidivism among drug and alcohol offenders. *Psychological Reports*, 64(1), 83-90.

Little, G.L., & Robinson, K.D. 1989b. Relationship of DUI recidivism to moral reasoning, sensation seeking, and MacAndrew alcoholism scores. *Psychological Reports*, 65(3), 171-174.

Lobel, A. 1986. *The Random House book of Mother Goose*. New York: Random House.

Lobel, D., & Spratto, G. 1983. *The nurse's drug handbook.* New York: John Wiley & Son.

Loizeaux, W. 1993. *Anna: A daughter's life*. New York: Arcade Publishing Co.

Long, A., & Smyth, A. 1998. In the palm of my hand: An exploration of a man's perception of becoming a father to a premature infant and the nursing care received in a NICU. *Journal of Neonatal Nursing*, 4(1), 13-17.

Luckner, K.R., & Weinfeld, I.J. 1995. Informed consent as a parent involvement model in the NICU. *Bioethics Forum*, 11(1), 35-41.

Lyon, J. 1985. *Playing God in the Nursery*. New York: W.W. Norton & Company.

Lyons, N.P. 1983. Two perspectives: On self, relationships, and morality. *Harvard Educational Review*, 53(2), 125-145.

Magezis, J. 1996. *Women's studies*. New York: NTC Publishing Group.

Mahowald, M.B. n.d. Disability, difference, and discrimination: A feminist standpoint. Unpublished paper.

Mahowald, M. 1998, February 27. Genetics and Women. Presentation at Nursing Ethics Clinical Rounds, Creighton University, Omaha, NE.

Mallow, G.E., & Bechtel, G.A. 1999. Chronic sorrow: The experience of parents with children who are developmentally disabled. *Journal of Psychosocial Nursing and Mental Health Services*, 37(7), 31-35, 42-43.

Mann, G.B. 1970. Ethical problems and solutions for clinical research in human nutrition. *Annals of the New York Academy of Science*, 169(2), 351-356.

Manning, P.K., & Cullum-Swan, B. 1994. Narrative, content and semiotic analysis. In N.K. Denzin & Y.S. Lincoln (Eds.). *Handbook of qualitative research* (pp. 463-477). Thousand Oaks, CA: Sage Publications.

Marchwinski, S. 1988. The dilemma of moral and ethical decision making in the intensive care nursery. *Neonatal Network*, 6(5) 17-20.

Martin, D. 1985. Withholding treatment from several handicapped newborns: Ethical-legal issues. *Nursing Administrative Quarterly*, 9(4), 47-56.

Martin, D.A. 1989. Nurses' involvement with ethical decision-making with severely ill newborns. *Issues in Comprehensive Pediatric Nursing*, 12(6), 463-473.

Martin, D.A. 1990 Termination of treatment decisions for handicapped infants. (Unpublished paper).

Martin, J.Q., & Park, M.M. 1999. Trends in twin and triplet births: 1980-97. *National vital statistics report*, 47(24). Hyattsville, MD: National Center for Health Statistics.

Marton, P., Minde, K., & Perrotta, M. 1981. The role of the father for the infant at risk. *American Journal of Orthopsychiatry*, 51, 672-679.

Mason, J.K. 1986. Parental choice and selective non-treatment of deformed newborns: A view from mid-Atlantic. *Journal of Medical Ethics*, 12, 67-71.

Maxwell, G.E. 1968. A problem with prematurity. *Journal of the American Medical Association*, 203(4), 304.

May, J. 1996. Fathers: The forgotten parent. *Pediatric Nursing*, 22(3), 243-46, 271.

May, K.A. 1989. Interview techniques in qualitative research: Concerns and challenges. In J.M. Morse (Ed.). *Qualitative nursing research: A contemporary dialogue* (pp. 171-182). Newbury Park, CA: Sage Publications.

McCain, G.C., & Deatrick, J.A. 1994. The experience of a high-risk pregnancy. *JOGNN - Journal of Obstetric, Gynecologic, and Neonatal Nursing*, 23(5), 421-427.

McCluskey-Fawcett, K., O'Brien, M., Robinson, P., & Asay J.H. 1992. Early transitions for the parents of premature infants: Implications for intervention. *Infant Mental Health Journal*, 13(2), 147-156.

McCormick, M.C. 1994. Survival of very tiny babies - Good news and bad news. *The New England Journal of Medicine*, 331(12), 802-803.

McCormick, M.C., Brooks-Gunn, J., Workman-Daniels, K., Turner, J., & Peckham, G.J. 1992. The health and developmental status of very-low-birth-weight children at school age. *The Journal of the American Medical Association*, 267(16), 2204-2208.

McCormick, M.C., & Richardson, D.K. 1995. Access to neonatal intensive care [Electronic version]. *The Future of Children*, 5(1). Retrieved March 26, 2001 from http://www.futureofchildren.org/LBW/11LBWMCC.htm.

McCormick, M.C., & Richardson, D.K. 2002. Premature infants grow up. *New England Journal of Medicine*, 346(3), 197-198.

McCormick, R.A. 1974. To save or let die: The dilemma of modern medicine. *Journal of the American Medical Association*, 229(2), 172-176.

McGettigan, M.C., Adolph, V.R., Ginsberg, H.P., & Goldsmith, J.P. 1998. New ways to ventilate newborns in acute respiratory failure. *Pediatric Clinics of North America*, 45(3), 475-509.

McHaffie, H.E. 1992. Social support in the neonatal intensive care unit. *Journal of Advanced Nursing*, 17, 279-287.

McHaffie, H. 1994. *Holding on?* Cheshire, England: Books for Midwives Press.

McHaffie, H.E., Cuttini, M., Brolz-Voit, G., Randag, L., Mousty, R., Duguet, A.M., Wennergren, B., & Benciolini, P. 1999. Withholding/withdrawing treatment from neonates: Legislation and official guidelines across Europe. *Journal of Medical Ethics*, 25(6), 440-446.

Meadow, W., Lantos, J.D., Mokalla, M., & Reimshisel, T. 1996. Distributive justice across generations: Epidemiology of ICU care for the very young and the very old. *Clinics in Perinatology*, 23(3), 597-608.

Mehren, E. 1991. *Born too soon*. NY: Doubleday.

Mellien, A.C. 1992. Ethical dilemmas in the care of premature infants. *Clinical Nurse Specialist*, 6(3), 130-134.

Menzel, P. 1990. *Strong Medicine*. New York: Oxford.

Merenstein, F.B., & Gardner, S.L. 1985. *Handbook of neonatal intensive care*. St. Louis, MO: Mosby.

Merenstein, G.B. 1994. Teamwork: The key to quality neonatal care. *Neonatal Network*, 13(6), 53-54.

Micro-preemies. 2000 August 21. *Nightline*. ABC News Home Video (#N000821-01).

Miles, M.S., Carlson, J., & Funk, S.G. 1996. Sources of support reported by mothers and fathers of infants hospitalized in a neonatal intensive car unit. *Neonatal Network*, 13(3), 45-52.

Miles, M.S., Funk, S.G., & Kasper, M.A. 1991. The neonatal intensive care unit environment: Sources of stress for parents. *AACN: Clinical Issues*, 2(2), 346-354.

Miles, M.S., Funk, S.G., & Kasper, M.A. 1992. The stress response of mothers and fathers of preterm infants. *Research in Nursing & Health*, 15, 261-269.

Miles, M.S., Holditch-Davis, D., & Shepherd, H. 1998. Maternal concerns about parenting: Prematurely born children. *MCN*, 23(2), 70-75.

Miller, L.H. 1984. Alternative approaches to measuring nursing: Gilligan's and Kohlberg's moral development scales. *Rehabilitation Nursing*, 9(5), 22-23, 26.

Millette, B.E. 1994. Using Gilligan's framework to analyze nurses' stories of moral choices. *Western Journal of Nursing Research*, 16(6), 660-674.

Minogue, B. 1996. *Bioethics: A committee approach*. Boston, MA: Jones and Bartlett Publishers.

Mitchell, C, 1986. Ethical issues in neonatal nursing. In D. J. Angelini, C.M.W. Knapp, & R.M. Gibes (Eds.). *Perinatal/ Neonatal Nursing: A Clinical Handbook* (pp. 429-437). Boston: Blackwell Scientific Publications.

Miya, P.A. 1989. Imperiled infants: Nurses' roles in ethical decision making. *Issues in Comprehensive Pediatric Nursing*, 12(6), 413-422.

Miya, P.A., Boardman, K.K., Harr, K.L., & Keene, A. 1991. Ethical issues described by NICU nurses. *Journal of Clinical Ethics*, 2, 253-257.

Miya, P., Pinch, W.J., Boardman, K., Keene, A., Spielman, M., & Harr, K. 1995. Ethical perceptions of parents and nurses in NICU: The case of Baby Michael. *JOGNN*, 24(2), 125-130.

Moore, K.N., & Day, R.A. 1993. Child care and family autonomy: Empowerment through a model for ethical decision making. *Humane Medicine*, 9(2), 131-140.

Morgan, K.P. 1987. Women and moral madness. *Canadian Journal of Philosophy*, 13(Suppl.), 201-226.

Moriarty, H.J., & Cotroneo, M. 1993. Sampling issues and family research: Recruitment and sampling strategies. In S.L. Feetham, S.B., Meister, J.M. Bell, & C.I. Gillis (Eds.). *The nursing of families: Theory/research/education/practice* (pp. 79-89). Newbury Park, CA: Sage

Morse, J. 1991, October 5-6. Neonate project consultation, transcribed notes from verbatim discussion. University of Alberta: Edmonton, Alberta, Canada (unpublished manuscript).

Morse, J.M., Solberg, S.M., Neander, W.L., Bottorff, J.L., & Johnson, J.L. 1990. Concepts of caring and caring as a concept. *Advances in Nursing Science*, 13(1), 1-14.

Moskop, J.C,. & Saldanha, R.L. 1986. The baby Doe rule: Still a threat. *Hastings Center Report*, 16(2), 8-14.

Munhall, P. 1980. Moral reasoning levels of nursing students and faculty in a baccalaureate nursing program. *Image*, 12, 57-61.

Muraskas, J., Carlson, M.J., Halsey, C., Frederiksen, M.C., & Sabbagha, R.E. 1991. Survival of a 280 gram infant. *New England Journal of Medicine*, 324, 1598-1599.

Muraskas, J., Marshall, P.A., Tomich, P., Myers, T.F., Gianopoulos, J. G., & Thomasma, D.C. 1999.Neonatal viability in the 1990s: Held hostage by technology. *Cambridge Quarterly of Healthcare Ethics*, 8, 160-170.

Murphy, C. 1976. Levels of moral reasoning in a selected group of nursing practitioners. (Unpublished dissertation. Teachers College, Columbia University). *Dissertation Abstracts International*, 38(02B), 0593.

Murray, T.H. 1985a. The final, anticlimactic rule on Baby doe. *Hastings Center Report*, 15(3), 5-9.

Murray, T.H. 1985b. Suffer the little children..." In T.H. Murray, & A.L. Caplan (Eds.). *Which babies shall live?* (pp. 71-82). Clifton, NJ: The Humana Press.

Murray, T.H., & Caplan, A.L. (Eds.). 1985. *Which babies shall live? Humanistic dimensions of the care of imperiled newborns*. Clifton, NJ: Humana Press.

Nair, I. 2000. Science and technology with care; Women's inclusion, education and decision making. Keynote lecture, Forum on Women in Science and Technology, Beijing +5 Women 2000 Conference. Retrieved March 12, 2001 from http://www.awis.org/nair.html.

The National Fathers' Network: A passionate voice for change. 1992-1993. *Family Centered Care Network*, 10(3), 2,7.

Nelson, H.L. 1992. Paternal-fetal conflict. *Hastings Center Report*, 22(2), 3.

Nelson, H.L., & Nelson, J.L. 1995a. Family. In W. T. Reich (Ed.). *Encyclopedia of bioethics* (pp. 801-808). New York: Simon & Schuster Macmillan.

Nelson, H.L., & Nelson, J.L. 1995b. *The patient in the family: An ethics of medicine and families*. New York: Routledge.

Newacheck, P.W. 1990. Financing the health care of children with chronic diseases. *Pediatric Annals*, 19(1), 60-63.

Newman, J. 2000. How old is too old to have a baby? *Discover* [Electronic version]. Retrieved March 19, 2001 from http://www.findarticles.com

Not so many are married with kids. 2001, May 15. *Omaha World Herald*, p. 6.

Novak, J. 1988. An ethical decision-making model for the neonatal intensive care unit. *Journal of Perinatal and Neonatal Nursing*, 1(3), 57-67.

Novak, J.C. 1990. Facilitating nurturant fathering behavior in the NICU. *Journal of perinatal and neonatal nursing*, 4(2), 68-77.

O'Donnell, J. 1990. The development of a climate for caring: A historical review of premature care in the United States from 1900 to 1979. *Neonatal Network*, 8(6), 7-17.

Olshansky, S. 1962. Chronic sorrow: A response to having a mentally defective child. *Social Casework*, 43(4), 191-193.

Overbay, J.D. 1996. Parental participation in treatment decisions for pediatric oncology ICU patients. *Dimensions of Critical Care Nursing*, 15(1), 16-24.

Padden, T., & Glenn, S. 1997. Maternal experiences of preterm birth and neonatal intensive care. *Journal of Reproductive & Infant Psychology*, 15(2), 121-140.

Palmer, C.E., & Noble, D.N. 1986. Premature death: Dilemmas of infant mortality. *Social Casework: The Journal of Contemporary Social Work*, 67(6), 332-339

Paneth, N. 1992. Tiny babies - Enormous costs. *Birth*, 19(3), 154-161.

Paneth, N.S. 1995. The problem of low birth weight. *The Future of Children*, 5(1), 19-34.

Paris, J.J., Ferranti, J., & Reardon, F. (2001). From the Johns Hopkins Baby to Baby Miller: What have we learned from four decades of reflection on neonatal cases? *The Journal of Clinical Ethics*, 12(3), 207-214.

Paris, J.J., & Schreiber, M.D. 1996. Physicians' refusal to provide life-prolonging medical interventions. *Clinics in Perinatology*, 23(3), 563-571.

Parse, R.R., Coyne, A.B., & Smith, M.J. 1985. *Nursing research: Qualitative methods*. Bowie, MD: Brady Communication Company.

Paterson, J.G., & Zderad, L.T. 1976. *Humanistic nursing*. New York: John Wiley & Sons.

Patton, M.Q. 1980. *Qualitative evaluation methods*. Beverly Hills: Sage Publications.

Peabody, J.L., & Martin, G.I. 1996. From how small is too small to how much is too much: Ethical issues at the limits of neonatal viability. *Clinics in Perinatology*, 24(3), 473-489.

Pence, G.E. 2000. *Classic cases in medical ethics*. Boston: McGraw-Hill.

Penticuff, J.H. 1982. Psychologic implications in high-risk pregnancy. *Nursing Clinics of North America*, 17(1), 69-78.

Penticuff, J.H. 1987. Neonatal nursing ethics: Toward a consensus. *Neonatal Network*, 6(5), 7-14.

Penticuff, J.H. 1988. Neonatal intensive care: Parental Prerogatives. *Journal of Perinatal and Neonatal Nursing*, 1(3), 77-86.

Penticuff, J.H. 1992. The impact of the child abuse amendments on nursing staff and their care of handicapped newborns. In A.L. Caplan, R.H. Blank, & J.C. Merrick (Eds.). *Compelled compassion* (pp. 267-284). Totowa, NJ: The Humana Press Inc.

Penticuff, J. H. 1993, September 13, 15. Neonate project consultation, transcription of verbatim telephone consultation. University of Texas at Austin: Austin, TX (unpublished document).

Penticuff, J.H. 1994. Nursing ethics and perinatal care. In A. Goldworth, W. Silverman, D.K. Stevenson, W.E.D. Young, & R. Rivers (Eds.). *Ethics and perinatology* (pp. 405-426). New York: Oxford University Press Inc.

People v. Messenger. No. 94-67694-FH. (Ingham County 30th Judical Circuit Court, Michigan 1995).

Petrinovich, L. 1998. Reproductive technologies. In *Human evolution, reproduction and morality* (pp. 271-305). Cambridge, MA: MIT Press.

Philipp, C. 1983. The role of recollected anxiety in parental adaptation to low birthweight infants. *Child Psychiatry and Human Development*, 13(4), 239-248.

Piaget, J. 1932. *The moral judgment of the child*. London: K. Paul, Trench, Trubner & Co., Ltd. Translated by Marjorie Gabain.

Pierce, D., & Frank, G. 1992. A mother's work: Two levels of feminist analysis of family-centered care. *The American Journal of Occupational Therapy*, 46(11), 972-980.

Pierce, S.F. 1998. Neonatal intensive care: Decision making in the face of prognostic uncertainty. *Nursing Clinics of North America*, 33(2), 287-297.

Piers, M.W. 1978. *Infanticide: Past and present*. New York: Morton.

Pillitteri, A. 1992. *Maternal and child health nursing* (pp. 423-424). New York: Lippincott.

Pinch, W.J. 1990. Looking back: Five families share their views of ethical decision making in the NICU. *Caring*, 9(12), 12-18.

Pinch, W.J. 1993. Investigator as stranger. *Qualitative Health Research*, 3(4), 493-498.

Pinch, W.J. 1996. Is caring a moral trap? *Nursing Outlook*, 44(2), 84-88.

Pinch, W.J., Producer, & Lenosky, C. Director. 1989. *Ethical dilemmas in NICU: The parents' perspective.* Produced at Biomedical Communications Department, Creighton University, Omaha, NE. (Seven-minute "trigger tape" video production).

Pinch, W.J., & Producer, Lenosky, C. Director. 1990. *I'm just the mother. Ethical dilemmas in NICU: The parents' perspective.* Produced at Biomedical Communications Department, Creighton University, Omaha, NE. Distributed by Health Sciences Consortium, Chapel Hill, NC (28 minute video production).

Pinch, W.J., & Parsons, M.E. 1993. Ethical decision making and the elderly patient's perspective. *Geriatric Nursing*, 14(6), 289-293.

Pinch, W.J., & Spielman, M.L. 1989a. Ethical decision making for high-risk infants: The parents' perspective. *Nursing Clinics of North America*, 24, 1017-1023.

Pinch, W.J., & Spielman, M.L. 1989b. Parental voices in the sea of ethical dilemmas. *Issues in Comprehensive Pediatric Nursing*, 12, 423-435.

Pinch, W.J., & Spielman, M.L. 1990. The parents' perspective: Ethical decision-making in neonatal intensive care. *Journal of Advanced Nursing*, 15, 712-719.

Pinch, W.J., & Spielman, M.L. 1993. Parental perceptions of ethical issues post-NICU discharge. *Western Journal of Nursing Research*, 15, 422-437.

Pinch, W.J. Ellenchild, & Spielman, M.L. 1996. Ethics in the neonatal intensive care unit: Parental perceptions at four years post discharge. *Advances in Nursing Science*, 19(1), 72-85.

Pinelli, J.M. 1981. A comparison of mothers' concerns regarding the care-taking tasks of newborns with congenital heart disease before and after assuming their care. *Journal of Advanced Nursing*, 6(4), 261-270.

Plaas, K.M. 1994. The evolution of parental roles in the NICU. *Neonatal Network*, 13(6), 31-33.

Polit, D.F., & Hungler, B.P. 1995. *Nursing research: Principles and methods*. Philadelphia: J.B. Lippincott Company.

Pope Pius XII. 1977. The prolongation of life. In J. Reiser, A.J. Dyck, & W.J. Curran (Eds.). *Ethics in Medicine: Historical and Contemporary Concerns* (pp. 501-504). Cambridge, MA: MIT.

Porter, F.L., Grunau, R.E., & Anand, K.J.S. 1999. Long-term effects of pain in infants. *Developmental and Behavioral Pediatrics*, 20(4), 253-261.

Porter, F.L., Wolf, C.M., & Miller, J.P. 1999. Procedural pain in newborn infants: The influence of intensity and development. *Pediatrics*, 104(1), 1e-10e.

Post, S.G. 1987 Parental duties toward severely impaired infants: An ethical analysis. *Linacre Quarterly*, 54(1), 61-76.

Post, S.G. 1997. The Judeo-Christian case against human cloning. *America*, 176(21), 19-22.

Pratt, M.W., Diessner, R., Hunsberger, B, Prancer, S.M., & Savoy K. 1991. Four pathways in the analysis of adult development and aging: Comparing analyses of reasoning about personal-life dilemmas. *Psychology and Aging*, 6(4), 666-675.

Probert, W., & Carson, R.A. 1984. Terminating artificial feeding for dying infants: Ethics, emotions, and societal impact. *Death Education*, 8, 405-412.

Queenan, J.T. 1985. *Management of high-risk pregnancy*. Oradell, NJ: Medical Economics Books.

Ragatz S.D., & Ellison P.H. 1983. Decisions to withdraw life support in the neonatal intensive care unit. *Clinical Pediatrics*, 22(11), 729-735.

Raines, D.A. 1996. Parents' values: A missing link in the neonatal intensive care equation. *Neonatal Network*, 15(3), 7-12.

Raines, D.A. 1998. Values of mothers of low birth weight infants in NICU. *Neonatal Network: Journal of Neonatal Nursing*, 17(4), 41-46.

Raines, D.A. 1999. Suspended mothering: Women's experiences mothering an infant with a genetic anomaly identified at birth. *Neonatal Network: Journal of Neonatal Nursing*, 18(5), 35-39.

Ramsey, P. 1970. *The patient as person*. New Haven: Yale University Press. (sometimes cited as the Beecher Lectures actually given in 1969 at Yale University before publication in this book form).

Ramsey, P. 1978. *Ethics at the edges of life*. New Haven: Yale University Press.

Ravin, A.J., Mahowald, M.B., & Stocking, C.B. 1997. Genes or gestation? Attitudes of women and men about biologic ties to children. *Journal of Women's Health*, 6(6), 639-647.

Rawls, J. 1958. Justice as fairness. *Philosophical Review*, 67, 164-194.
Raymond, J.G. 1993. *Women as wombs: Reproductive technologies and the battle over women's freedom*. New York: HarperCollins.
Reaney, P. 2001, July 3. Test-tube babies show no emotional problems. Retrieved July 7, 2001 from http://www.changesurfer.com.
Recer, P. 2000a. Premature babies and pain. Retrieved September 1, 2000 from http://more.abcnews.go.com/sections/living/dailynews/premiepain000728.html.
Recer, P. 2000b: Prematurity problems. Retrieved September 1, 2000 from http://more.abcnews.go.com/sections/living/dailynews/preemie0808.html
Reedy, N.J., Minogue, J.P., & Sterk, M.B. 1987. The critically ill neonate: Dilemmas in perinatal ethics. *Critical Care Nursing Quarterly*, 10(2), 56-64.
Reich, W.T. 1987a. Caring for life in the first of it: Moral paradigms for perinatal and neonatal ethics. *Seminars in Perinatology*, 11(3), 279-287.
Reich, W.T. 1987b. Models of pain and suffering: Foundations for an ethic of compassion. *Acta Neurochirurgica, Supplement*, 38(Suppl.), 117-122.
Reich, W.T. 1987c. A theory of compassion. Society for Health and Human Values Annual Meeting, November 6-8. Abstract.
Reich, W.T. 1989. Speaking of suffering: A moral account of compassion. *Soundings*, 72(1), 83-108.
Reich, W.T. 1990. Compassion: The spirituality of health care ministry. Society for Health and Human Values Annual Meeting, November 9-11. Unpublished paper.
Reich, W.T. 1991. The case: Denny's story. *Second Opinion*, 17(1), 41-56.
Reiser, S.J. 1993. The birth of bioethics. View the third. *Hastings Center Report*, 23(6), S13-S14.
Resnick, P.J. 1969. Child murder by parents: A psychiatric review of filicide. *American Journal of Psychiatry*, 126(3), 325-334.
Rest, J. 1975. Recent research on an objective test of moral judgment: How the important issues of a moral dilemma are defined. In D.J. DePalma & J.M. Foley (Eds.). *Moral development: Current Theory and research* (pp. 75-93). New York: John Wiley & Sons.
Rest, J. 1976. Developmental psychology as a guide to value education: A review of "Kohlbergian" programs. In D. Purpel & K. Ryan (Eds.). *Moral education...it comes with the territory* (pp. 252-274). Berkeley, CA: McCutchan Publishing Corporation.

Rest, J.R., Turiel, E., & Kohlberg, L. 1969. Level of moral development as a determinant of preference and comprehension of moral judgment made by others. *Journal of Personality*, 37, 225-252.

Reverby, S. 1987. *Ordered to care: The dilemma of American nursing, 1850-1945*. New York: Cambridge University Press.

Rich, A. 1976. *Of woman born*. New York: W. W. Norton & Co., Inc.

Rich, J.M., & DeVitis, J.L. 1985. *Theories of moral development*. Springfield, IL: Charles C. Thomas, Publisher.

Richardson, D.K. (2001). A woman with an extremely premature newborn. *JAMA,* 286(12), 1498-1505.

Richardson, S. 1998. Thirteen ways of looking at a baby. *Discover*, 19(5), 80.

Rickham, P.P. 1969. The ethics of surgery in newborn infants. *Clinical Pediatrics*, 8(5), 251-253.

Rikli, J.M. 1995. Parenting the premature infant: Potential iatrogenesis from the neonatal intensive care experience. *Online-Journal-of-Knowledge-Synthesis-for-Nursing*, 3(doc 7, Online #31), 1-21.

Roach, M.S. 1987. *The human act of caring: A blueprint for health professions*. Toronto, Canada: Canadian Hospital Association.

Robb, C. 1980, October 5. Vive la difference. *Boston Globe Magazine*, pp. 11, 69-72, 74, 76, 78-80.

The Robert Wood Johnson Foundation. 1985. *Special report, number three*. Princeton, NJ: The Foundation.

Robertson, B. 1983. Lung surfactant for replacement therapy. *Clinical Physiology*, 3(2), 97-110.

Robinson, E.L.E, Nelson, H.L, & Nelson, J.L. 1997. Fluid families: The role of children in custody arrangements. In H.L. Nelson (Ed.). *Feminism and families* (pp. 90-101). New York: Routledge.

Rogers, A., & Gilligan, C. 1988. Translating the language of adolescent girls: Themes of moral voice and stages of ego development (Monograph No. 6). Cambridge, MA: Harvard Graduate School of Education, Project on the Psychology of Women and the Development of Girls.

Rose, P. 1995. Best interests: A concept analysis and its implications for ethical decision-making in nursing. *Nursing Ethics*, 2(2), 149-160.

Rosenthal, E. 1991, September 29. As more tiny infants live, choices and burdens grow - smallest survivors: Dilemmas of prematurity. *The New York Times*, pp. 1, 26.

Rosser, S.V. 1994. *Women's health - Missing from U.S. medicine.* Bloomington, IN: Indiana University Press.

Rostain, A. 1986. Deciding to forgo life-sustaining treatment in the intensive care nursing: A sociologic account. *Perspectives in Biology and Medicine*, 30(1), 117-134.

Rothman, B.K. 1986. *The tentative pregnancy: Prenatal diagnosis and the future of motherhood.* New York: Viking.

Rothman, B.K. 1992. The frightening future of baby-making: The new reproductive technologies may turn out to be the breast implants of tomorrow. *Glamour*, 90(June), 210-213+.

Rottman, C.V.B. 1986. Ethics in neonatology: A parents' perspective. (Doctoral dissertation, Case Western Reserve University, 1985). *Dissertation Abstracts International*, 42(12A), 3877.

Rue, V.M. 1985. Death by design of handicapped newborns: The family's role & response. *Issues in Law and Medicine*, 1(3) 201-225.

Rushton, C. 1994. Moral decision-making by parents of infants who have life-threatening congenital disorders. (Doctoral dissertation, The Catholic University of America). *Dissertation Abstracts International*, 55(03B), 0822.

Rybash, J.M., Hoyer, W.J., & Roodin, P.A. 1983/84. Responses to moral dilemmas involving self versus others. *International Journal of Aging and Human Development*, 18(1), 73-77.

Rybash, J.M., Roodin, P.A., & Lonky, E. 1981. Young adults' score on the Defining Issues Test as a function of a "self" versus "other" presentation mode. *Journal of Youth and Adolescence*, 10(1), 25-31.

Sabat, S. R. 2001. *The experience of Alzheimer's disease: Life through a tangled veil.* Malden, MA: Blackwell Publishers Inc.

Sabbeth, B.F., & Leventhal, J.M. 1984. Marital adjustment to chronic childhood illness: A critique of the literature. *Pediatrics*, 73(6), 762-768.

Saigal, S. 2000. Follow-up of very low birthweight babies to adolescence [Electronic version]. *Seminars on Neonatology*, 5(2), 107-118.

Saigal, S., Feeny, D., Rosenbaum, P., Furlong, W., Burrows, E., & Stoskopf, B. 1996. Self-perceived health status and health-related quality of life of extremely low-birth-weight infants at adolescence. *JAMA*, 276(6), 453-459.

Saigal, S., Stoskopf, B.L., Feeny, D., Furlong, W., Burrows, E., Rosenbaum, P.L., & Hoult, L. 1999. Differences in preferences for neonatal outcomes among health care professionals, parents, and adolescents. *JAMA*, 281(21), 1991-1997.

Saigal, S., Szatmari, P., Rosenbaum, P., Campbell, D., & King, S. 1990. Intellectual and functional status at school entry of children who weighed 1000 grams or less at birth: A regional perspective of birth in the 1980s. *The Journal of Pediatrics*, 116(3), 409-416.

Sandelowski, M. 1986. The problem of rigor in qualitative research. *Advances in Nursing Science*, 8(3), 27-37.

Sandelowski, M. 1993. Rigor or rigor mortis: The problem of rigor in qualitative research revisited. *Advances in Nursing Science*, 16(2), 1-8.

Sandelowski, M. 1999. Culture, conceptive technology, and nursing. *International Journal of Nursing Studies*, 36, 13-20.

Sanders, M.R., Donohue, P.K., Oberdorf, M.A., Rosenkrantz, T.S., & Allen, M.C. 1995. Perceptions of the limit of viability: Neonatologists attitudes toward extremely preterm infants. *Journal of Perinatology*, 15(6), 494-502.

Satariano, H.J., Briggs, N.J., & O'Neal, C. 1987. Discharged from neonatal intensive care: How satisfied are parents? *Pediatric Nursing*, 13(5), 352-353, 357.

Sauer, D.J.J. 1992. Ethical decisions in neonatal intensive care units: The Dutch experience. *Pediatrics*, 90(5), 729-732.

Savage, T.A., Durand, B.A., Friedrichs, J., & Slack, J.F. 1993. Ethical decision making with families in crisis. In S.L. Feetham, S.B. Meister, J.M. Bell, & C.L. Gilliss (Eds.). *The nursing of families: Theory, research, education, and practice* (pp. 118-126). Newbury Park, CA: Sage Publications.

Scharer, K., & Brooks, G. 1994. Mothers of chronically ill neonates and primary nurses in the NICU: Transfer of care. Neonatal Network, 13(5), 37-47.

Scharf, P. (Ed.). 1978. *Readings in moral education*. Minneapolis, MN: Winston Press, Inc.

Schlomann, P. 1992. Ethical considerations of aggressive care of very low birth weight infants. *Neonatal Network*, 11(4), 31-36.

Schlomann, P., & Fister, S. 1995. Parental perspectives related to decision-making and neonatal death. *Pediatric Nursing*, 21(3), 243-247, 254.

Schraeder, B.D. 1980. Attachment and parenting despite lengthy intensive care. *MCN*, 5(1), 37-41.

Scully, D. 1994. *Men who control women's health: The miseducation of obstetrician-gynecologists*. New York: Teachers' College Press, Columbia University.

Scully, T., & Scully, C. 1987. The Baby Doe dilemma: To treat or not to treat. In *Playing God: The New World of Medical Choices* (pp. 194-229). New York: Simon and Schuster.

Seidel, J.V., Kjolseth, R., & Seymour, E. 1988. *The Ethnograph: A user's guide* (Version 3.0). Littleton, CO: Qualis Research Associates.

Seideman, R.Y., & Kleine, P.F. 1995. A theory of transformed parenting: Parenting a child with developmental delay/mental retardation. *Nursing Research*, 44(1), 38-44.

Self, D. 1987. A study of the foundations of ethical decision-making of nurses. *Theoretical Medicine*, 8, 85-95.

Service Merchandise Co. Inc. Catalogue, C0017 AX, 1997.

Shaevitz, M.H. 1984. *The superwoman syndrome*. New York: Warner Books, Inc.

Shaw, A. 1973. Dilemmas of 'informed consent' in children. *New England Journal of Medicine*, 289, 885-894.

Shelp, E.E. 1986. *Born to die? Deciding the fate of critically ill newborns*. New York: The Free Press.

Sherer, D.M., Abramovicz, J.S., Bennett, S.L., Mercier, C.E., & Woods, J.R. 1992. Case report: Survival of an infant with a birthweight of 345 grams. *Birth*, 19(3), 151-161.

Sherwin, S. 1992. *No longer patient: Feminist ethics & health care*. Philadelphia: Temple University Press.

Shields, S.A. 1984. "To pet, coddle, and 'do for'": Caretaking and the concept of maternal instinct. In M. Lewin (Ed.), *In the shadow of the past: Psychology portrays the sexes* (pp. 256-273). New York: Columbia University Press.

Shields-Poë, D., & Pinelli, J. 1997. Variables associated with parental stress in neonatal intensive care units. *Neonatal Network*, 16(1), 29-37.

Shiono, P.H., & Behrman, R.E. 1995. Low birth weight: Analysis and recommendations. *The Future of Children*, 5(1). Retrieved March 27, 2001from: htttp://futureofchildren.org/LBW/02LBWANA.htm.

Silverman, W.A. 1979. Incubator-baby side shows. *Pediatrics*, 64(2), 127-141.

Silverman, W.A., 1981. Mismatched attitudes about neonatal death, *Hastings Center Report*, 11(6), 12-16.

Silverman, W.A. 1982. Russian roulette in the nursery--again. *Pediatrics*, 69(3), 380-381.

Silverman, W.A. 1992. Overtreatment of neonates? A personal retrospective. *Pediatrics*, 90(6), 971-976.

Simpson, T.J. 1999. Response to "Neonatal viability in the 1990s: Held hostage by technology" by Jonathan Muraskas et al. and "Giving 'Moral distress' a voice: Ethical concerns among neonatal intensive care unit personnel" by Pam Hefferman and Steve Heilig (CQ Vol. 8, No2). *Cambridge Quarterly of Healthcare Ethics*, 8, 524-526.

Sims-Jones, N. 1986. Ethical dilemmas in the NICU. *The Canadian Nurse*, 82(4), 24-26.

Singer, L.T., Salvator, A., Guo, S., Collin, M., Lilien, L., & Baley, J. 1999. Maternal psychological distress and parenting stress after the birth of a very low-birth-weight infant. *JAMA*, 281, 799-805.

Sise, C.B. 1988. Maternal rights versus fetal interests: An ethical issue with nursing implications. *Journal of Professional Nursing*, 4(4), 262-267.

Smith, D. 1974. On letting some babies die. *The Hastings Center Studies*, 2(2), 37-46.

Smith, E.D. 1986. Infant care review committee and ethical decision making. *Nursing Administration Quarterly*, 10, 44-50.

Smith, J.F. 1996. Communicative ethics in medicine: The physician-patient relationship. In S.M. Wolf (Ed.). *Feminism and bioethics: Beyond reproduction* (pp. 185-215). New York: Oxford University Press.

Snarey, J., & Lydens, L. 1990. Worker equality and adult development: The kibbutz as a developmental model. *Psychology and Aging*, 5(1), 86-93.

Sparks, R.C. 1988. *To treat or not to treat*. Mahwah, NJ: Paulist Press.

Special Education Staff. 1992-1992. *Nebraska special education statistical report*. Lincoln, NE: Nebraska Department of Education, Special Education Office.

Stein, S. 1994, December 11. The cruelest choice: Medicine is forcing some parents to decide the fate of their severely premature babies. *Chicago Tribune Magazine*, pp. 16-22.

Steinbock, B. 1984. Baby Doe Jane in the Courts. *Hastings Center Report*, 14(1), 13-19.

Steinfels, M.O.B. 1978. New childbirth technology: A clash of values. *Hastings Center Report*, 8(1) 9-12.

Sternlof, K.R. 1999. Magnetic resonance imaging. *Gale encyclopedia of medicine.* Retrieved July 22, 2001 from http://www.findarticles.com/cf_dls/g2601/0008/2601000863/p1/article.jhtml

Stetler, C.B. 1994. Refinement of the Stetler/Marram model for application of research findings to clinical practice. *Nursing Outlook*, 42(1), 15-25.

Stevenson, D.K. & Goldworth, A. 1999. Commentary: "Neonatal viability in the 1990s: Held hostage by technology." *Cambridge Quarterly of Healthcare Ethics*, 8, 170-172.

Stewart, A.L., Rifkin, L., Amess, P.M., Kirkbride, V., Townsend, J. P., Miller, D.J., Lewis, S.W., Kingsley, D.P.E., Moseley, I.F., Foster, O., & Murray, R.M. 1999. Brain structure and neurocognitive and behavioral function in adolescents who were born very preterm. *Lancet*, 353, 1653-1657.

Stewart, J.A.D. 1998. Best interests and persistent vegetative state [letter to the editor]. *Journal of Medical Ethics*, 24, 350.

Stinson, R., & Stinson, P. 1979. On the death of a baby. *Atlantic Monthly*, 244(1), 64-66, 68-70, 72.

Stinson, R., & Stinson, P. 1981. On the death of a baby. *Journal of Medical Ethics*, 7, 5-18.

Stinson, R., & Stinson, P. 1983. *The long dying of Baby Andrew*. Boston: Little, Brown.

Strauss, A., & Corbin, J. 1990. *Basics of qualitative research*. Newbury Park, CA: Sage.

Strong, C. 1983a. Defective infants and their impact on families: Ethical and legal considerations. *Law, Medicine & Health Care*, 11(4), 168-172, 181.

Strong, C. 1983b. The tiniest newborns. *Hastings Center Report*, 13(1), 14-19.

Strong, C. 1984. The neonatologist's duty to patient and parents. *Hastings Center Report*, 14(4), 10-16.

Success and failure. 1969. *British Medical Journal*, 3(671), 607-608.

Sudia-Robinson, T.M., & Freeman, S.B. 2000. Communication patterns and decision making among parents and health care providers in the neonatal intensive care unit: A case study. *Heart & Lung*, 29(2), 143-148.

Swanson, K.M. 1990. Providing care in the NICU: Sometimes an act of love. *Advances in Nursing Science*, 13(1), 60-73.

Swanson, K.M. 1991. Empirical development of a middle range theory of caring. *Nursing Research*, 40(3), 161-166.

Swanson-Kauffman, K.M. 1986. A combined qualitative methodology for nursing research. *Advances in Nursing Science*, 8(3), 58-69.

Swigart, B., Lidz, C., Butterworth, V., & Arnold, R. 1996. Letting go: Family willingness to forgo life support. *Heart & Lung*, 25(6), 483-494.

Swyter, J.L. 1984. Ethical dilemmas in medicine: An anthropological approach. (Doctoral dissertation, The American University). *Dissertation Abstracts International*, 45(03A), 0882.

Szawarski, Z. 1990. A report from Poland: Treatment and non-treatment of defective newborns. *Bioethics*, 4(2), 143-153.

Tanaka, Y., Takei, T., Aiba, T., Masuda, K., Kiuchi, A., & Fujiwara, T. 1986. Development of synthetic lung surfactants. *Journal of Lipid Research*, 27(5), 475-485.

Tanner, L. 2000. Premature babies at risk. Retrieved September 1, 2000 from http://more.abcnews.go.com/sections/living/dailynews/premature000814.html.

Task Force on Technology-dependent children releases report. 1988. *Capitol Update*, 6(9), 6.

Tavris, C. 1992. *The mismeasure of woman*. New York: Simon & Schuster.

Taylor, S.J., & Bodgan, R. 1984. *Introduction to qualitative research methods: The search for meanings*. New York: John Wiley & Sons.

Teel, C.S. 1991. Chronic sorrow: Analysis of the concept. *Journal of Advanced Nursing*, 16(11), 1311-1319.

Tesch, R. 1990. *Qualitative research: Analysis types & software tools*. New York: The Falmer Press.

Thorne, A., & Robinson, C. (1989). Guarded alliance: Health care relationships in chronic illness. *Image: Journal of Nursing Scholarship*, 21(3), 153-157.

Thurman, S.K., & Korteland, C. 1989. The behavior of mothers and fathers toward their infants during neonatal intensive care visits. *Children's Health Care*, 18(4), 247-251.

Tong, T. 1995. Feminist perspectives and gestational motherhood. In J.C. Callahan (Ed.). *Reproduction, ethics and the law* (pp. 55-79). Bloomington: Indiana University Press.

Tooley, M. 1983. *Abortion and infanticide*. New York: Oxford University Press.

Tooley, W.J., & Phibbs, R.H. 1976. Neonatal intensive care: The state of the art. In A.R. Jonsen & M.J. Garland (Eds.). *Ethics of newborn intensive care* (pp. 11-15). University of California, Berkeley: Institute of Governmental Studies.

Trachtenbarg, D.E. & Golemon, T.B. 1998. Office care of the premature infant: PartII. Common medical and surgical problems. *American Family Physician*. Retrieved from: http://www.aafp.org/afp/09805ap/tracht.html.

Trafford, A. 2001, July 24. 'Miracle' birth is nothing worth celebrating. *The Washington Post*, p. HE9. Retrieved July 24, 2001from http://washingtonpost.com.

Trause, M.A., & Kramer, L. 1983. The effects of premature birth on parents and their relationships. *Developmental Medicine and Child Neurology*, 25(4), 459-465.

Travelbee, J. 1969. *Interventions in psychiatric nursing: Process in the one to one relationship*. Philadelphia: F.A. Davis.

Triplets are born to Norfolk couple. 1988, March 31. *Omaha World Herald*, p. 43.

Turiel, E. 1974. Conflict and transition in adolescent moral development. *Child Development*, 45, 14-29.

Turnbull, A.P., & Turnbull, H.R. 1990. *Families, professionals, and exceptionality: A special partnership*. Columbus: Merrill.

Turnbull, H.R. (Ed.). 1985. *Parents speak out: Then and now*. Columbus: C.E. Merrill.

Turnbull, H.R. 1986. Incidence of infanticide in America: Public and professional attitudes. *Issues in Law & Medicine*, 1(5), 363-389.

Tyson, J. 1995. Evidence-based ethics and the care of premature infants [Electronic version]. *Future of children*, 5(1), 197-213. Retrieved June 7, 2001 from http://www.futureofchildren.org/LBW/13LBW TYS.htm

U.S. Office of Technology Assessment. 1987. Neonatal intensive care for low birth weight infants: Costs and effectiveness (NTIS order #PB88-158902). Washington, DC: U.S. Government Printing Office. Retrieved June 5, 1996 from http://www.wws.princeton.edu.

van der Heide, A., van der Maas, P.J., van der Wal, G., de Graaff, C.L.M., Kester, J.G.C., Kollee-Louis, A.A., de Leeuw, R., & Holl, R.A. 1997. Medical end-of-life decisions made for neonates and infants in the Netherlands. *Lancet*, 350(9073), 251-255.

van Eys, J. 2001. Commentary: Humanity and personhood. *The Pharos*, 64(2), 11.

Vohr, B.F. 2000a, November. Neurodevelopmental outcomes and resource utilization of ELBW infants. Presentation at Children's Hospital Omaha, NE.

Vohr, B.F. 2000b, November. Outcomes of twins and triplets. Powerpoint Presentation. Brown University School of Medicine, Providence, RI.

Walker, L.J. 1989. A longitudinal study of moral reasoning. *Child Development*, 60, 157-166.

Walters, J.W. 1988. Approaches to ethical decision making in the neonatal intensive care unit. *American Journal of Disabled Children*, 142, 825-830.

Walters, L. (Ed.). 1975. *Bibliography of bioethics*. Detroit, MI: Gale Publishing Co.

Waltman, P.A., & Schenk, L.K. 1999. Neonatal ethical decision making: Where does the NNP fit in? *Neonatal Network*, 18(8), 27-32.

Walwork, E., & Ellison, P.H. 1985. Follow-up of families of neonates in whom life support was withdrawn. *Clinical Pediatrics*, 24(1), 14-20.

Watchko, J.F. 1983. Decision making on critically ill infants by parents. *American Journal of Disabled Children*, 137, 795-798.

Watson, J. 1985. *Nursing: Human Science and human care. A theory of nursing*. Norwalk, CN: Appleton-Century-Crofts.

Watson, V.B. 1996. *Miracle Heidi: When doctors couldn't...God could!* Bedford, TX: Sterling Press International.

Weber, F.J. 1976. *Who shall live? The dilemma of severely handicapped children and its meaning for other moral questions*. New York: Paulist Press.

Weber, R.P. 1985. *Basic content analysis*. Beverly Hills: Sage Publications.

Weir, R. 1984. *Selective nontreatment of handicapped newborns*. New York: Oxford University Press.

Weir, R.F. 1992. Life and death decisions in the midst of uncertainty. In A.L. Caplan, R.H. Blank, & J.C. Merrick (Eds.). *Compelled compassion* (pp. 1-33). Totowa, NJ: The Humana Press, Inc.

Weir, R.F. 1994. Withholding and withdrawing therapy and actively hastening death II. In A. Goldworth, W. Silverman, D.K. Stevenson, W.E.D. Young, & R. Rivers (Eds.). *Ethics and perinatology* (pp. 172-183). New York: Oxford University Press Inc.

Weir, R.F. 1995. Infants: Ethical Issues. In W.T. Reich (Ed.). *Encyclopedia of bioethics* (pp. 1206-1214). New York: Simon & Schuster Macmillan.

Weis, C.M., & Fox, W.W. 1999. Current status of liquid ventilation. *Current Opinion in Pediatrics*, 11(2), 126-132.

Wertz, R.W., & Wertz, D.C. 1977. *Lying-in: A history of childbirth in America*. New York: The Free Press.

West, C. 2001. *Race matters*. New York: Random House, Vintage Books.

What is early intervention? 1996. KidSource OnLine, Inc. Retrieved March 26, 2001from http://www.kidsource.com/kidsource/content/early.intervention.html.

White, C.B. 1988. Age, education, and sex effects on adult moral reasoning. *International Journal of Aging and Human Development*, 27(4), 271-281.

Whitney, S. 1998, June 11. Bioethics and technology. Message posted to: mcw-bioethics@post.its.mcw.edu

Wildes, K.W. 1995. *Critical choices and critical care: Catholic perspectives on allocating resources in intensive care medicine*. Dordrecht: Kluwer Academia Publishers.

Willing, R. 2000, November 29. Who decides whether a baby lives or dies. *USA Today*, 1A-2A.

Wingert, P. 1988. Two babies on the brink of life: One mother's poignant account of her experience. *Newsweek*, 111(20), 68-69.

Wolf, S. 1996a. Gender, feminism and death. In S. Wolf (Ed.). *Feminism and bioethics: Beyond reproduction* (pp. 282-317). New York: Oxford University Press.

Wolf, S.M. (Ed.). 1996b. *Feminism & bioethics: Beyond reproduction*. New York: Oxford University Press.

Wretmark, A.A. 1993. *Perinatal death as a pastoral problem*. Stockholm: Graphic Systems.

Wright, B.A. 1979. Atypical physique and the appraisal of persons. *Connecticut Medicine Supplement*, 43(10), 19-24.

Wright, K. 1998. Human in the age of mechanical reproduction. *Discover*, 19(5), 75-81.

Wynia, M. (2002, February 5). The cost of children. Message posted to: mcw-bioethics@post.its.mcw.edu

Zachary, RB. 1968. Ethical and social aspects of treatment of spina bifida. *Lancet*, 2(2562), 274-276.

Zaner, R.M., & Bliton, M.J. 1991. Decisions in the NICU: The moral authority of parents. *Children's Health Care*, 20(1), 19-25.

Zelizer, V.A. 1985. *Pricing the priceless child: The changing value of children*. New York: Basic Books.

Zewe, C. 1998 December 21. World's first octuplets struggle for survival [On-line]. Retrieved March 19, 2001from http://cgi,cnn.com/US/9812/21/octuplets.02/.

INDEX

L

M

ABOUT THE AUTHOR

Winifred J. Ellenchild Pinch is currently a full professor at Creighton University, Omaha, Nebraska. She holds a primary appointment in the School of Nursing with joint appointments in the Center for Health Policy and Ethics and the School of Medicine. She received a diploma in nursing from Harrisburg Hospital School of Nursing in Pennsylvania. She obtained a baccalaureate degree from Temple University in Philadelphia and holds masters degrees from both the State University of New York at Buffalo (Education) and Creighton University (Nursing). Dr. Pinch's interest in bioethics began when she was a graduate student at Boston University where she obtained her doctorate degree. She was a special student at Harvard Divinity School for one year. In addition to her project on the ethics of high-risk newborns, she also participated in research projects examining the healthy elderly's perception of ethical decision making, confidentiality and mothers with AIDS/HIV infection, the implementation of the patient self-determination act (PSDA), a meta-analysis of quantitative research studies in nursing ethics, and the status of ethics committees in state nursing associations. Dr. Pinch has a strong interest in feminist bioethics, the ethics of care, and moral develop-ment. She is currently working as a team member on a project focusing on ethics, palliative care, and Alzheimer's Disease. Dr. Pinch is a member of the American Nurses Association, the Midwest Nursing Research Society, American Society for Bioethics and Humanities, and Sigma Theta Tau International.